RUTH PERIN STRYKER, R.N., B.S.

Director of Nursing Education, American Rehabilitation Foundation, Minneapolis, Minnesota. Formerly Administrative Assistant Nursing Service, St. Barnabas Hospital, Minneapolis, Minnesota.

BACK TO NURSING

W. B. SAUNDERS COMPANY
Philadelphia and London

W. B. Saunders Company: West Washington Square,
Philadelphia, Pa. 19105

12 Dyott Street
London, W.C.1

Reprinted January, 1967

BACK TO NURSING

 Library of Congress catalog card number 66-18504.

This book is dedicated to the Refreshers whom I have known. Regardless of background, their motivation and perseverance have proved that it can be done excellently.

Preface

In 1960, 1961 and 1962, St. Barnabas Hospital in Minneapolis, Minnesota, offered a refresher course to a total of 125 nonpracticing registered nurses who had been out of nursing from five to thirty years. Some were graduates of diploma schools no longer existing and some had master's degrees from top universities. They had only two things in common: a sense of inadequacy and a sincere desire to return to work. While our courses were geared to the needs we anticipated, each one was enriched by additional suggestions and comments from members of the previous class.

Because there continues to be a demand for refresher courses and because it is often difficult for communities to provide adequate courses, it is felt that a book based on the needs elicited from these courses would be worthwhile. Building upon these experiences, this book attempts to guide independent study for the nonpracticing nurse who wishes to return to hospital nursing and needs to know where to begin.

We found that the nurse who has not practiced nursing for many years needs more than an orientation, no matter how long it might be. Some nurses can readjust to hospital work after a slow orientation, but they suffer from a lack of historical and perceptual understanding of why and how nursing has changed and what future directions might be expected. Our "Refreshers" were no less frightened of their first renewed patient contact because of this background, but they were willing to postpone immediate adjustment for a wider background. They were motivated by the excitement of returning to a career which they had long desired and were reassured by the knowledge that more time and more study would provide future satisfactions.

Our course was not all-inclusive and a major part of the work was done by the nurse who spent many hours reading the "Bib. List." It is the aim of this book to gather facts which will help the nurse to refresh herself, to give her survey information and to provide a guide to clinical readings. It can be used in conjunction with a refresher course and includes material which we taught our nurses and material which they taught us. It is hoped that it will help prepare the nonpracticing nurse for hospital employment and orientation.

Although this book was primarily designed for the refresher nurse returning to a hospital, it perhaps will interest the practicing nurse who is often so absorbed in her work that she does not see beyond her job. It is also hoped that it may give the new graduate an understanding of the daily revolutions occurring in her new profession, thus giving her a hint of what to expect if she is in need of refreshing later on. In addition, perhaps the nonpracticing nurse will use the book as a link to her profession.

RUTH PERIN STRYKER

Acknowledgments

No book is written alone. Casual suggestions become the inspiration for larger thoughts. Special interest is often a source of inspiration as well as direct help. The author is particularly grateful for the singular contributions made by John D. Foley, Loretta Mathiowetz and the late William Raney.

In addition, for many useful suggestions I am indebted to Shirley Asklund, Lorraine Botts, Rosalie Burton, Elvera Carleton, Mary Conroy, Evelyn Dressel, Helen Hayden, Anita Goldbarg, Sylvia Kupchs, Dorothy Marlow, Grace Mateo, Marjorie Person, Emil Schleicher, Virginia Schmidt and Judith Yates.

I am especially grateful to my mother who has spent many a weary hour just listening.

RUTH PERIN STRYKER

Table of Contents

1
Stages of Refreshing 1

2
Sociological, Economic and Technical Advances Affecting Nursing 5

3
Changes in Hospitals Today 14

4
Present Patterns of Nursing Service 27

5
Nursing Education Programs of Today 48

6
Responsibilities of Personnel Supervised by the Registered Nurse 63

7
The Registered Nurse at Work in a Hospital 76

8
Teaching Today's Patient 92

9
Diagnostic Laboratory and X-ray Examinations 107

10
Major Changes in Dietary Service 118

11
Care of the Patient's Skin 135

12
Care of the Patient With Anoxia 146

13
Care of the Operative Patient 162

14
Care of the Patient Needing Rehabilitation 174

15
Prevention of Hospital Infections 187

16
Guides for Administering Medications 195

17
Fluid and Electrolyte Balance 212

18
Common Types of New Equipment and Supplies 225

19
Major Changes in Care of the Mother and Infant 243

20
Major Changes in Pediatric Care 261

21
Major Changes in Care of the Psychiatric Patient 274

22
Back to Nursing 288

23
Beyond the Present 299

INDEX 305

1

Stages of Refreshing

When you embark upon a program of "refreshing" yourself, you cannot make up for every deficiency and learn every modern concept which has developed since you last practiced nursing. Nonetheless, you can learn some of the important influences in health care, the effects upon nursing and the areas in which nursing is developing and expanding. Thus, you will perhaps gain insight into the reasons why some things have occurred.

This book is designed to give the nurse a background of the rapid and radical changes which affect the nursing profession and to provide a guide for those who wish to return to work in a hospital, in particular. Refreshing has three stages: First, you must understand the changes and you will need an orientation to changing roles and new goals. Second, you need up-to-date knowledge required by the clinical area where you will perform your work. This would include a review of old learning. Third, you must learn new procedures. Most refreshers consider the latter stage to be the only one to be dealt with. Keep in mind that this stage is only one of your goals. One of the greatest mistakes made by refreshers and employers is to consider the learning of skills as the only aspect of refreshing. Taken in stages, refreshing becomes a series of steps, not a gigantic obstacle to be overcome. This book deals mainly with the first stage: acquaintance with changes in emphasis and some of the reasons for such changes.

Many times you will find that something is not as new as it may seem; it may really be something old in a new setting or an adaptation of something you once learned. Be prepared for many pleasant surprises. You will find fewer new things than you expect. The patient still has a disease and needs both physical and psychological care. He still responds to kind, thoughtful care. He still may not be able to void and he still has pain after surgery. He may lie on a high-low bed, use an intercom system and have a pillow speaker for his T.V. He may be catheterized by using a disposable set rather than requiring a nurse to set up a tray which will need to be washed, reset and autoclaved. He may receive Levo-Dromoran instead of codeine for his pain. In preparing the hypodermic, no elaborate procedure is needed to sterilize a 2 cc. syringe, no forceps is handled, no forceps solution needs daily changing, and no can for alcohol sponges is required. The nurse of today prepares a hypodermic by removing a cover from a sterile disposable syringe with an attached needle, withdrawing the desired dose of medicine from a single dose vial and picking up an individually wrapped alcohol sponge. These are but a few examples of simple adaptations which you will learn when you return to work.

Do not be concerned with learning gadgets and procedures initially. Even if you have taken a refresher course with clinical experience, procedures and equipment vary among hospitals so that many of these things will have to be learned during your orientation period at the hospital which employs you. Most hospitals provide a formal orientation of one or two weeks followed by one or two weeks to allow a newly employed graduate to gain experience while working with other personnel. No beginning refresher should have less time than this. Very few nurses are plunged into a nursing station to shift for themselves and to be responsible for many patients without the aid of some orientation. No nurse should have this experience. Any refresher returning to work should have it clearly explained how much time she will have for orientation and from whom she will get her help. It is important for the refresher to know that institutions vary greatly in the amount and kind of orientation provided.

Someone with experience should be available to you during most of this period. In larger institutions, the in-service director will at least start with you. A supervisor or head nurse will ultimately be concerned about your performance and will help you. In any case, you need competent persons available to show you new things as they come about and to answer your questions as they arise.

Before any of this occurs, however, you must have enough background knowledge to present yourself to a hospital for employment and orientation. To be employed without knowing the influences which make things different is likely to make you resistant and critical. It can well prevent you from working to your own potential when you do go back to work.

You also should be an intelligent spokesman in your community for your profession. Orientation to procedures does not give you this. What is your answer when a neighbor says, "The cost of hospitalization these days is highway robbery?" If you see a young graduate inserting a nasal tube for the first time in her life, do you say, "Nursing education has gone to the dogs?" Once you understand the goals and influencing factors, you will be able to answer intelligently, enter into some of nursing's many spirited issues and contribute to the activities which you feel are important.

As you read this book, I hope that you will consider going back to nursing. If not, I hope that it will at least stimulate you to contribute to nursing in some other way. Whether you have a refresher course or not, you will need time to read and study. If you can devote two hours a day to studying for about a month or two, you will find you have much information to start you off.

Suggested readings are included at the end of each chapter to give you a resource for reading now or later. They provide a guide for you to bridge some of the gaps in your knowledge. It is not expected that you will read all the suggested readings. You should, however, try to read one from each section. In areas of your special interest, you will undoubtedly want to read more. Look at the bibliographies of the articles you read. There you will find still more resources from which to draw.

Where will you find these references if there is no refresher course offered in your vicinity? If there is a school of nursing nearby, try to obtain permission to use their library for a few months. Explain to them what you are doing. It is quite likely that they will be more than happy to help you. If there is no college or school, go to your nearest hospital and find out if they have any of these references in the hospital library or nursing office, as the case may be. If you have neither one of these facilities, go to your nearest library and see if they can be of help to you.

Even if library resources are available to you, it will be most helpful to have at least some up-to-date material in your home. The following might be considered minimal:

1. Subscribe to a nursing journal. See Chapter 23 for a listing.
2. Purchase a book which describes procedures, such as *Bedside Nursing Techniques in Medicine and Surgery* by Audrey L. Sutton, published by W. B. Saunders Co., West Washington Square, Philadelphia, Pennsylvania, 19105. The 1964 edition costs $8.00.
3. Purchase a current textbook on nursing care, such as *Medical-Surgical Nursing* by Kathleen Shafer and others, published by C. V. Mosby Co., 3207 Washington Boulevard, St. Louis, Missouri, 63103. The third edition (1964) costs $9.00.
4. Look in the attic for your medical dictionary. If it is not there or if it is too old, you might want to purchase Dorland's Pocket *Medical Dictionary*, published by W. B. Saunders Co., West Washington Square, Philadelphia, Pennsylvania, 19105. The 20th edition costs $4.50.

A refresher has a real contribution to nursing. There is a give and take between the nurse of yesterday and the nurse of today. Neither must apologize for her age or stage of knowledge. Today's nurses are well educated, young and dedicated, but they often lack the maturity and experience which comes from age and personal experience. Yesterday's nurses may need re-education, but they possess the philosophy and maturity which comes from living. The patient truly gains when he is attended by personnel with this combination of educations, insights and experiences. Today's graduates and yesterday's graduates have much to learn from each other.

With this in mind, may you gain both pleasure and satisfaction in renewing an old acquaintance—nursing.

SUGGESTED READINGS

Reese, Dorothy E., Siegel, Stanley E., and Testoff, Arthur: The Inactive Nurse. *American Journal of Nursing*, November, 1964, p. 124.

Stryker, Ruth P.: A Refresher Course—A Series of Surprises. *Nursing Outlook*, April, 1962, p. 232.

Tabler, Madeline: Welcome Back to Nursing. *Nursing Outlook*, September, 1965, p. 67.

2

Sociological, Economic and Technical Advances Affecting Nursing

Additions to the body of knowledge of nursing and the resulting changes in nursing practice do not take place in a vacuum. Economic expansion, technological advances, new educational methods, physiological research, sociological developments, psychological insights, governmental support, new legislation and industrial participation all alter or modify the work of the nurse and her fellow workers every day. The forward progress of nursing has been so greatly influenced by all these factors that it is impossible to understand without at least an awareness of what they are. The patient may be the recipient of up-to-date care, but his care is often influenced by institutional adaptations and personnel adjustments to the many changes. A nurse in today's community, whether or not she is employed, should not only comprehend the changes that affect her profession but also be able to interpret them with some insight. In this chapter, there can only be an attempt to mention some of the more outstanding impacts upon nursing.

ECONOMIC CHANGES

Where has the good old nurse gone? She has not gone. She has merely been absorbed in the cultural changes and economic advances of the nation. Like everyone else, she works a 40-hour week (in most parts of the country), and five days a week instead of seven. She is just beginning to be paid a salary commensurate with her growing knowledge and skill. In general, working conditions for nurses have improved, but greater effort is still needed in this area. In this decade, no one would expect a young girl who is graduating from high school to become a nurse if she were to work a seven-day week at less than subsistence pay. However, it is important to remember that economic inflation has affected everyone's salary as well as the cost of living, so that this financial problem is not peculiar to nursing. It is also important to be aware of the fact that our culture does not expect a young girl to spend her life dedicated to an all-consuming cause. At present this is reserved mainly for women in religious orders. This does not mean that a young woman takes her work any less seriously. It merely means that she has time to develop herself in other facets of her life as well.

Why are hospital costs so high? Two major factors are responsible. The first is inflation. For example, a new car once cost $700, but this is not true today. Second, the increased cost of services as well as the increased number of services available at a hospital are expensive to provide. About 70 cents of every dollar spent by a hospital is expended on salaries. About 12 cents is spent for supplies and equipment. The rest of the dollar is spent on food, laundry, etc., or is accounted for by depreciation.

Hospital costs are often compared with hotel costs. This is like comparing apples with oranges, when one explores the differences between the two. About 40 per cent of a hospital staff are professional or technical personnel. This includes nurses, dietitians, medical technologists, laboratory technicians, medical records librarians, physical therapists, occupational therapists, x-ray technicians, pharmacists, administrative personnel and others. Only about 10 per cent of the personnel in a hotel can usually be classified as professional. Aside from the type of personnel employed, the kinds of equipment required by a hospital are very costly. A $25,000 x-ray machine is not an unusual expense. Microscopes, operating room equipment, whirlpool tubs, autoclaves, brain wave machines and food transportation carts are only a few items which are not needed by a hotel. Even the required type of bed is very different. It is important to be aware of these distinctions because many nurses are called upon to answer the question, "Why can't a hospital be businesslike and operate at the cost of a hotel?" There is a difference!

Few people know that the average patient stay has been shortened from about 21 days to about 6 days. It is interesting to note that the cost of each patient illness is approximately the same as it was 20 years ago. The cost per day is obviously higher, but the cost per illness is about the same. As a result of this, the loss of time and pay from work is less per illness.

Few hospitals are heavily endowed, as they were in the past. A hospital can no longer run in the red and expect some benefactor to take care of the deficit at the end of each year. A hospital must run like a business financially and be in the black at the end of the fiscal year. Increased services, increased salaries and fewer private subsidies are helping the cost of hospitalization to become commensurate with services rendered.

Who pays the bill? About 60 per cent of the money paid to a hospital for services rendered comes from insurance companies. Between 1953 and 1963, insurance company payments for health care rose by 250 per cent. Basically, this is prepaid hospitalization, because the patient carries his insurance to protect himself in case of illness. The types and kinds of hospital and medical insurance are many, but they continue to cover more and more services. Naturally, as the coverage of an insurance policy increases, so does its premium rate. At the present time the major source of financial worry about health expenses in most families is the fear of a catastrophic illness, which would last many months or years and could literally wipe out a family's savings. Study of answers to this problem continues.

THE HOSPITAL COMMUNITY

Who are some of the people providing service to patients today? Housekeeping maids, dietary technicians, purchasing agents, hospital administrators, personnel directors, admitting officers, business office personnel, EEG. technicians, physical therapists, pharmacists and laboratory and x-ray technicians are only a few of them. Twenty years ago, most of these jobs either were performed by nurses or else they were not performed at all. These are not nursing jobs, but frequently the distinctions still have to be made. These are some of the jobs which nurses should give up with enthusiasm, as they prevent us from nursing.

Where is the spirit of nursing? First of all, over twice as many patients are being treated in hospitals each day as were treated each day 20 years ago. A doubled hospital census, a shorter patient stay and a shorter work week for the nurse all contribute to make interpersonal relations between nurse and patient so brief and so infrequent that both are aware that something is missing. Depersonalization is not usually the result of indifference on the part of personnel; it is many times the result of economic and scientific advancement. If a nurse works from 7:00 A.M. to 3:30 P.M. on Monday, has Tuesday and Wednesday off and works from 3:00 P.M. to 11:30 P.M. on Thursday and Friday, and if a patient enters the hospital at 4:00 P.M. on Monday and goes home at 2:00 P.M. on Friday, he and that nurse have had a chance to meet on only one afternoon of the patient's stay. Practicing nurses may feel a sense of failure if they are unaware of some of the real reasons for their problems. When people talk about the good old days, they fail to see that this particular problem did not exist when the nurse worked a 12-hour day and a seven-day week and the patient stayed 21 days. Obviously, the good old days were not that good. Other answers are needed. One of nursing's main concerns today is demonstrated by the study of ways to lessen the impact on patient care caused by fewer patient contacts.

Expense

Item	%
Salaries	67.5%
Supplies	11.5
Food	4.2
Laundry Service	1.9
Equipment repairs	.3
Heat, water, light and power	2.5
Depreciation	4.3
Services purchased	3.4
Other expenses	4.4
	100.0%

Income

Item	%
Blue Cross	21.7%
Industrial Commission	5.2
Welfare patients	4.4
Commercial insurance	24.1
Paid on discharge	18.0
Credit extended — Deferred payments	7.2
Other	19.4
	100.0%

Contributions to the health of the community

Total patients admitted	13,542
Total patient days	87,147
Average length of stay in days	6.4
Out patient visits	21,540
Emergency room visits	11,348
Births	1,973
Operations	6,345
X-ray procedures	28,694
Laboratory procedures	137,565
Physical therapy treatments	13,388
Pharmacy issuances	191,838
Electroencephalograms	863
Total meals served	465,381
Total employees (full time equivalent)	619.2
Total student nurses enrolled	117
Total interns and residents	17
Total X-ray students enrolled	15
Total auxiliary membership	337
Volunteers — average monthly	199
Total volunteer services (in hours)	19,571

Figure 2–1. *Hospital expenses and income. (From Annual Report 1964, St. Barnabas Hospital, Minneapolis, Minnesota.)*

Where has the good old submissive patient gone? He is also with us, but he is far better educated about his illness and is paying a great deal more for the treatment of it. Keeping the patient uninformed and in helpless ignorance is a thing of the past. Public health education, medical reports in popular magazines, popular medical books, educational literature put out by special foundations and even advertisements make the hospitalized patient far better informed today than he was at any time in the past. When he is ill, he expects to know what his medicines are and what they will do for him. Medical workers must work together with their patients. When the patient asks why he has a footboard, we need a better answer than, "because the doctor ordered it." This will be discussed in more detail in Chapter 8.

In general, the atmosphere of a hospital reflects the many changes in our culture and society in general.

COMMUNITY SERVICES

Community and governmental interest (local, state and federal) in the nation's health has increased and may be expected to increase. A new service becomes available to the public as it is proved to be beneficial. Research and treatment facilities are backed by private endowments, private enterprise, community agencies and government. Most volunteer agencies are devoted to one disease or a group of related diseases. The American Cancer Society, for instance, is engaged in research and public education for the prevention of that disease. An organization may change its emphasis as knowledge unfolds. Although the Kenny Rehabilitation Institute started out as a facility for poliomyelitis victims, the reduced incidence of that disease has been responsible for altering the focus of this institution. It now cares for persons with strokes, spinal cord injuries, cerebral palsy, multiple sclerosis and other neuromuscular diseases. Long overdue attention is at last being paid to the treatment and rehabilitation of our mentally ill. These services contribute to the health of the community, not just the individual, so that we all have reason to support any agency which provides good up-to-date services. Vocational rehabilitation, recreational programs for various age groups and organizations devoted to a particular disease also exist in most areas.

The movement to provide clean, cheerful, safe nursing home services is something which will also continue to grow. The life span of the human being continues to lengthen and is estimated to be 130 years by the year 2000 A.D. Looking to future health needs, care of the aged obviously becomes a rather urgent one.

It is impossible even to list the kinds of community facilities which are available, because they are so numerous. If you are interested in the details of a particular area, call your local public health nurse or local health department to obtain a roster or directory, as the case may be.

TECHNICAL ADVANCES

Advanced surgical skills are developing at such a rapid rate that before the ink is dry on one report, another even more fantastic procedure has been perfected. The artificial kidney, the heart pump, organ banks and the use of plastic and Dacron for vein grafts are only a few examples of developments which permit hitherto unheard of surgical procedures. No nurse can expect to be conversant with all these developments. Only if she were assigned to an area where such a specialized piece of equipment is used or such a procedure performed, could she be expected to learn about it. No practicing nurse or physician can know the details of all new advances. Each of us must be responsible, however, for knowing the things within our particular work area. Outside of this, we can try to stay abreast of new developments, in general. The refresher soon finds that the use of informational resources is her most valuable tool.

The field of biomedical engineering is also new and growing. The pacemaker is an excellent example of a product of work in this field. This is a remarkably manufactured 3- by 3-inch little bundle of transistor batteries and wires encased in Teflon and silicone rubber. It is sewed inside the patient to give impulses to a heart which has a conduction system disorder. It gives years of life to persons who would otherwise die.

What will electronic inventions do to nursing? At the present time, we have inklings and some knowledge. Some hospitals have begun to use computers. Computers can transmit physician's orders, take care of business office operations, plan hour schedules for personnel, store the patient's record and store other information for future use. This one technical invention may do more to give the nurse more time to be with her patients than any other one thing. Computers cannot replace nurses. They will do some of the nurse's clerical tasks, but cannot replace the services which require human attributes.

Patient monitoring devices often give the public the impression that the nurse will be looking at a monitoring screen rather than at the patient. This is not true. These devices do not give treatments, bathe patients or provide them with emotional support. If anything, the nurse is needed more because of these machines.

LEGISLATION AFFECTING HEALTH CARE

Major legislation concerning health care has been passed in the last decade. The Nurse Training Act of 1964 is of particular interest to nurses. The first substantial amount of federal funds made available for recruitment and training of nurses was in 1943, when the U.S. Cadet Corps was established. The 1964 act provides funds for education of nurses at the baccalaureate level and beyond for administrators, supervisors, teachers and nurse specialists. It also makes funds available to schools for projects designed to improve their programs of edu-

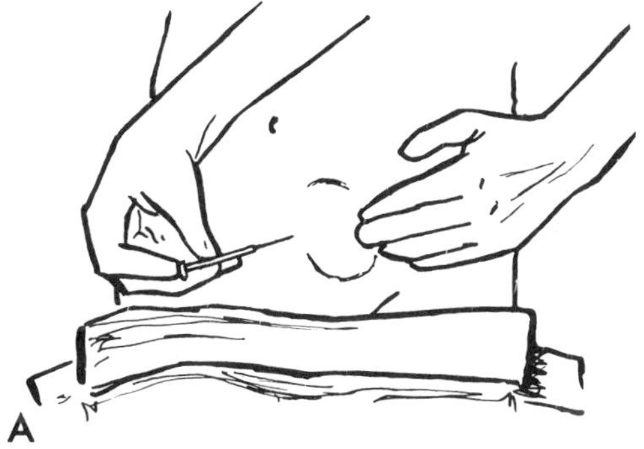

After implantation, the controls are easily located by palpation. Adjustment of rate and/or current is made by percutaneous needle insertion with a standard "Keith" skin needle of triangular cross-section, then turning to the desired new position.

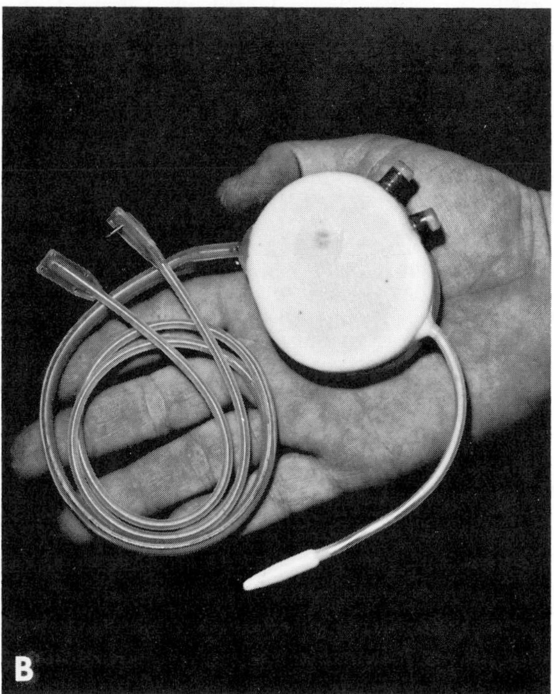

Figure 2–2. *Implantable pacemaker. (Medtronic, Inc., 3055 Highway 8, Minneapolis 8, Minnesota.)*

cation, for construction and renovation of building facilities and for loans to student nurses. The Division of Nursing of the United States Public Health Service administers this act.

Other legislation which has a direct effect on health care includes the equal pay for comparable work bill signed by President Kennedy in 1963, the Health Professions Act of 1963, various bills controlling the sale and distribution of drugs and the bill creating the Administration on Aging, and the Hill-Burton legislation. Funds are also now available for research and treatment of many specific diseases.

In 1965, the Medicare bill was passed by Congress. This bill provides specified health care to persons over 65 years of age, regardless of their financial status, and has expanded programs for medically needy children and mothers. Many private insurance plans are reconstructed around these benefits. It is administered by the Secretary of the Department of Health, Education, and Welfare. This bill will make a need for more hospitals, more outpatient facilities and more nursing homes. This, in turn, will increase the demand for nurses and other health workers.

SUMMARY

Cultural, sociological, economic and technical changes are all interrelated. Changes in available health care have been dramatic in the past decade. Although this has been a very brief survey of what is happening around us, it is important that we at least be aware of these things as we step inside one of today's hospitals—in our next chapter.

REFERENCES

American Women. Report of the President's Commission on the Status of Women, 1963.

Becker, Harry: Medicare: What it Means, What it Covers, How it Works. *Modern Hospital,* August, 1965, p. 27.

Boyle, Rena: Federal Legislation: Its Impact on NLN's Accrediting Programs. *Nursing Outlook,* March, 1965, p. 34.

The Division of Nursing U.S.P.H.S. *American Journal of Nursing,* July, 1965, p. 82.

Dreves, Katharine Densford: 1933–1952 Measuring Up. *Three Score Years and Ten 1893–1963,* National League for Nursing, 1963.

Freemen, John R.: You Can Too Learn to Live With Unions. *Modern Hospital,* November, 1964, p. 95.

Health Insurance Payments on the Increase. *American Journal of Nursing,* July, 1965, p. 34.

Hess, Arthur E.: Medicare: Administrative Authority and Its Limitations. *Hospitals,* September 1, 1965, p. 53.

Hungler, Bernadette P.: What Every Patient Needs. *American Journal of Nursing,* October, 1964, p. 112.

Leone, Lucile Petry: The Attack on Heart Disease, Cancer,and Stroke—Is Nursing Ready? *American Journal of Nursing,* May, 1965, p. 68.

McClenahan, J. Everett: Utilization Review Under Medicare. *Hospitals,* September 1, 1965, p. 55.

Nursing Concern in Health Insurance for the Aged. A Statement from the American Nurses' Association, September, 1965, p. 120.

Pamphlets on Nurse Training Act of 1964 published by the U.S. Department of Health, Education, and Welfare, Public Health Service, Division of Nursing, Washington, D.C., 20201. Nurse Training Act of 1964, No. 1154, Professional Nurse Traineeship Program, No. 1154-1, Project Grants For Improvement in Nurse Training, No. 1154-2, Payments to Diploma Schools of Nursing, No. 1154-3, Nursing Student Loan Program: Information For Schools, No. 1154-4, Construction Grants Program For Schools of Nursing, No. 1154-5.

Paulsen, Dorothy: Patients Give Tests, Too. *American Journal of Nursing,* August, 1962, p. 58.

Snyder, James D.: Medicare—Its Impact on Hospital. *Hospital Management,* September, 1965, p. 39.

Toward Quality in Nursing—Needs and Goals. Report of the Surgeon General's Consultant Group on Nursing, U.S. Department of Health, Education, and Welfare, Public Health Service, Publication No. 992, February 1963.

Williamson, Kenneth: Medicare: Vast New Resource in Health and Welfare. *Hospitals,* September 1, 1965, p. 39.

3

Changes in Hospitals Today

The basic roles of the hospital, to provide patient care, to conduct programs of education and to conduct research, continue to expand. In order to function in these roles, the hospital has been called upon to perform many other services and to expand its facilities, which traditionally have not been associated with hospitals of the past.

In order to be more specific, let's take a tour through a modern hospital with full accreditation by the American Hospital Association. Since no one hospital has all the facilities which we will describe, our hospital will be a composite of up-to-date hospitals of various kinds and sizes.

A hospital must be part of a community and its services should be based upon the needs of that community. Whenever an institution expands in size or increases its number of services without consideration of its neighboring institutions, it dilutes the quality of health care offered in the area and the patient is the loser. Community planning will prevent duplication of costly facilities and promote cooperative rather than competitive services.

INCREASED NUMBER OF ANCILLARY SERVICES

As we enter our fully air-conditioned hospital, notice how the bustle in the lobby reminds you of a hotel. Observe the shops and services which you ordinarily do not associate with a hospital. Volunteer women are delivering flowers and selling toys, negligees and glassware in the Gift Shop. Others are serving lunches in the Coffee Shop. If the volunteer group belongs to the Women's Auxiliary Council of the American Hospital Association, they will probably be wearing cherry-colored smocks. The proceeds from their volunteer services go to the hospital for particular projects such as research, student scholarships or specialized equipment.

A small flower shop, a beauty shop, a barber shop, a branch bank and a library are down the hall. I am sure you would find that you could receive dry cleaning service through this hospital even though it does not have a dry cleaning shop. Are these unnecessary luxury services? No. They are services which all of us have come to use more and more, so that we expect them wherever we are. A shampoo, set and manicure after seven weeks of a dangerously acute illness is not a luxury. A patient who recently had this service said that it was therapeutic. I agree.

The Housekeeping Department has taken over many chores formerly performed by nurses. The nurse no longer mops the floor, dusts her patient's bed, changes the linen when a patient goes home or cleans the station refrigerator. In our hospital, the housekeeping maids can be recognized by their pink dresses. Although the color of the uniform varies from hospital to hospital, the role of the department is similar.

INCREASED PARAMEDICAL SERVICES

Notice the chapel with its doors open to all faiths, regardless of the religious affiliation of the hospital. It is used by patients, families and personnel 24 hours a day. Rabbis, priests and Protestant ministers attend to the spiritual needs of patients of their own faith.

Illness is rarely an isolated factor in a family's life. It may produce additional dilemmas, such as financial burdens, employment loss, need for care of dependents, social adjustments or any one of many other difficulties. A social worker can coordinate services and advise patients and families with multiple problems. That is the function of our Social Service Department.

The Dietary Department has changed. Special carts keep food at the proper temperature. The hot food stays hot and the cold food stays cold. Large stainless-steel refrigerators and instant frozen food cookers are only a few of the many improvements which provide patients with better food service.

The X-ray Department is larger and busier. Greater skill and knowledge are required of its employees. More and more diseases can be identified by x-ray because of progress in the sensitivity of new types of film, new "cameras" with high speed action and better developing methods. Powerful x-ray, cobalt and radioactive isotope treatments are performed in the X-ray Department.

The Laboratory also has new equipment to expedite diagnosis. As an example, the auto-analyzer determines and records the results of blood chemistries faster than a medical technologist would have dreamed a decade ago. More precise and sensitive methods and equipment permit analysis of very small amounts of blood. These "micro" blood determinations on infants were impossible when a larger amount of blood had to be obtained by venapuncture to make the analysis.

The Physical Therapy Department and the Occupational Therapy Department have both expanded greatly because more patients need one or both services. We have a mock-up kitchen in which the handicapped or postcoronary housewife may practice. Crafts and hobbies can relax the mind and exercise muscles needing rehabilitation. Whirlpool tubs and many other restorative devices are available. Increased numbers of physicians are studying to become physiatrists. These specialists supervise, prescribe for and evaluate the patient who may benefit from physical therapy.

Research is done at this private hospital; it is no longer the sole prerogative of the large university hospital. Most private urban hospitals encourage at least one medical researcher to work under its auspices. This adds prestige to an institution, provides an outlet for medical curiosity and attracts patients who require the most current knowledge about their particular condition.

We have a large Outpatient Department. Patients who come to this private center are treated by medical interns and residents under the supervision of a teaching physician. This department also provides emergency care for patients whose physicians are on the staff of the hospital. An office building for physicians is going up across the street so that private patients can better utilize the hospital diagnostic facilities.

AUTOMATION AND MECHANICAL DEVICES

No one would want to abolish the many devices in which patients are served by automation. Nonetheless, users of automatic devices must keep in mind that depersonalization accompanies automation. Depersonalization occurs whenever the number of contacts between patients and personnel, as well as between personnel of various departments, are reduced. This is immediately recognized by anyone who has worked in a small hospital or "in the good old days."

Notice the large number of dumbwaiters: for the Pharmacy, the Laboratory, the Dietary Department. Some equipment is delivered directly to a department on a conveyor belt. When everything from the equipment room is delivered to the station via dumbwaiter, you do not know or even recognize personnel from the equipment room. However, this was not true when someone delivered it to you or when you went to the equipment room to get it. The dumbwaiter and conveyor belt exemplify the kind of equipment which keeps nursing personnel from running errands, but this convenience also serves to isolate departments within an institution.

The pneumatic tube is another device which keeps personnel from leaving their work areas. Messages, orders, charges, charts, small items, etc., can be sent and received via the pneumatic tube. Like all automatic devices, it is not perfect; it needs maintenance and inspection at regular intervals. In addition, it is not free from human error. For example, drug orders may arrive in the Chaplain's Office if someone has sent a tube incorrectly. The sender must set the tube dial so that it is sent to the appropriate department.

Our hospital uses a closed circuit paging system which almost eliminates the public paging system. With this system, personnel and physicians who are likely to be paged carry a small transistor radio in their pockets. When someone wants one of them, a call is placed to the operator who sends a signal which is received only by the person being called. The person receiving the signal then presses a button and receives his message.

Electrically powered beds contribute to patient comfort and safety. The patient learns to raise and lower the head and foot of his bed by using the buttons on a control switch. They enjoy this device a great deal. Often a patient wants to change his position slightly or at frequent intervals. He would not do so if he had to call the nurse every time he wished to lower the head of his bed an inch or two. New beds can also be placed in the high position as well as the low position. This is a safety feature. Beds are placed in the high position (the height of most hospital beds in 1952) whenever a nurse makes the bed or performs a treatment.

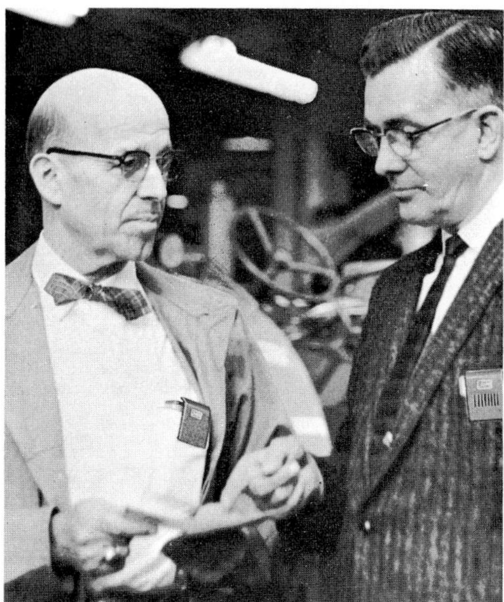

Figure 3–1. *Key personnel wear page receivers in their pockets for rapid transmission of messages. (Courtesy L. F. Johnson Company, Waseca, Minn.)*

This prevents back injury and fatigue to nursing personnel. When the nurse leaves her patient, she places the bed in the low position (the height of beds in most homes). Thus, the patient can get in and out of bed more easily and the old-fashioned step stool is eliminated. If the patient were to fall out of bed, he would fall such a short distance that he would be less likely to sustain an injury of any consequence.

The Medical Records Department continues to participate more actively in keeping the patient's chart as well as statistical analysis. Dictating machines are seen on each floor and in the operating room. These machines are used by the physician and are connected to a recording device in the Medical Records Department. Doctors can dictate admission notes, progress notes, histories, physical examinations, discharge records and operating room reports immediately. By the next day, the typewritten record is sent to the nursing station, where it is placed in the patient's chart. Far less time is spent in this way than would have been spent in deciphering the doctor's handwriting! Our hospital has an extension number so that the physician can telephone his dictation when he is outside the hospital. Patient records are microfilmed if they are seven years old. This saves precious storage space.

Various types of machines help to compile statistics, which enable a hospital to know the trends of its patient population and which can help in mass research data in other areas. This contributes to future planning of the individual hospital as well as research.

Time clocks have been installed on each floor. They are becoming a common sight in most hospitals. Punch-coded time cards are used in order to save many man hours in the Payroll Department and to provide an accurate record of hours worked by employees.

In our intensive care area, monitoring devices provide a continuous check on patient's blood pressure, pulse, temperature and heart activity. These machines are used only for acutely ill patients. Though the nurse can keep track of her patient from outside his room, the purpose of the machine is not to lessen the number of patient contacts with the nurse. It is used to keep track of his physical signs at a frequency and in detail which constant attendance could not accomplish. His other physical needs and his emotional needs are not ignored by use of this machine. It is merely an additional tool for caring for a patient with acute needs.

Our hospital is presently studying the use of computers. Some hospitals use computers to transcribe doctor's orders, to make charges, to remind nurses to give pills, to store records, to compute bills and to do many other clerical chores. With further research and development of programs for these machines, more hospitals will be using them.

HOSPITAL ADMINISTRATION

The fifth largest industry in the United States is the hospital industry. Because of the growing business and financial complexity of

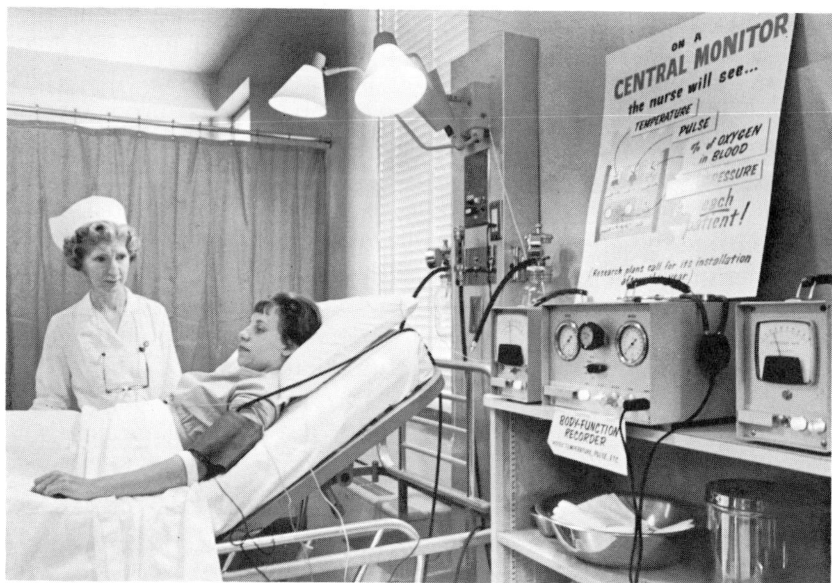

Figure 3–2. Electronic device for monitoring vital signs of patient. (From George, Joyce Holmes: Electronic Monitoring. American Journal of Nursing, *February, 1965, p. 68.)*

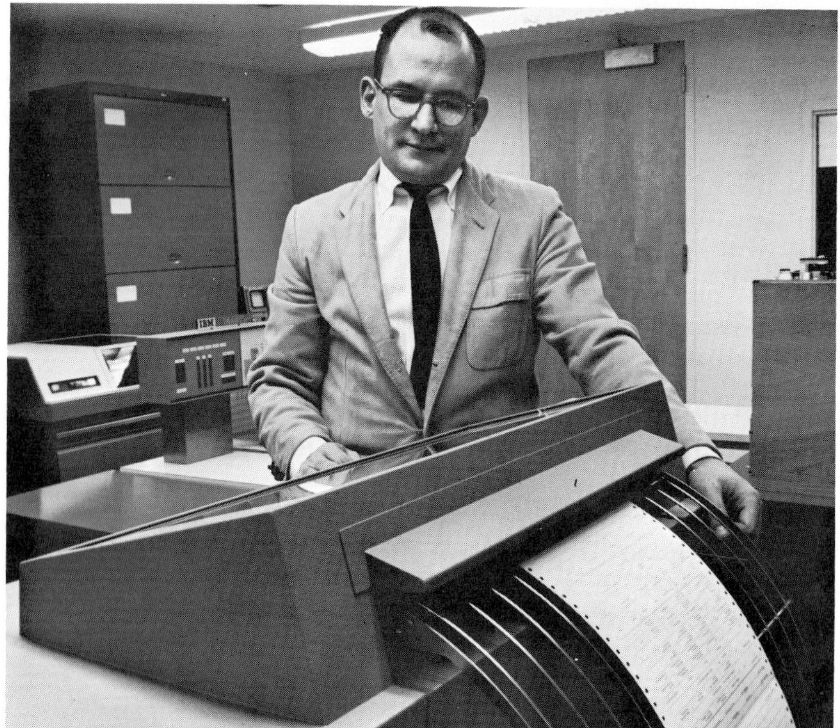

Figure 3–3. Computer used to interpret electrocardiograms. As cardiogram tapes on unit at right are fed into the computer, they are stored in system's disk memory unit (left), computed and printed on special form. (From Cordes, Donald W.: Computer Allows a Routine ECG for Every Admission. Modern Hospital, *April, 1965, p. 111.)*

managing a hospital, fewer nurses and doctors sit behind the hospital director's desk. At this desk in our hospital is a man with undergraduate work in business administration and postgraduate work in hospital administration. He assists in solving interdepartmental problems and advises on collective bargaining activities with labor groups. He works with the Board of Governors in planning for the future, and with the medical staff in seeking and maintaining high medical standards. He helps to bring the hospital budget within a realistic goal and constantly seeks ways of operating the hospital in the black, while providing quality service in many growing spheres. He must keep abreast of many subjects and needs expert departmental supervisors to advise him and to keep him apprised of their needs and problems. Judicious selection of new directions for better patient care becomes his ultimate responsibility. The hospital administrator combines a service organization with business know-how.

PROGRESSIVE PATIENT CARE

Progressive patient care has been completely adopted by a few hospitals and in part by many. This provides medical and nursing facilities to the patient according to the degree of his illness rather than the type of illness. Personnel and facilities increase and decrease according to the needs of the patient. When progressive patient care is properly functioning in a hospital, one receives the least amount of nursing care when one is least ill and the most nursing care when one is sickest. There are five stages of progressive patient care (P.P.C.). All five stages may be found in a hospital in which the concept is wholly adopted, or the community may provide care for the phases in different types of institutions. Few patients require all five stages of care. When P.P.C. is found in a hospital, specialties, such as orthopedics, urology, medicine, etc., may no longer be found and staffing patterns will alter according to the needs of the patients in each section.

The first stage of P.P.C. is self-help or minimal care. Patients who require little assistance are located in one section of the hospital. They are usually hospitalized for diagnostic tests or simple treatments. The patient requires very little physical care. These patients walk to and from hospital departments unassisted by personnel. They get dressed and eat in a special dining room or in the employee cafeteria. There is usually about one nurse for every 20 patients. The nurse is there to provide general supervision of care and to see that the patient receives his medications, proper instructions for examinations and convalescent treatments.

The second stage of P.P.C. is intermediate care. A section of the hospital houses patients who are recovering from an acute illness, who require only a moderate amount of nursing care or do not require continuous observation. These patients constitute a large percentage of a hospital's total case load.

The third stage of P.P.C. is intensive or special care. This is the phase of P.P.C. which has recently been adopted by many hospitals. The units vary in size, according to the total number of beds in the hospital in which the unit is located. One nurse for every two patients is usually considered a desirable nurse-patient ratio. This may fluctuate up or down depending on the requirements of the patients. These units provide care for the acutely ill patient who needs constant vigilance and frequent treatments. As a result, private duty nurses are less frequently used in the care of the acutely ill patient not only because intensive care personnel are highly skilled in caring for this type of patient but also because the equipment within the unit is specialized. This equipment is thus centralized for emergency care.

Some insurance plans cover the additional costs for patients in these areas. The rates for intensive care are usually higher because of the additional personnel and equipment, just as the rates for minimal care are usually lower because there is virtually no equipment except that which you would find at a hotel. Some hospitals, however, charge similar rates allowing the low cost area to balance the high cost area.

A fourth phase of P.P.C. is convalescent or long-term care. Patients with chronic diseases and those who require rehabilitative and restorative care are housed on the convalescent floor. A great deal of physical therapy and occupational therapy time is devoted to these patients.

The fifth phase of P.P.C. is extended or home care. This care is sometimes given by hospital personnel after the patient has gone home. In this event, a nurse and/or a physical therapist (employed by the hospital) visits the home to see that the patient understands the instructions he received when he left the hospital and also to see whether it is possible for him to carry out such orders. It is often very difficult to adapt instructions to home equipment. Such visits usually are concerned with initial home adjustment problems and are rarely of a long-term nature. This particular phase of P.P.C. can also be handled in other ways. If the physician feels that some of this belongs in his realm of responsibility, he may wish to make home visits. This may or may not be in conjunction with visits by other personnel. A public health agency may be available for referral of such patients for whom supervision is needed. Like everything else, consideration of total community facilities may help to clarify the boundaries and need for this service and to determine the wisest source. Our hospital has developed a system for identifying and referring patients in need of follow-up and/or home care.

OTHER FACILITIES

As we enter the operating room (O.R.), notice the shoe baths and the synthetic floor mats which remove lint to lessen the possibility of infection. Right next to the O.R. is the postanesthesia room (P.A.R.) or recovery room. Immediately following surgery, the patient is taken to the P.A.R. until he awakens from his anesthesia. Personnel with specialized knowledge and life-saving devices are within inches. A medical anesthesiologist and a nurse anesthetist are nearby in case of emergency. After surgery, the patient does not leave the room until his blood pressure is stable and he is nearly awake. Because visitors are not allowed in this area, it is important for a hospital to provide a method for keeping relatives informed of the patient's condition during his stay in the P.A.R.

The Central Service Department (C.S.R.) has changed character in many ways. It now dispenses many disposable items which were once hand-prepared. Parenthetically, disposing of disposables has become a major job of hospitals. Chemical cleaning agents and new machines easily wash equipment which used to require many man hours. Furthermore, the C.S.R. provides services to many departments other than the nursing department. Because of these things, it is becoming less common to have it administered by a nurse. At our hospital, a nurse works in the C.S.R. to advise on special trays and nursing treatments and to coordinate nursing procedures, but the C.S.R. is administered by the Purchasing Department. At some hospitals, the office of Hospital Administration directs its activities. In any case, the person in charge needs much knowledge which is non-nursing.

New architectural designs of hospitals can be seen from the outside as well as from the inside. There are many concepts and opinions about the shapes and sizes of units which provide maximum visibility of the patient, nearness to the patient, easy access to equipment and reduction of fatigue of personnel. Ours is the offset cross design in which patients are in each arm with supplies and equipment at one end. There are many other designs, such as the rectangle, with equipment and records at the center of one of the long sides. Circular units locate the nursing station, records and equipment at the center so that all patients are equally distant from this center area. The pros and cons of various shapes provide material for many lively debates.

The type of patient being served helps to determine how effective an architectural design is and how important some of the advantages and disadvantages are. Research is presently being conducted to identify some of the variables which exist. Other trends in building include the addition of nursing home wings onto acute private hospitals and the addition of psychiatric wings in private facilities. Hill-Burton funds have provided great impetus to hospital building.

Expansion also occurs in the form of satellite hospitals. A satellite hospital is a small hospital which is generally managed by a larger hospital in another area. Some satellites are over 100 miles away from the larger hospital, while others may be only a few blocks away as is the case at our hospital. There are advantages, such as sharing equipment, purchasing, managing personnel, and policy and procedural development. Another trend is for hospitals to share services. In such an event, total merger is not required. Two hospitals sharing one laundry rather than each having its own laundry is an example of such sharing.

Certain highly specialized facilities are not at our hospital and can be seen only in certain institutions. A hyperbaric chamber for the treatment of certain diseases is an example. It is expensive and personnel require special knowledge. Although they will increase in numbers, they most likely will not become part of every hospital. Chemists, physicists, biologists`and engineeers will continue to contribute to the treatment of disease. For such complex developments communities will need to share their facilities.

The places we have visited are only a few of the highlights of the modern hospital. Every area we have visited is a subject unto itself so it has been possible only to briefly mention some of them.

Before we leave our hospital, it should be mentioned that one of a hospital's major functions is almost unnoticeable—that of education. The student nurse is in evidence, and so are interns and residents. Though nursing and medical education is an accepted part of the hospital, other fields of education are not so evident. The hospital provides a field experience to many different groups, such as postgraduate nurses, hospital administrators, medical social workers, dietitians, x-ray technicians, the general public, such as visitors, and volunteers, seminary students, the press, and many others. The Nursing Department participates in a majority of such educational programs.

THE TEAM APPROACH

Because scientific knowledge continues to unfold at a phenomenal pace, more and more men and women in the health fields are seeking areas of specialization. Man recognizes that his abilities have limitations and as a result, new health occupations develop and expand. This has created the need for a team approach to patient care. One of the functions of a hospital is to provide continuity of patient care through a team of persons. This approach minimizes the separateness of specialization and pools resources for quality care. It also requires a sound organizational structure and attention to communications among those participating in the care of a particular patient.

With all these gadgets, all these people and all these services, what does the nurse do and how can she function in such a complex social system? She has adapted herself remarkably well. She has tried to maintain part of her old image and at the same time she has adopted a new image in the midst of many opposing forces. We will discuss some of these things in our next chapter.

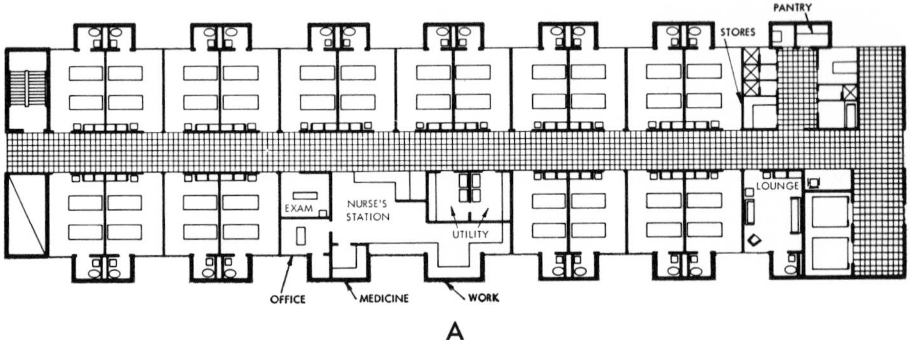

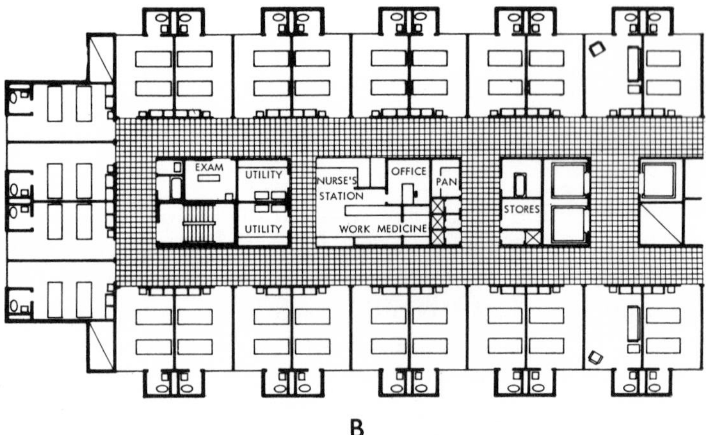

Figure 3–4. *Architectural designs for nursing units. A, Single-corridor 40-bed unit. B, Double-corridor 44-bed unit. C, T-shaped 40-bed unit. D, Circular 24-bed unit. (From McLaughlin, Herbert: What Shape Is Best for Nursing Units?* Modern Hospital, *December, 1964, p. 85.)*

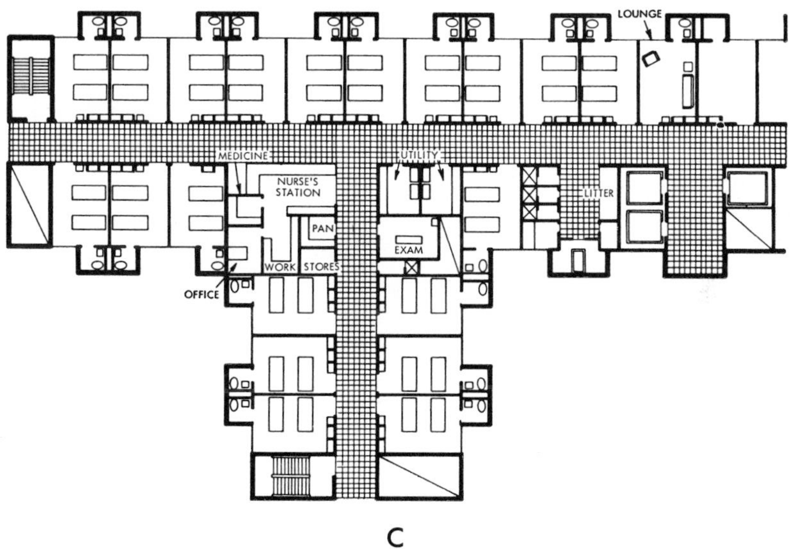

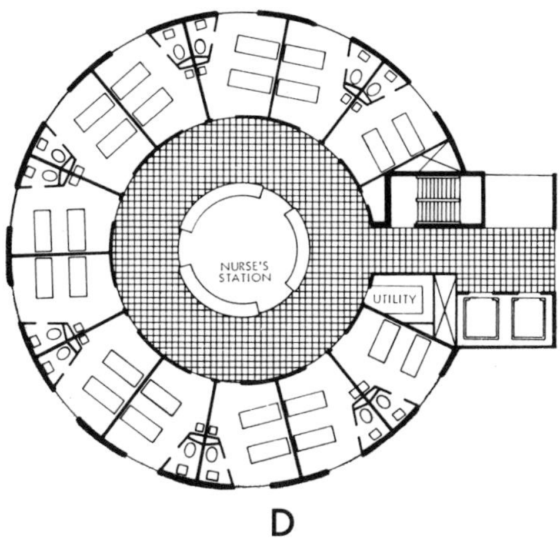

Figure 3–4. *(Continued)*

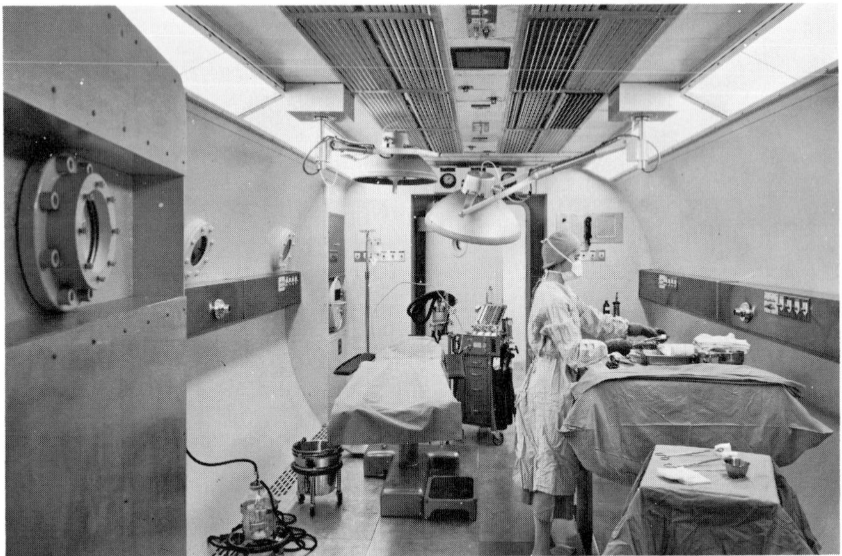

Figure 3–5. *Hyperbaric chamber. This view of the main chamber of the unit at Mount Sinai Hospital, New York, shows the medical and surgical equipment that permits treating a cyanotic baby or performing complex cardiovascular surgery. Every effort has been made to eliminate the possibility of fire or explosion, the two greatest hazards. (From McKillop, N.: The High Pressure Oxygen Chamber: Therapeutic Tool or Status Symbol,* Hospitals, *December 16, 1964, p. 59.)*

REFERENCES

Abdellah, Faye G., Meyer, Burton, and Roberts, Helen: Nursing Patterns Vary in Progressive Care. *Modern Hospital,* August, 1960, p. 85.

Abdellah, Faye G.: Progressive Patient Care. *Hospital Management,* June, 1960, p. 102.

Brown, Esther Lucile: *Newer Dimensions of Patient Care.* Part 2, Improving Staff Motivation and Competence in the General Hospital, New York, Russell Sage Foundation, 1962.

Brown, Ray E.: The General Hospital Has a General Responsibility. *Hospitals,* June 16, 1965, p. 47.

Burling, T., Lentz, E. M., and Wilson, R. N.: *The Give and Take in Hospitals.* New York, G. P. Putnam's Sons, 1956.

Colman, Douglas J.: The Key Issues. *Hospitals,* January 1, 1965, p. 30.

Coronary Care Units. U.S. Department of Health, Education, and Welfare, Public Health Service Publication No. 1250, 1964.

George, Joyce Holmes: Electronic Monitoring of Vital Signs. *American Journal of Nursing,* February, 1965, p. 68.

Juzwiak, Marijo: Glimpse of the Future: The Friesen Hospital. *R.N.,* October, 1964, p. 67.

Kelly, Cordelia W.: Dimensions of Professional Nursing. New York, Macmillan Co., 1962.

Letourneau, C. V.: Planning For Hospital Central Service. *Hospital Management,* January, 1964, p. 46.

McKillop, William: The High Pressure Oxygen Chamber: Therapeutic Tool or Status Symbol. *Hospitals,* December 16, 1964, p. 59.

McLaughlin, Herbert: What Shape is Best for Nursing Units? *Modern Hospital,* December, 1964, p. 85.

Nursing Service Without Walls. Department of Hospital Nursing and Department of Public Health Nursing, National League for Nursing, 10 Columbus Circle, New York, 1963.

Perspectives For Nursing. Report of the Committee on Perspectives, National League for Nursing, 1965.

Sloan, Raymond P.: *This Hospital Business of Ours.* New York, G. P. Putnam's Sons, 1952.

Zwald, Robert L.: Role of Central Service in the Hospital Organization Chart. *Hospital Management,* January, 1964, p. 93.

4

Present Patterns of Nursing Service

After describing various influences on nursing, it will be helpful now to review some of the adaptations to these influences made by the hospital nurse. It is impossible to describe all of them, as there are many variations among types and kinds of hospitals. Nonetheless, there have emerged general patterns which are changing the responsibilities of nursing personnel and which profoundly affect patient service. We need to examine each change closely to decide whether it indicates authentic progress and improvement in the scope of patient care.

NEW INSIGHTS BREAK OLD PATTERNS

Interest in modern psychological findings is evidenced in many ways. Enormous sales of books about popularity, happiness and release from tension demonstrate this. More profound books by students of psychology have also enjoyed a large circulation. The patient benefits whenever the knowledge of his nurse goes beyond the organic aspects of his condition.

Insights into patient behavior and reaction to illness and knowledge of physiological responses to illness can increase our therapeutic influence. The older nurse needs to become aware of some of the principles of psychology and techniques of helping patients to express themselves. She needs to be tolerant of her patient's feelings. She needs to realize that a patient may "hint around" at his problem, and she must listen for this. If the nurse explores patient conversation, if she listens to unspoken as well as spoken words and if she is uncritical of disconcerting behavior, she will be better able to help her patient.

Some patients desire a great deal of solitude; others do not. When a nurse visits her patient, she is wise to remember that there is a difference between loneliness and solitude. She must try to refrain from interpreting patients' behavior through her own reactions. We all too often listen to ourselves rather than to the other person.

Knowledge of humanities and social sciences helps us to focus our attention away from procedures and equipment. This provides a much needed balance at a time when we need to master the operation of so many machines and gadgets. Continued education makes one acutely aware of the fact that learning is a never ending process, regardless of the profession one chooses or the amount of education attained. Part of being prepared to perform a job is knowing that only a continuing curiosity and satisfaction of that curiosity will protect one from becoming outdated educationally. Along with this, we need a varied background so that we can best judge when to embrace new concepts, when to discard old ones and when to keep what we have. It may comfort the refresher to know that some employed nurses also need to refresh themselves.

Nurse-doctor relations have altered. The nurse is less often seen as the "handmaiden" of the doctor. Nurses are becoming more and more reluctant to perform only in the area of physician's orders. The nurse can identify many areas in which she performs independently. This actually means that she functions both dependently and independently. Dependent functions result from physician's prescribed orders. Independent functions result from observations and needs of patients as judged to be necessary by the nurse. At the same time, there is also a growing desire on the part of physicians to have nurses perform more of their functions. Misunderstandings may occur if the physician and nurse see these areas very differently. This will be discussed further a little later.

Attitudes within hospitals have changed. There is far greater permissiveness in almost all hospitals. Procedures and policies are beginning to be looked upon as sensible guides to methods rather than rules which can never be broken. Let us take two examples, both related to visiting regulations. A 90-year-old woman was admitted to our hospital with a broken hip. She was also blind and lived at a home for the blind. The only friend who was physically able to visit her used a seeing eye dog to get around. She was allowed to visit regularly with her canine friend at her side. On one other occasion, a woman dying of cancer asked to see a two-month-old grandchild whom she had never seen. The mother of the child brought her infant to the bedside, and the patient's wish was fulfilled. Indiscriminate breaking of rules is not permitted, but judicious breaking of rules by persons with proper knowledge and authority can prevent them from being unreasonable. Personnel are encouraged to use their own judgment rather than to depend upon someone else's decisions. If a rule cannot be satisfactorily interpreted in a majority of instances, it needs study.

In "Tenderness and Technique," Dr. Genevieve Meyer investigated the transition of values in nursing. She classified nurses in her study as "ministering angels" at one extreme, "efficient professionals" at the other and placed the "modern integrationist" between the two. This study describes the nurse's image in her own mind. Other studies identify changes in the image of the nurse in the patient's mind. Such studies give us further knowledge of ourselves.

A division of labor has led to a gap between the patient and the nurse. This in turn has led to uneasiness on the part of both the nurse and the patient. Nurse-patient contacts have decreased in number and in duration all too frequently. Mobility of nursing tasks has been toward administrative functions. The nurse has taken on more and more responsibilities. She has taught simpler tasks to unskilled workers, but unfortunately, many of the so-called simpler tasks are closely and intimately related to the patient. Patient dissatisfaction has often resulted, and the nurse has found her job frustrating and less rewarding. It has become increasingly apparent that more profound and more complicated insights are often gained during the performance of a simple task and that patients need to see more of their nurses.

Some changes in nursing service have occurred because of a personnel shortage due to increasing duties and responsibilities. Physicians no longer find time to perform tasks, such as taking blood pressures, starting intravenous fluids and changing dressings—to mention only a few. Nurses have often been very willing to accept additional work from physicians and other disciplines. This has tended to fragment the performance of nursing. In an effort to adjust, the nurse has shed some of her duties and created new jobs within the nursing department. Without judging their worth or describing variations among hospitals, we will look at the more common jobs and duties expected of these jobs. Along with the tasks, we will briefly describe the qualifications expected of persons who are to fill these positions. The American Nurses' Association statements on functions, standards and qualifications of the Director of Nursing Service are found on pp. 33–36, of the Supervisor on pp. 36–39, of the Head Nurse on pp. 39–44, and of the general duty nurse on pp. 44–66.

ROLES OF VARIOUS PERSONNEL

Director of Nursing Service

The Director of Nursing Service usually has a bachelor's or a master's degree from a university. She is responsible for recruitment and selection of qualified personnel, growth of her department, evaluation of its progress and coordination of activities with other departments. She must constantly look for new ways of upgrading nursing care. These job responsibilities are similar in most hospitals, but in addition, she is often assigned many other tasks, especially at small hospitals or in rural areas.

Assistant Director of Nursing

A nursing service department may have several assistant directors or none, depending upon the size of the hospital. In the latter case, these duties are incorporated into other positions. The assistant may also have a bachelor's or a master's degree. She may be responsible for in-service education, which usually includes on-the-job training of non-professional workers, orientation of new employees, education geared to new products and procedures and continuing development of personnel. She may work in method improvement projects, help to interview and select personnel, coordinate the purchase of new supplies and supervise staffing. The scope of these positions varies according to the duties delegated by the Director of Nursing Service and the organizational structure of the institution.

Supervisor

This particular job is better described by its duties than by its job title as the person with these responsibilities at some hospitals is called an Assistant Director of Nursing Service. The supervisor is responsible for analyzing and evaluating patient care and for assisting head nurses to develop and to solve patient care problems in several areas of the hospital. She interprets policies and delegates responsibility. She must guide and evaluate her head nurses. One essential duty is to recommend staffing and equipment needs for her patient areas to the director. The supervisor needs to be skilled in problem solving and must be able to provide the director with information which will help her to carry out the objectives of the nursing department. The supervisor is called upon to take on additional administrative duties when she is asked to represent the director on evenings, nights and weekends. Supervisors have a variety of background experience and education. I know of one institution in which the majority of supervisors are diploma graduates, but two have bachelor's degrees and one has a master's degree.

Head Nurse

At the present time, most head nurses are graduates of a hospital school of nursing. The head nurse has duties similar to those of the supervisor, but in only one nursing area rather than several areas. She is responsible for the immediate and direct planning and implementation of patient care. She is "on the scene," so to speak. This particular job is undergoing more changes than almost any other in the nursing department. In many instances, the majority of duties have become clerical and administrative. Effort to remedy this situation is being considered in many places. In hospitals in which the head nurse has been released from her pencil, patient care is thought to have improved. Whenever the head nurse gains additional time, she has a better opportunity to function as described on pp. 39–44. The head nurse is usually the person who has the most experience to offer, as well as knowledge of good generalized or specialized care. Some hospitals have even changed the title of the job when they wish to take away some of her clerical and administrative duties. Whether the hospital changes her title or not, it is what she can do with her time that makes the difference to the patient.

One of the tasks which can be taken away from the head nurse is that of transcribing physician's orders. This can be done by someone trained on the job. Nurses who are physically unable to do bedside nursing are often well suited to such a task. Lay persons can also be trained to do it. In any case, removal of this task from the head nurse on a 40-bed station of acutely ill patients can give her as much as five more hours a day to be with her patients and personnel. Basically, the job of the head nurse (regardless of the job title) should be to supervise patient care. If she can do this, she is available to both her patients and her personnel, providing better care for the patients on her unit.

The Registered Nurse

The registered nurse (R.N.) is responsible for the immediate treatments and needs of the patients assigned to her. Without explaining details of the team system in this chapter, it can generally be said that it is a method whereby several persons care for a group of patients. A station may have two or three teams, depending upon its size. An R.N. is responsible for about 15 patients who are cared for by a nurse aide, a licensed practical nurse (L.P.N.) or licensed vocational nurse (L.V.N.) and herself. This means that the R.N. gives direct care to some of her patients but not necessarily to all of them. She may give direct care to the patients with acute and complicated illnesses. She is also responsible for the patients who are cared for by the others. In this setting, the R.N. has become a supervisor of the nursing care given by several persons to several patients. A future chapter will describe this vital position in more detail and describe some of the variations.

OTHER PERSONNEL

With increasing numbers of patients and increasing numbers of responsibilities, nursing departments have shifted duties and reassigned tasks to other personnel. Increased numbers of practical nurses are now available. They are trained to care for the subacute, convalescent and chronically ill patient. They assist R.N.'s in the care of patients with more complicated and acute conditions. Chapter 6 has further details.

Nurse aides were originally added to nursing staffs to do housekeeping chores, to pass linen and order supplies. Today their duties have greatly expanded, and they give a great deal of direct patient care. Orderlies may be employed to care for male patients. Ward secretaries are assigned clerical duties. Duke University is conducting a two-year experimental course to train physician's assistants who will be trained to perform simple medical tasks under a physician's supervision.

Some institutions have what is called a staffing secretary. This is a lay person who schedules hours for nursing personnel and finds replacements when there is illness. Ward manager positions have been developed to take over the administration and coordination of non-nursing services to patients. Messengers, transportation personnel and many other jobs or regrouping of similar jobs are positions which the refresher may encounter. Before judging these positions, one needs to know their purpose, their function and their relationship to other jobs in order to learn if they accomplish their main purpose—better utilization of trained personnel.

LOOKING TO THE FUTURE

Changes in nursing service include the use of lay persons who are trained on the job, redistribution of duties and responsibilities of the registered nurse, increased numbers of licensed practical nurses and many other adaptations which have been made by individual institutions. There are many needs yet to be met. Many hospitals are truly short of help. Labor-saving devices are needed. Simplified procedures are required to meet changing concepts. Better distribution of personnel and spacing of work loads need to be introduced. More non-nursing duties need to be identified and removed from personnel educated to take care of patients.

It is often very difficult to give up old ways and old habits. It is a necessity, however, for the improvement of patient care. Once an institution is geared to change, it is less likely to meet resistance when it attempts innovations. Once change is thought of as a matter of development, it becomes a way of life and is both welcomed and expected by personnel.

The refresher will encounter many unfamiliar job titles. As an example, the title of nurse specialist or clinical specialist implies that the individual has advanced educational preparation in a clinical specialty. In-service education, workshops or postgraduate work at a university may be the source of such advanced preparation. Individual institutions attempt to correlate job specifications with educational requirements, but job titles and job specifications may vary greatly.

If the refresher examines nursing service job descriptions, she will also notice overlapping of job responsibilities. Although this is partly unavoidable, further clarifications will be developed in the future.

Research in nursing education, nursing practice and patient care has increased greatly in the past decade. As a result, the nursing profession at last is beginning to receive important tools and insights, which can be used to provide better patient care. Studies of factors which contribute to success in nursing, criteria for measuring patient care and patient satisfaction, elements of nurse satisfaction, etc., will continue to influence our future decisions about ways of providing optimum care to our patients.

Before we discuss more details of patient care, it is important to have a general understanding of the types of nursing educational programs available. Future patient care will be greatly influenced by graduates entering today's many kinds of educational programs. The refresher will be working alongside these young women, and it will help her to know a little bit about their education.

A.N.A. STATEMENT OF FUNCTIONS, STANDARDS AND QUALIFICATIONS OF THE DIRECTOR OF NURSING SERVICE*

Definition of Position

A director of nursing service is a registered professional nurse who is responsible for providing and improving the nursing service for patient care to meet the objectives of the hospital or similar institution.

An assistant and/or associate director of nursing service is a registered professional nurse whose responsibilities for specific function are assigned to her by the director of nursing service.

Qualifications for the Director of Nursing Service

Personal and Professional

- Evidence of good health and grooming, appropriate manner and conduct
- Ability to work effectively with others
- Demonstrated leadership ability
- Integrity, imagination, initiative and evidence of self-improvement
- Demonstrated ability in applying the principles of administration in an organization
- Recognition of civic responsibility of nursing
- Participation in professional organizations

Professional Preparation and Experience

- Broad knowledge of nursing
- Licensure to practice nursing
- Advanced educational preparation necessary, with a master's degree in nursing service administration desirable

*From Functions, Standards and Qualifications for Practice. American Nurses' Association, 10 Columbus Circle, New York 19, N.Y., February, 1963.

Progressive nursing experiences, such as experience as a head nurse or supervisor

Functions and Standards for the Director of Nursing Service

A. To provide for Nursing Care of Patients
- Determines the kind and amount of nursing care needed to achieve the objectives of the institution
  - Utilizes the objectives and policies of the institution as related to patient care in the establishment of departmental policies
  - Interprets departmental policies
  - Utilizes results of research studies
  - Interprets the nursing service to hospital administration
- Develops a nursing organization structure
  - Prepares, maintains and interprets organizational charts
  - Keeps lines of communication direct and open
- Assigns responsibility and delegates authority
  - Provides for maximum utilization of nursing personnel resources
  - Avoids duplication and overlapping of duties of personnel
  - Delegates authority proportionate to the assigned responsibility
  - Provides for development and revision of nursing procedure and departmental policy manual
- Analyzes and evaluates nursing care
  - Explores objective evidences of nursing care, such as hours of nursing care, reports from personnel, and information regarding patients' opinions
  - Makes patient rounds
  - Participates in establishing criteria for nursing care through research
  - Reviews with personnel the policies and procedures of nursing care
- Relates the responsibilities and authority within the nursing service to other hospital departments
  - Interprets nursing service to other departments
  - Encourages the contribution of nursing personnel to over-all hospital activities
  - Encourages planning for patient care within the health team

B. To Provide Personnel for Nursing Care of Patients
- Defines qualifications for personnel
  - Establishes criteria for each position within the nursing service
  - Provides written job descriptions for all categories of personnel
- Appoints personnel and maintains staffing
  - Evaluates qualification of applicants
  - Assigns and reassigns personnel to meet needs
  - Develops a recruitment program
- Provides opportunities for growth and development of personnel
  - Recognizes personal and professional abilities
  - Maintains a program of inservice education
  - Develops and carries out a guidance and counseling program
  - Constantly prepares personnel for increasing levels of responsibility through development of their potential
- Analyzes and evaluates performance of personnel
  - Explores the evidence of personal traits, abilities and degree of performance
  - Maintains and utilizes performance reports for personnel development
  - Terminates services of unsatisfactory employees
- Coordinates activities of personnel within the nursing service and with other departments
  - Promotes and maintains harmonious relationships between nursing personnel and personnel in other departments
  - Sets an example of loyalty

C. To Provide for Personnel Policies Which Will Allow for Job Satisfaction and Growth of Personnel
- Participates in the planning of personnel policies for employees
  - Interprets to hospital administration the needs and interests of nursing personnel
  - Utilizes the knowledge of current trends and research in analyzing policies
  - Supports policies which allow for job satisfaction and growth
- Develops programs for implementation of personnel policies
  - Provides for departmental orientation, guides and manuals
- Implements the established policies
  - Insures that personnel policies are clearly defined in writing
  - Provides the means for communicating personnel policies to nursing personnel
  - Modifies and interprets established policies according to the needs of the nursing service
- Analyzes and evaluates the effectiveness of personnel policies
  - Establishes and maintains adequate records of nursing employees
  - Reviews policies with nursing personnel

D. To Provide Adequate Physical Environment for Patients and Personnel in the Nursing Service
- Plans for allocation and utilization of space and equipment
  - Encourages participation of nursing personnel in planning physical environment
  - Interprets patient and nursing needs to hospital administration
  - Recommends modification of existing environment to meet needs of patients and nursing personnel
- Initiates the means by which planning for optimum physical environment can be obtained
  - Assigns responsibility for group planning
  - Provides for communication to nursing personnel
- Analyzes and evaluates the effectiveness of existing physical environment
  - Utilizes knowledge of current trends and research in evaluation
  - Provides for continuous review of needs by maintaining a system of records and reports
- Plans with other departments which contribute to the physical environment for the coordination of activities and services
  - Assist in providing means for interdepartmental planning

E. To Provide a Budget Which Will Allow for Adequate Personnel, Supplies, Equipment and Physical Facilities
- Plans the nursing service budget in cooperation with hospital administration
  - Provides for participation of nursing personnel in budget planning
  - Interprets and justifies nursing needs to hospital administration and makes recommendations
  - Utilizes research findings in establishing needs
- Compiles and prepares a statement of budget
  - Determines needs for personnel, supplies, equipment and physical facilities based upon past experience and future plans
- Applies approved budget to the nursing service
  - Interprets budget to personnel
- Reviews expenditures and needs and makes appropriate recommendations for changes
  - Utilizes records of expenditures
  - Provides for continuous review of needs

Evaluates expenditures in terms of effectiveness and economy
Establishes priorities within the nursing service
Explores priority needs with personnel

F. To Provide Means and Methods by Which the Nursing Personnel Can Work with Other Groups in Interpreting the Goals of the Hospital and Nursing Service to the Patient and the Community

Plans with hospital administration in determining the need for interpreting nursing service
Utilizes knowledge of community interests and needs
Plans content and methods of interpreting the nursing service
Defines public relations programs which explain hospital services and policies to the patient such as admission procedures, visiting hours, patient teaching programs, responsibilities of personnel, research and education
Encourages participation of personnel in interpreting needs and interests of nursing service
Assigns responsibilities to personnel for participation in public relations programs
Provides the means for communication, group planning and participation
Participates in hospital activities related to the community
Analyzes and evaluates the effectiveness of the interpretation of nursing service
Utilizes information obtained from patient contact, opinionnaires and hospital personnel
Utilizes knowledge of current trends and research

FUNCTIONS, STANDARDS AND QUALIFICATIONS FOR THE SUPERVISOR

Definition of Position

A supervisor of nursing service is a registered professional nurse who is assigned the responsibility of providing and improving nursing service to two or more organized nursing units or to a specialized area (such as operating room or outpatient department).

Qualifications for the Supervisor of Nursing Service

Personal and Professional
Evidence of good health and grooming appropriate manner and conduct
Ability to work effectively with others
Demonstrated leadership ability
Integrity, imagination, initiative and evidence of self-improvement
Demonstrated ability in applying principles of administration in an organization
Recognition of civic responsibility of nursing
Participation in professional organizations

Professional Preparation and Experience
Broad knowledge of nursing and ability to apply necessary skills and techniques
Licensure to practice nursing
Advanced educational preparation necessary with a baccalaureate degree in nursing desirable
Progressive nursing experiences such as experience as a team leader, assistant head nurse or head nurse

Functions and Standards for the Supervisor of Nursing Service

A. To Provide for the Nursing Care of Patients Within the Units
- Plans the kind and amount of nursing care in relation to the objectives of the nursing service
  - Interprets objectives of the institution related to patient care
  - Interprets and utilizes departmental policies
  - Utilizes the results of research study
  - Studies needs and interprets these to the director of nursing service
- Organizes the nursing service within her units in conformity with the total nursing service organizational structure.
  - Interprets organizational structure
- Assigns responsibilities and delegates authority
  - Provides for maximum utilization of skills and abilities of personnel
  - Avoids duplication and overlapping of duties
  - Delegates authority proportionate to the assigned responsibilities
  - Assists with the development and revision of nursing procedures and departmental policy manual
  - Ascertains that each employee is accountable to only one person for assigned responsibilities
- Continuously evaluates nursing care
  - Assembles and makes available information regarding number of nursing care hours, reports from personnel and patients
  - Makes patient rounds
  - Assists in planning nursing care
  - Participates and encourages others to participate in establishing criteria for nursing care through research
- Coordinates nursing activities within her units in relationship to the total nursing service
  - Acts in liaison capacity in interpreting nursing care within the unit
  - Promotes conformity to departmental policies and procedures
- Coordinates the efforts of the health team in planning patient care

B. To Assist the Director of Nursing Service in Providing Personnel for Nursing Care of Patients Within the Units
- Determines the qualifications of personnel for unit staffing
  - Assists in establishing criteria for each position
  - Participates in the formulation and revision of written job descriptions for personnel
- Recommends personnel for appointments to positions
  - Evaluates qualifications of applicants
  - Assigns and reassigns personnel within units to meet needs
  - Assists head nurses in making assignments and staff adjustments to meet unit needs
  - Supports the recruitment program
- Participates in promoting growth and development of personnel
  - Recognizes personal and professional abilities
  - Encourages participation in and contributes to inservice education programs
  - Guides, counsels and supports the head nurses
  - Reviews and interprets job classification to nursing personnel
  - Encourages the development of initiative, confidence and loyalty of personnel
- Analyzes and evaluates the performance of head nurses and reviews the evaluation of all other personnel
  - Confers with head nurses in evaluating personnel as needed
  - Explores evidences of personal traits, abilities and degree of performance

Maintains and utilizes performance reports for personnel development
Recommends termination of services of unsatisfactory employees
Recommends personnel for advancement

Coordinates nursing activities within her units as related to the total nursing service

Promotes harmonious relationships of personnel
Sets example of loyalty to unit personnel and to administration

C. To Assist in the Planning and Implementation of Personnel Policies Which Will Allow for Job Satisfaction and Growth of Personnel Within the Units

Plans the implementation of policies within her units and makes recommendations for policy revision

Interprets needs and interests of nursing personnel to the director of nursing service
Utilizes knowledge of current trends and research in analyzing policies and making recommendations
Supports policies which will allow for job satisfaction and growth

Organizes the program for implementation of policies

Establishes orientation programs and ward conferences

Interprets and implements policies

Provides means for communicating policies to personnel
Guides head nurses in implementing policies
Encourages and participates in group discussion, providing better understanding and practice of policies

Analyzes and evaluates the effectiveness of policies

Interprets need for and use of records to personnel
Evaluates with head nurses the method and use of records

D. To Assist in Providing an Adequate Physical Environment for Patients and Personnel Within the Units

Assists the director of nursing service in planning for allocation and utilization of space and equipment

Interprets to personnel plans for providing optimum environment
Guides head nurses in providing and maintaining optimum environment
Recommends modification of existing environment to meet needs of patients and personnel

Initiates the means by which planning for optimum physical environment can be obtained

Defines methods of establishing optimum environment
Assumes responsibility for leadership in group planning and participation
Provides communication to personnel and to the director of nursing

Analyzes and evaluates the effectiveness of existing physical environment

Utilizes observation and confers with head nurses and other departments to determine needs of the environment in regard to: noise, control, equipment maintenance, cleanliness, adequacy of safety measures

Assists in planning with other departments which contribute to the physical environment for the coordination of activities and services

Contributes to planning information gained from own observation, patients, and personnel contacts

E. To Assist With the Establishment of a Budget Which Will Allow for Adequate Personnel, Supplies, Equipment and Physical Facilities Within the Units

Participates in budget planning with the director of nursing service

Interprets the purpose of the budget and over-all budget planning to head nurses

Encourages participation of personnel in budget planning
Interprets and justifies nursing needs to director of nursing service
Prepares budget recommendations with head nurses
Determines needs for personnel, supplies, equipment and physical facilities based upon past experience and future plans
Implements the approved budget
Interprets budget to head nurses and personnel
Continuously reviews with head nurses the expenditures and needs and makes appropriate recommendations for changes
Utilizes records of expenditures
Evaluates the utilization of personnel, supplies, equipment and physical facilities to provide for effectiveness and economy
Establishes priorities
Explores priority needs with personnel

F. To Assist the Director of Nursing Service in Providing Means and Methods by Which the Nursing Personnel Can Work With Other Groups in Interpreting the Goals of the Hospital and the Nursing Service to the Patient and the Community
Plans with director of nursing service in determining the need for interpreting nursing service
Utilizes knowledge of community interests and needs
Assists in defining content and methods of interpreting the nursing service
Interprets to personnel the public relations programs which explain hospital services and policies to the patient, such as admission procedures, visiting hours, patient teaching programs, responsibilities of personal, research and education
Encourages participation of personnel in interpreting needs and interests of nursing service
Assigns responsibilities to personnel in implementing a program of public relations within her units
Provides means for communications, group planning and participation
Stimulates participation in patient teaching and community programs
Participates in hospital activities related to the community
Evaluates program of public relations within her units
Utilizes information obtained from nurses, patients and other hospital personnel
Gives direction and guidance to personnel as needed

FUNCTIONS, STANDARDS AND QUALIFICATIONS FOR PRACTICE FOR THE HEAD NURSE*

A head nurse is a professional nurse who is responsible for an organized hospital unit within which nursing care is directly and/or indirectly provided.

Functions and Standards

Patient Care

1. Plans to meet total nursing needs of patients
    a. Creates a sensitivity in the staff to patient needs and resources encouraging recognition of the patient as an individual

*Functions, Standards and Qualifications for Practice. Prepared by the Committee on Functions, Standards and Qaulifications for Practice, Head Nurses Branch, A.N.A. General Duty Nurses Section, American Nurses' Association, February, 1963.

   b. Develops awareness of and stimulates the utilization of all available resources in planning patient care
   c. Encourages and utilizes observations and suggestions of staff in planning for patient care
   d. Evaluates, with the staff, the physical, emotional, spiritual, social and economic needs and resources of each patient
   e. Interprets to and plans with professional and departmental groups in developing the patient care plan
2. Allocates the type and amount of care to meet the individual needs of each patient
   a. Develops a staffing pattern within the nursing unit to meet needs of patients on a 24-hour basis
   b. Assigns staff to meet patient's needs
   c. Provides for maximum utilization of nursing skills in determining composition of the group members
   d. Delegates to general duty nurses the responsibility for optimum utilization of nursing skills
   e. Interprets to supervisors and/or nursing service administrators the quality and quantity of nursing care required in the unit indicating ratio of professional and nonprofessional staff necessary
3. Supervises all nursing activities related directly and indirectly to patient care
   a. Observes quality and effectiveness of care given by all personnel
   b. Directs nursing personnel within the unit
   c. Coordinates all services of the hospital related to patient care in the unit
4. Evaluates the effectiveness of patient care
   a. Observes, with cooperation of nursing group, the response of patients to all medical and nursing care
   b. Recognizes effect of interpersonal relationships on the patient's well-being
5. Promotes the improvement of patient care
   a. Provides for conferences and guides in the development of a nursing care plan for each patient
   b. Communicates to the physician patient's needs, preferences and progress
   c. Recognizes and utilizes contribution of family and visitors in planning for patient care
   d. Coordinates contribution of professional, departmental and educational groups for the most effective patient care
   e. Provides for continuity of nursing care
6. Gives direct nursing care to patients when judged advisable
   a. Utilizes patient contact in teaching the patient and personnel, in establishing rapport, and observing and evaluating patient's needs and care
   b. Applies knowledge, skill and judgment in giving patient care when indicated
7. Is responsible for the execution of doctor's orders
   a. Participates in developing effective methods of implementing doctor's orders
   b. Delegates responsibility to qualified members of the nursing staff
   c. Interprets to personnel physician's orders and care anticipated
   d. Gains cooperation of patient, family and visitors in execution of the physician's plan of care
   e. Performs within framework of accepted hospital policies

   f. Understands and abides by the nurse and medical practice acts in the state
8. Is responsible for the accurate reporting and recording of patient's symptoms, reaction and progress
   a. Participates in developing methods and tools for improving skills in observing, reporting and recording
   b. Cooperates in developing skills of personnel in recognizing and reporting pertinent information through established channels
   c. Promotes accurate recording of medications and treatments and comprehensive, meaningful reporting and recording
9. Promotes and participates in patient education and rehabilitation
   a. Recognizes individual patient's needs for health teaching
   b. Plans within the concept that patient rehabilitation is influenced by contacts and activities occurring from day of admission
   c. Plans for maximum utilization of teaching opportunities
   d. Assists in orientation of the patient toward active and effective cooperation in therapy and rehabilitation
   e. Fosters patient, family, visitors and staff attitudes that are conducive to effective rehabilitation.
10. Interprets community resources available for continuity of patient care
   a. Becomes familiar with available community resources
   b. Stimulates patient, family and staff awareness of community resources and encourages their effective utilization in planning for patient care
   c. Provides for continual rehabilitation of patient through utilization of hospital and community resources

Unit Management

1. Plans for an environment that is conducive to the physical, spiritual and emotional well-being of patients and personnel
   a. Participates in planning and confers with nursing service and other departments
   b. Creates an awareness of factors that contribute to an optimum environment
   c. Enlists the participation of personnel in planning and providing for a safe and wholesome environment
   d. Recognizes importance of and promotes positive health in personnel assigned to unit staff
2. Participates in formulating, interpreting and implementing objectives and policies of nursing service
   a. Evaluates the effectiveness of existing policies and procedures
   b. Provides opportunity for participation of the unit staff in reviewing and evaluating effectiveness of existing policies and procedures
   c. Cooperates with nursing service administration and unit staff in initiating, formulating and revising objectives, policies and procedures
   d. Provides orientation to existing objectives, policies and procedures
   e. Conforms to and promotes acceptance of established objectives, policies and procedures
3. Promotes good interpersonal relationships
   a. Develops a sense of personal worth and recognizes each person as an individual
   b. Is aware of the needs and resources of all personnel
   c. Develops an attitude of understanding and tolerance
   d. Acts in good faith with unit personnel and administration
   e. Develops staff morale

   f. Creates an atmosphere of understanding and tolerance
   g. Maintains harmonious relations with other departments and allied professions
4. Evaluates the effectiveness of nursing service in the unit
   a. Utilizes patient contact and contributions of personnel in appraising the degree to which patient needs are being met
   b. Analyzes assignments and evaluates ability of staff to complete assignment effectively
   c. Observes functioning of unit plan for patient care and its effect upon the patient
   d. Maintains records and information which substantiate the evaluation of effectiveness of nursing service
   e. Participates in developing and formulating criteria and methods for evaluating nursing service
   f. Appraises effectiveness of own administrative abilities and techniques
5. Promotes the improvement of nursing service in the unit
   a. Provides an opportunity for group conferences and encourages contributions from the unit staff in planning for improving nursing service
   b. Utilizes and interprets to nursing service own suggestions and the suggestions of staff for improvement of services
6. Evaluates the work performance and attributes of nursing personnel
   a. Observes work performance and the effect on the patient
   b. Participates in the development of criteria by which a person is evaluated
   c. Evaluates self and seeks constructive suggestions
   d. Confers with supervisor and/or nursing service administrator and staff for purposes of evaluating the individual objectively
   e. Encourages self-evaluation, counsels and guides individual members of the staff
   f. Maintains periodic written evaluation records
7. Plans for and participates in the continuous learning experiences of nursing personnel
   a. Participates with unit personnel and nursing service in planning for the over-all inservice education program
   b. Orients new staff and maintains an ongoing orientation for personnel in the unit
   c. Allocates time for educational purposes and ward conferences, recognizing the inherent value to patient care
   d. Provides opportunities for learning experiences for staff
   e. Utilizes all means and opportunities for teaching
8. Promotes personal growth and development of personnel
   a. Keeps abreast of current nursing trends and developments
   b. Encourages staff to keep abreast of nursing trends and developments
   c. Recognizes potentials for growth and stimulates development of the individual
   d. Recognizes that increasing and varying the type of responsibility and experience allocated to staff contributes to development of the individual
   e. Creates staff interest and participation in education, studies and research
   f. Encourages active participation in nursing organization
9. Participates with supervisor and/or nursing service administrator in planning for the unit budget

a. Assists in determining needs for personnel, supplies, equipment and physical facilities
b. Encourages suggestions from staff for budget planning
c. Interprets and justifies budgetary requests to nursing service administrators
d. Interprets the budget to personnel and enlists their cooperation
e. Promotes optimum utilization of personnel, supplies and equipment

Institutional Objectives

1. Coordinates the service of the nursing personnel in the unit with other hospital departments
   a. Utilizes and orients staff to the proper channels of communication
   b. Channels effectively communication between the staff, other personnel and hospital departments
   c. Interprets to other departments the individual patient's needs, correlating all services to improve patient care
   d. Interprets, within the unit, services and requirements of other departments
   e. Promotes harmonious relationships with other departments
2. Cooperates in over-all educational and research programs
   a. Assists in planning for and contributes to learning experience of the student
   b. Refers suggestions to existing nursing education department for consideration in curriculum planning
   c. Participates in planning for medical research when it relates to patient care
   d. Participates in orientation of other educational disciplines within the hospital
   e. Participates in and assists with planning for studies and research
3. Participates with administration in establishing standards of patient care, policies and objectives
   a. Assists in interpretation of nursing requirements for the improvement of patient care
   b. Contributes to formulation and review of policies, program and objectives interpreting the nursing implications
   c. Participates in planning physical facilities
   d. Recommends modification of existing facilities to meet needs of patients and personnel
4. Interprets hospital objectives and policies to staff and patient, family and community
   a. Evidences a spirit of loyalty to the hospital
   b. Develops an awareness of and fosters good public relations
   c. Cooperates in enlisting support in achieving the hospital goals
   d. Promotes acceptance of change in hospital policy

Qualifications for Practice for a Head Nurse

Professional

1. Graduation from a state-accredited school of nursing
2. Currently licensed to practice professional nursing
3. Additional educational preparation is desirable
4. Progressive experience in the nursing field with at least one year's experience as a general duty nurse
5. Active participation in the professional nursing organization

Personal

1. Accepts, understands and abides by *The Code for Professional Nurses.* (Adopted by the A.N.A. House of Delegates, May 1950, Revised 1956)
2. Possesses those personal qualities desired in a professional nurse

3. Maintains optimum physical and emotional health
4. Demonstrates knowledge and competence in area of practice
5. Exercises good judgment
6. Possesses the ability to recognize and understand the common needs of all individuals
7. Possesses qualities of leadership
8. Demonstrates knowledge of and ability to apply principles of administration, personnel supervision and teaching
9. Communicates in an effective manner
10. Maintains an up-to-date knowledge of current trends and new developments
11. Applies to the current situation new concepts, knowledge and skills gained from education and experience

FUNCTIONS, STANDARDS AND QUALIFICATIONS FOR PRACTICE OF GENERAL DUTY NURSES

A general duty nurse is a registered professional nurse, employed by a hospital or an institution, who is responsible for the direct and/or indirect total nursing care of the patient.

Functions of the General Duty Nurse

I. The general duty nurse is aware of the total nursing needs of the patient and is responsible for seeing that they are fulfilled
   A. Prepares, administers and supervises a patient care plan for each patient in the group for which she is responsible
      1. Makes a detailed evaluation of his physical needs, habits and resources
      2. Evaluates his spiritual, emotional, social and economic needs, habits and resources
      3. Becomes familiar with available resources, personnel and physical facilities of the hospital and community
      4. Cooperates and shares responsibility with general duty nurses, the head nurse, supervisor, attending physician and other personnel
      5. Communicates and acts as liaison between patient, family, physician, hospital personnel and community agencies
      6. Interprets to the patient that he himself is the most effective resource in promoting successful therapy and rehabilitation
      7. Applies knowledge of drugs, other therapeutic methods and diagnostic tests based on understanding established principles and precautions
   B. Applies scientific principles in performing nursing procedures and techniques through constant evaluation in the light of nursing and medical progress
   C. Performs therapeutic measures prescribed and delegated by medical authority*
      Recognizes the need for and participates in the interpretation of treatment to the patient, especially forms of therapy which may seem radical or unusual to the patient or family
   D. Continuously evaluates symptoms, reactions and progress
      Observes, records and reports to the appropriate person symptoms, reactions and progress

*For the nurses' legal protection, there should be a written order signed by the physician for prescribed therapeutic measures.

E. Assists in patient education and rehabilitation, including the promotion of mental and physical health
F. Assists in the provision of optimum physical and emotional environment
G. Teaches and directs nonprofessional nursing personnel for whom she or he is assigned responsibility

II. The general duty nurse participates in the administration of nursing service in a general or special hospital
A. Interprets philosophy, aims and policies of hospital administration to:
1. Patients and family
2. Hospital personnel
3. Allied health groups
4. Community
B. Participates in intra- and inter-departmental activities designed to assist the hospital and nursing administration in improving the service of the hospital
C. Establishes and maintains good interpersonal relationships
D. Coordinates the objectives and aims of nursing service
E. Assumes responsibility for contributing to the educational program of any student who is having clinical experience under the nurses' guidance
F. Contributes to the improvement of nursing care

III. Fulfills community obligation as a citizen and a nurse
A. Assumes responsibility for professional growth and development
B. Assumes responsibilities and obligations of citizenship

Standards for the General Duty Nurse

Standards Related to Patient Care

1. Participates in planning, directing and coordinating total patient care
2. Observes patient and renders indicated nursing care
3. Considers the patient's needs and preferences
4. Knows the patient as an individual and becomes familiar with his background and history
5. Safeguards integrity of the individual and family
6. Applies knowledge of nursing skills and exercises judgment in the delegation of duties, recognizing throughout the importance of nurse-patient relationship
7. Understands the provision of the nurse practice acts of the state in order to recognize the legal aspects of nursing
8. Interprets the needs of the patient for whom she or he is responsible to all personnel participating in patient services and providing the opportunity for them to cooperate in planning for total patient care
9. Keeps informed and relates the basic illness with the new developments and current therapeutic measures for total patient care
10. Recommends methods by which patient may cooperate most effectively toward successful therapy and rehabilitation
11. Utilizes available resources with relation to needs of patient
12. Communicates with the family and visitors necessary in preparing the nursing care plan and for its effective execution
13. Recognizes and utilizes opportunities for health teaching of patient, relatives and visitors

Standards Relating to Nursing Service

1. Utilizes improved channels and methods of communication
2. Teaches and directs other nursing personnel
3. Promotes a sense of personal worth in all personnel by recognizing their contribution to total care of the patient
4. Participates in revising procedures and techniques. Exercises sound judgment in adapting nursing procedures to individual patient needs

5. Follows rules of established procedures
6. Understands and participates in the development of policies
7. Actively participates in formulating the criteria for, and assists in, the evaluation of the nursing service program
8. Assists in plans for development of an evaluation program for all nursing personnel
9. Continuously evaluates the nursing program, herself, and other nursing personnel
10. Participates in inservice programs, including on-the-job learning
11. Contributes in scheduled ward discussion groups, scheduled conferences with other departments, scheduled meetings with the director of nursing service and her assistants

Standards Relating to the Individual

1. Conducts herself at all times so as to reflect credit on her profession
2. Recognizes the importance of example
3. Practices good health habits
4. Increases ability for self-expression
5. Continues formal education
6. Attends workshops and institutes conducted by consultants in the field of nursing service
7. Participates in research
8. Promotes the organization of general duty nurses in the hospital

Standards Related to the Community

1. Assumes responsibility for knowledge of, progress in, and utilization of community resources such as:
   a. Health groups
   b. Civic groups
   c. General education groups
   d. Nursing recruitment
   e. Others
2. Actively participates in nursing organizations (the American Nurses' Association and the National League for Nursing) and the interpretation of their role in the community
3. Recognizes and utilizes the privilege of citizenship

Qualifications for Practice for the General Duty Nurse

Professional

1. Graduation from a state accredited school of nursing and holding a current license to practice professional nursing
2. Evidence of interest in continuous professional growth

Personal

1. Appreciation of the value of professional general duty nursing in the care of the patient
2. Maintenance of optimum physical and emotional well-being
3. Competence in the area of practice in which the nurse functions
4. Ability to plan for and evaluate total nursing care
5. Possession of personal qualities which make it possible for the nurse to maintain good interpersonal relationships. Examples of these are kindliness, sympathy, understanding, interest in and respect for people as individuals, good judgment, integrity, loyalty and sense of humor.
6. Evidence of knowledge and ability to use recognized channels of communication
7. Evidence of knowledge of new trends and developments in the field of nursing based on research
8. Interest in the profession of nursing as evidenced by membership and active participation in professional nursing organizations
9. Demonstrated interest and willingness to participate in community affairs

SUGGESTED READINGS

Barrett, Jean: The Head Nurse's Changing Role. *Nursing Outlook,* November, 1963, p. 800.

Hassenplug, Lulu Wolf: The World of Nursing—2000 A.D. *American Journal of Nursing,* August, 1962, p. 101.

REFERENCES

A.N.A. Statements of Functions, Standards and Qualifications for Practice. American Nurses Association, 10 Columbus Circle, New York 19, N.Y., February, 1963.

Barabas, Mary Helen: *Contemporary Head Nursing.* New York, Macmillan Co., 1962.

Barrett, Jean: The Head Nurse's Changing Role. *Nursing Outlook,* November, 1963. p. 800.

Batte, Allen O.: Quasi-Experimental Research Designs in Nursing. *Nursing Outlook,* October, 1964, p. 31.

Brown, William King: An Administrator s View of the Head Nurse s Work. *Nursing Outlook* November, 1963, p. 798.

Burling, T., Lentz, E., and Wilson, R.: *The Give and Take in Hospitals.* Chapter 7, The Nursing Profession—A Study of Change. New York, G. P. Putnam's Sons, 1956.

Calender, Tiny M.: *Unit Administration.* Philadelphia, W. B. Saunders Co., 1962.

Forman, Alice M., and Brown, Myrtle Irene: *The Utilization of Research Findings in the Improvement of Nursing Care of the Aging* American Nurses Foundation, Inc., April, 1963.

Freeing the Nurse to Nurse. *American Journal of Nursing,* March, 1964, p. 72 (Cynthia Henderson, reporter).

Harder, Helen I.: Steward Program Provides Administrative Assistants for Nurse-Supervisor. *Hospital Topics,* November, 1963, p. 75.

Hartman, Jane: Floor Managers Share Responsibility in this Food Distribution System. *Modern Hospital,* February, 1963, p. 124.

Hassenplug, Lulu Wolf: The World of Nursing—2000 A.D. *American Journal of Nursing,* August, 1962, p. 101.

Hospital Personnel. Report of a Personnel Research Project, U.S. Dept. of Health, Education, and Welfare, Public Health Service Publication No. 930-C-9, October, 1964.

Houtz, Duane T.: The Unit Manager Plan Provides Administrative Control of Wards. *Modern Hospital,* August, 1962, p. 75.

Hughes, Everett, Hughes, Helen MacGill, and Deutscher, Irwin: *Twenty Thousand Nurses Tell Their Story.* Philadelphia, J. B. Lippincott Co., 1958.

Levine, Eugene: Some Answers to the Nurse Shortage. *Nursing Outlook,* March, 1964, p. 30.

Levine, Eugene: Turnover Among Nursing Personnel in General Hospitals. *Hospitals,* September 1, 1957, p. 50.

Mercadante, Lucille T.: An Organizational Plan for Nursing Service. *Nursing Outlook* May, 1962, p. 305.

Mercadante, Lucille T.: Unit Manager Plan Gives Nurses Time to Care for the Patients. *Modern Hospital,* August, 1962, p. 73.

Meyer, Genevieve Regge: *Tenderness and Technique.* Institute of Industrial Relations, University of California, Los Angeles, 1960.

Nahm, Helen: Nursing Dimensions and Realities. *American Journal of Nursing* June, 1965, p. 96.

Perrodin, Cecilia M.: *Supervisions of Nursing Service Personnel.* New York, Macmillan Co., 1959.

Sellew, Gladys, and Furfey, Paul H.: *Sociology and Social Problems in Nursing Service* Philadelphia, W. B. Saunders Co., 1946, Chapters XV & XVI.

Wilson, Janis M.: Transporting Patients Through a Centralized Service. *American Journal of Nursing,* September, 1962, p. 72.

5

Nursing Education Programs of Today

Since World War II, changes in nursing education have been rapid. Some have been experimental, some have created new problems, some have shed conventional plans, many are just emerging. Changes in general education, as well as changes resulting from technological advances and the desire of nurses to upgrade patient services and their profession have all had their influence on nursing education. Time and attention are being devoted to the identification and development of nursing theory.

Vocational, technical and professional are adjectives used to distinguish the background, education and functions of various levels of nursing care. Neither our educational programs nor our functions are as clearly differentiated as our terminology. In spite of this, these terms describe future goals as well as some present practice.

PRACTICAL NURSE EDUCATION

Practical nursing education prepares the practical or vocational nurse. The number of persons graduating from these programs increased from about 3000 to more than 16,000 between 1950 and 1960. Approximately three fourths of all state-approved programs are under the control of educational agencies, such as state or local boards of education or vocational education. A few are within college or university control, and the other one fourth are mainly under the control of hospitals. Whenever a course is administered by an educational agency, contractual agreements are made with patient care centers for clinical practice.

Practical nursing education is aimed at preparing persons to give care under the supervision of a professional nurse or physician in situations which are mainly free of scientific complexity. These persons are

also prepared to assist the professional nurse in caring for patients in situations which are more complex. About two thirds of them have a high school diploma, while only about half of them were high school graduates ten years ago. Most courses are one year in length, providing clinical experience and classroom instruction in the major specialties. Courses vary greatly in the amount of practice and classroom teaching. Assignment of duties after graduation varies almost more. Unfortunately, the latter often varies with the number of registered nurses available rather than the type of education which the practical nurse has had. The graduate is eligible to take an examination to become a licensed practical or vocational nurse as designated by her state. This is a terminal program of education, as further education cannot be built upon it.

ASSOCIATE DEGREE EDUCATION

The associate of arts degree was first granted in 1954 to nurses from a junior college pilot program under the direction of Mildred Montag. Methods used in these pilot schools have had a profound effect on all forms of nursing education, as a description of other programs will reveal. By the end of 1964, there were over 100 programs for nurses in community and junior colleges. About 50 per cent of the content of these courses is devoted to general education and about 50 per cent is devoted to nursing education. The aim of these courses is to produce a graduate who can give safe, effective patient care at the bedside. State boards of nursing worked with these programs and often had to alter laws because of rigid time and curriculum requirements.

Many of these programs are dead-end in terms of future college education. If the nurse wishes to continue her education, she is likely to find that few, if any of her credits count toward a baccalaureate degree unless they meet certain specified conditions. Graduates are eligible to take licensure examinations for registration and are considered technical nurses in the strict sense.

Junior colleges are springing up all over the country. These two-year colleges, usually without resident facilities because most are community agencies, serve two functions. They enroll academic students who eventually wish to graduate from a four-year college, and they enroll students who come to obtain vocational and technical training. Some are considered dead-end programs. When a student graduates with an associate of arts degree, he may or may not be eligible to enter college with advanced standing. Programs within these schools vary. Some are preparatory for further study while others complete a course in some specialized technical skill. The advantage of the community college for the latter group of students is that they can obtain a rather broad liberal arts background along with a skill.

Dr. Edmund J. Gleazer, Jr., Executive Director of the American Association of Junior Colleges, states,

> The community college has its most productive development not when it is conceived of as the first two years of the baccalaureate program, nor when seen as grades thirteen and fourteen, but as an institution in its own right—a new kind of college, standing between the high school and the university, offering broad programs of experience of value in and of themselves, neither post-high school as such nor pre-college as such.*

From this statement, it is clear that the position of the nurse graduating from a junior college will vary with the particular institution where her program exists.

DIPLOMA SCHOOL EDUCATION

Approximately 80 per cent of all registered nurses graduate from a diploma school of nursing. With few exceptions, these schools are administratively controlled and financed by a hospital. Nursing education is historically related to hospitals in which a great deal of teaching revolved around apprenticeship learning.

Throughout the past 20 years, many diploma schools have made major changes. Class hours were increased, faculties developed and were better qualified, college affiliation for the basic social and physical sciences was sought, and general standards were raised. Other schools, however, either could not or did not make such changes. Thus, the educational differences among hospital schools of nursing vary greatly.

Clinical experience at some schools is beginning to be dissociated from the Nursing Service Department. When this is done, there are two major adjustments which must be made. First of all, the hospital must learn to staff its institution without utilizing students. Student assignments and hours are scheduled by the clinical instructor, who relates the student's experience to her education rather than to the staffing needs of the hospital. As a result of this, the hospital must hire more employees to replace student help for patient service. It is then unable to subsidize the school enough to make up for these employees, so tuition rates must rise. Patient rates cannot be increased, since this would penalize the patients in a hospital which conducts a nursing school. The student can no longer have an inexpensive education.

Some educators feel that more faculty per student is required when clinical time is reduced, so that the quality of the clinical experience can be that much better by making more instructor time vital. Therefore, faculty costs also rise. As one aspect of a program improves, others also improve, such as library and classroom facilities, and counseling and health services.

There has been a great deal of controversy about diploma schools of nursing. Educators agree that education should be under the control

*From Dapper, Gloria: Spokesman for the Two-Year College. *Saturday Review,* December 19, 1964, p. 55.

of an educational institution rather than a service agency. Some schools of nursing have removed themselves from the administrative and financial control of the hospital and formed a school separate from the hospital. Whether this is done or not, financial aid to nursing education has long been needed. Discussion of some of the legislation which has affected nursing is found in Chapter 2.

Diploma programs vary in length. The traditional three-year program comes in many forms. Some are 36 months long. Some are 27 months long (three academic years of nine months each). There are new two-year diploma programs which may be on a calendar year of 12 months. If one looks at a program in terms of time, one will find that a three-year program may be 27 months in length and a two-year program may be 24 months in length. The trend is toward shortening diploma programs rather than lengthening them.

Diploma graduates are considered technical nurses rather than professional nurses, although they are more frequently referred to as professional nurses. In everyday usage it is more common to find that persons refer to any R.N., regardless of her education, as a professional nurse.

A diploma graduate may or may not find that her credits have value at a college or university if she wishes to study for a degree later on. This varies with the college, courses in her school of nursing and other factors which will be discussed later. In any case she is eligible to take state board examinations for her licensure as a registered nurse at the end of diploma programs of varying length and with varying content.

BACCALAUREATE EDUCATION FOR NURSING

Baccalaureate education for all professional nurses is a long-term goal of the nursing profession. It is based on the premise that professional education is preceded by liberal education. Nursing students would be expected to meet the same standards of performance and eligibility as the college or university expects of all its students.

The graduate with a baccalaureate education in nursing would have a broader foundation on which to base her nursing education and eventually her nursing decisions. Students will learn principles for making a nursing diagnosis. They will learn how to select, apply and evaluate their nursing care, and they will have learned to better understand patient behavior. They also have a foundation for study on the master's level.

These programs also vary a great deal. In some programs the student spends her first two years studying liberal arts courses and then enters nursing which is somewhat segregated from the rest of the college. In other programs nursing is integrated with other college courses throughout the four or five years required to obtain the degree. Clinical experience is usually limited in time but is very selective, so that the student can gain the maximum amount of meaning and learning from her observation of a particular patient, condition or institutional area. This always includes public health.

The graduate of a college nursing program is also eligible to take examination for licensure. They are more likely to be prepared to assume a beginning position in *any* field of nursing rather than a beginning position in hospital nursing only. Another goal of baccalaureate education is to prepare its graduates for postgraduate education.

BACCALAUREATE EDUCATION FOR GRADUATES OF DIPLOMA AND ASSOCIATE DEGREE PROGRAMS

Educational changes require experimentation and sometimes radical changes to create meaningful alterations in the status quo. As a result, there may be wide swings of the pendulum, creating real controversy. Such swings often lead to clarification of goals as well as improved quality of service, whether it be to the student or to the patient.

Whenever a college accepts a registered nurse in a program of collegiate education, it is faced with the job of evaluating the previous education of the applicant. Because there is such a wide discrepancy in the quality of instruction given to these graduates, transfer of blanket credits is not feasible. In terms of college education, the background of a nurse from a small hospital school of nursing where nurses and staff physicians gave most of the lectures as opposed to a graduate from a diploma program at a large medical center is quite likely to be very different. On the other hand, individual differences in learning might make the difference between these two students less significant than might be suspected.

It has been recommended by those who have reviewed and set standards for such programs that any transferred credits be from courses with the same characteristics and standards as those defined by collegiate schools of nursing. This includes admission requirements of students based on the evaluation of previous education which is sometimes done by examination. They further recommend that these nurses should obtain a substantial foundation in general education, physical, biologic, behavioral and medical sciences from persons qualified to teach in the respective disciplines. In addition, they suggest that they receive an upper division major in nursing which utilizes these disciplines and lays the foundation for graduate study in nursing.

This is the long way to higher education and should be avoided whenever possible. When someone wishes to become a nurse, selection of a program requires testing and counseling to match each student to the appropriate program.

NON-NURSING DEGREES

There are many nurses who have non-nursing degrees. There is the nurse who was an elementary school teacher and later obtained a diploma in nursing. There is the nurse who is a diploma graduate who takes a baccalaureate degree in sociology. There are colleges without a nurse on their faculty offering a degree with a nursing major. The student does not take any course in nursing in her college program, yet her transferred credits are enough to give her a major in nursing. Nurse educators feel that a degree such as this should be supplanted by a degree with another major, as the college is not offering a degree on the basis of standards they have set.

Many nurses take postgraduate degrees in non-nursing programs. They may major in psychology, sociology, industrial relations or some physical science. Nurse educators, however, feel that the bachelor's degree for the R.N. should be founded upon a nursing major.

POSTGRADUATE EDUCATION FOR NURSES

Another trend in nursing education is to discourage specialization on the bachelor's level. A nurse is expected to obtain a good general education in the humanities, social sciences and nursing in her undergraduate study. Her postgraduate program can then be devoted to a specialization.

There are 37 programs on the National League for Nursing (N.L.N.) 1965-1966 accredited list for master's degrees. The specialties which are offered include teaching, administration, public health, psychiatric nursing and other clinical specialties.

DISTINCTIONS STILL NEEDED

One of the principle needs for the future is to better distinguish the vocational, the technical and the professional nurse from one another. Both curricula and functions need clearer distinctions, especially between the latter two.

Some people look upon diploma and baccalaureate educations as a kind of ladder by which one type of program prepares a graduate for another type of program. Nursing services often use various types of personnel interchangeably for the same function. These things make it difficult to see any very clear differences between various levels of nursing and nursing care.

Another thing which often clouds the issue is the basis on which students select various programs. The length of the course often becomes a criterion in the student's selection of a program rather than the quality, depth of content or goal of a particular program. It is hoped that greater attention will be paid to A.N.A. functions and N.L.N. guidelines for both the education and utilization of nurses in the future.

SELECTING A NURSING EDUCATION PROGRAM

Young men and women who wish to enter nursing need to seek the counsel of someone who knows about the kinds of available nursing programs. High school counselors need to have adequate information in order to be of the greatest benefit to their students. Program selection should be made on the basis of an attempt to match the program with the abilities and aspirations of the potential student. Ignorance, impatience and/or a need to earn a living in a short period of time often interferes with proper matching of student with program. Nevertheless, any student of college potential should be guided carefully. This is easier said than done because high school age is a young age to make rather far-reaching decisions about the future. Students in diploma and associate degree programs may be well matched in terms of their goals immediately following graduation, but long-range goals are often neglected. Those who may wish to assume leadership positions in the future or desire further education will find that their choice was not expedient in the long run.

More men are entering the profession, as a result of better salaries and working conditions. The increase in numbers of men entering nursing is a healthy influence and needs to be encouraged.

Another source of students is among persons over 35 years of age. Many schools of nursing have had age limits for students. The usual work pattern of women is to marry after a brief period of work, to raise a family and then to return to work for many years. At this time a woman either seeks a new career or re-enters a career which she left at the time of her marriage. Tenure studies demonstrate that employees in the older age group are more stable than those in the younger group. This is also true of refreshers. When they return to nursing, they usually stay for many years. Junior colleges have often encouraged this age group to enter their programs.

High school and college counselors can help in the selection of an appropriate program for a particular student. It is, however, up to all of us in the profession to make our knowledge available to young people and to those working with persons who aid in program selection.

CHANGES IN TEACHING METHODS

There are many misconceptions about newer teaching methods. One often hears the statement that students are just not learning what they used to. When we talk about nursing education, the implication usually is that this is not good. When we talk about a child in grade school, we are often astounded at what the child has learned. With just a moment's thought, it suddenly becomes obvious that if grade school and high school teaching includes things the past generation received in college, changes must be made.

Another misconception is that visual aids and machines are replacing teachers. Teaching aids have been and are being developed which enable the teacher to teach more material to more students in less time. Teaching aids do not replace teachers; they supplement them and assist them in their immense task. The following will merely highlight some of the changes in teaching utilized in nursing education:

Programed Learning

Programed learning is a self-teaching technique which enables a student to go at his own rate of speed. Each step of the course is planned around a so-called "frame." Each frame increases in complexity based upon the previous frame. Before a student goes on to a new frame he is tested. A book or machine may be used, and the student can make and correct errors which are revealed only to him.

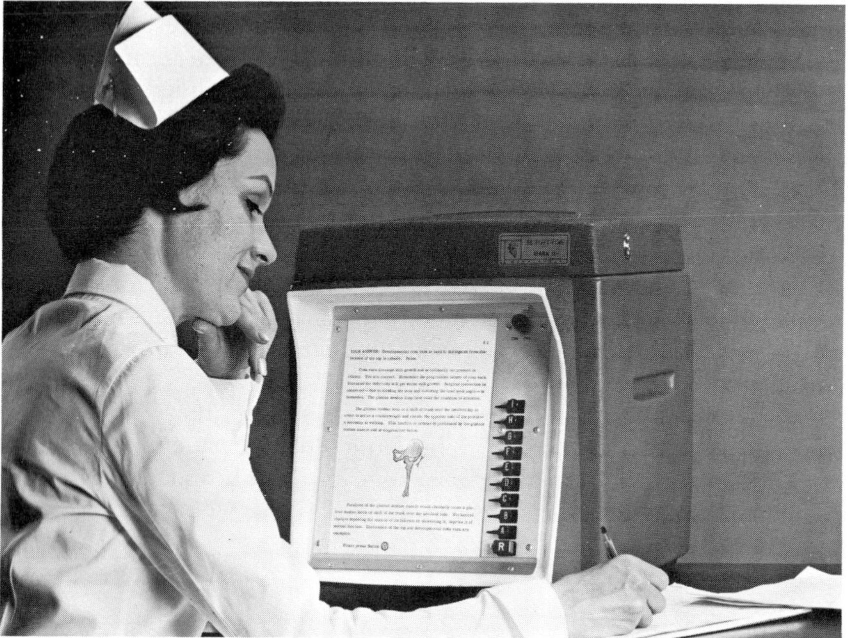

Figure 5–1. *Autotutor teaching machine. (Courtesy United Science Industries, Educational Division, Galeto, Calif.)*

Programed learning can be used in elementary education as well as postgraduate medical education. A course is usually planned with a behavioral psychologist who is concerned with steps in the learning process and a person who knows the field in which the course is being programed.

The student must remain active throughout a program because he must respond to questions at frequent intervals. Studies on learning by this method reveal that almost all students can be expected to learn at least 90 per cent of the material contained in the course.

Television

Television can be used in several different ways. A closed-circuit television system can be installed in a hospital and used by the clinical instructor for student observation in the clinical area. At Montefiore Hospital in New York City, a study was done in which clinical instructors monitored students in several different rooms, rotating at regular intervals. The instructor was also able to talk to the student without the patient hearing the conversation.

Another use of television is in the teaching of courses such as anatomy, physiology, chemistry, psychology, etc. This was first done by the Video Nursing Education program in St. Paul where five Twin City hospital schools of nursing utilized the courses. Instructors visited each hospital at specified intervals so that teacher contact was not lost. One of the advantages of televised teaching is that it can be re-used and updated as necessary by the use of videotape. Expert teachers can therefore be available to students whenever the program is scheduled. Repetitious teaching is avoided. Televised education also ensures that each student sees and hears the same thing. It permits larger classes for some things. In a class on passive range of motion, for instance, no one's view is blocked because the camera is positioned so that hard-to-see techniques are visible to all students.

At the University of Mississippi, videotapes have been made so that students can see themselves with their patients. Students, rather than instructors, were asked to evaluate their own care after reviewing the tapes.

Television has also been used for teaching interviews, patient monitoring and "visit vision." The latter enables patients to see and sometimes talk to visitors who must remain in the hospital lobby rather than come to the room, such as children or friends with colds.

Tape Recorder

The tape recorder can be used in many different ways. It can merely tape lectures which can be used for students who miss lectures or it can be made for a lecture which needs to be repeated by a person who cannot come as often as is desired. Tapes are also used for patient teaching. A script can be prepared with patient statements. Time can be allowed for student responses. Afterwards, they can be played back and evaluated by student and instructor.

Clinical Experience

Clinical experience is more likely to be referred to as clinical observation periods or laboratory periods in today's nursing programs. As nursing education departs from apprenticeship learning, clinical experience becomes more important rather than less.

In most baccalaureate and associate degree programs and in some diploma programs, clinical learning is divorced from day-by-day needs of nursing service. The clinical instructor controls assignments which are related to course content. In this way needless repetition is avoided. Chores which are not conducive to learning are avoided, and non-nursing tasks are not assigned. At the end of most educational programs, the nurse is prepared to enter nursing at a beginning level of nursing. She is not expected to be an expert practitioner at the time she graduates.

This is not as incompatible with practice as it may appear on the surface. To take thousands of T.P.R.'s and to make hundreds of beds takes valuable time which could be used to better advantage. To learn to do both of these things with some skill does not take long. We expect nurse aides to learn much more than this in two weeks. It certainly should not require the nurse a longer time to learn than an aide, nor does it seem reasonable to call such repetition a form of education.

Clinical experience in most of today's programs has been greatly reduced. It is also somewhat less procedure-oriented. A student is expected to understand the purpose of a procedure and the principles underlying it, and to make an adaptation which is safe and most comfortable for her patient. With this philosophy, procedures become less rigid. Skill training is still important but it is not all-important.

Regrouping of Content

By changing course content, altering the sequence of courses and using patient-centered rather than disease-centered approaches, repetitive course content has been eliminated by many programs. This is a long painstaking process but a vital and rewarding one. Congenital deformities might serve as an example of a curriculum problem. They used to be included in many courses such as pediatrics, obstetrics and surgery. They were then repeated according to system, orthopedics, urology, neurology, etc. Symptoms, diseases and general principles can be identified and then combined to minimize this kind of repetition.

(Text continued on page 60.)

1	1 In the early history of drug preparation, medicines were administered in the form of powders or brews made from herbs, roots and other parts of plants. There was no way of knowing exactly *how much* medication a patient was receiving, because no standards had been set for accurately weighing and measuring drugs. Today, when a physician prescribes a drug, he is assured of the accuracy of the dosage because there are universally accepted standards or systems for the measurement of drugs.
2 system measurement	2 A universally accepted standard which assures accuracy in the weighing and measuring of drugs is called a _______________ of _______________.
3 apothecaries'	3 In the United States we now use two systems of measurement in preparing and administering drugs. Of the two, the *apothecaries'* system is the older. It was brought to the United States from England during the colonial period. A system of measurement brought to the United States in the eighteenth century, and still used today in the preparation and administration of drugs, is the _______________________ system.
4 metric	4 Another system by which drugs are weighed and measured is the *metric* system. This system is more convenient than the apothecaries' system, and it is the one used in the official listings of drugs. Since most drugs are prepared and dispensed from an official listing, the system most frequently used in the weighing and measuring of drugs is the _______________________ system.

Figure 5–2. *A sample program. (From Part One of Keane, Claire B., and Fletcher, Sybil M.:* Drugs and Solutions. *W. B. Saunders Co., 1965.) Read with left side covered.*

5

apothecaries' } (either
metric } order)

5

Two systems used for weighing and measuring drugs in the United States are the ________________ system and the ________________ system.

6

household

6

When drugs are administered in the home, they must often be measured in some household article such as a teaspoon or a tablespoon. These articles are not always standard in size, however, and they should be used only if the drug is prescribed according to a unit of measure from the household system.

A system of measurement sometimes used for the administration of drugs in the home is called the ________________ system.

7

apothecaries'
metric

7

The administration of drugs would be much simpler if all drugs were prescribed, weighed, measured, and dispensed according to one universal system of measurement. However, even though the apothecaries' system is gradually being replaced by the metric system, each system is in current use, and the nurse must be familiar with both.

Many times a physician will prescribe a dosage of a drug using the apothecaries' system, when the drug is dispensed according to the units of the metric system. When this happens, the nurse must be able to translate, or *convert*, from units of measure in the ________________ ________ system to units of measure in the __________ ________________ system.

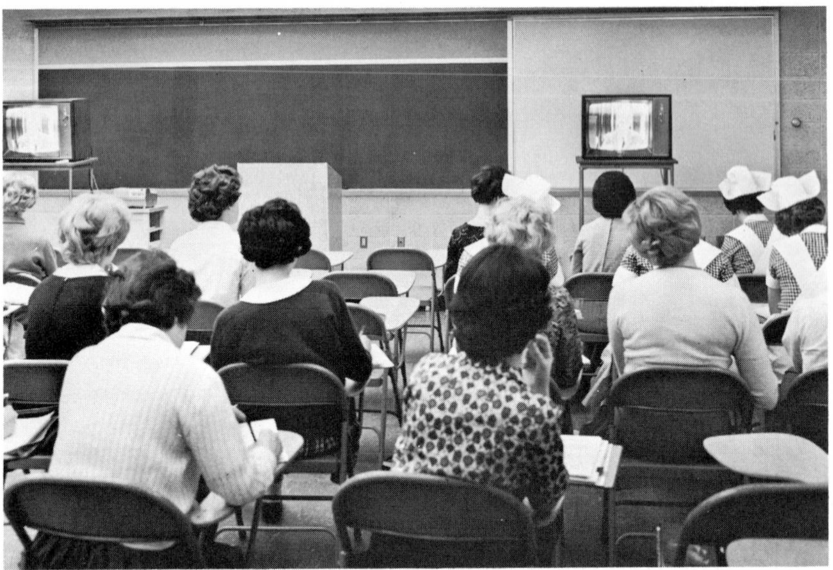

Figure 5–3. *Televised education class. (Courtesy St. Barnabas Hospital.)*

The use of doctor's lectures has been greatly reduced. Past experience has demonstrated that although the doctor's lecture is often vitally interesting, it does not help the student to learn nursing care. Therefore, the emphasis in all nursing courses is on nursing care, not medical care.

Curricula are planned so that content goes from simple to more complex concepts, from the normal to the abnormal and from generalizations to specific situations by transfer of learning. It is impossible, regardless of time, to teach everything so that these concepts are vital. The latter statement should encourage refreshers.

SUMMARY

Changes in nursing education programs will continue so that what is new today does not become stale tomorrow. New programs are not shortened old programs. Actual content has been rearranged, weeded out and refocused. New teaching aids are used along with a generous amount of time devoted to shared student experience and problem-solving discussions.

The emergence of junior college programs has done much to stimulate examination of all existing programs. Clinical facilities are selected and arranged by the college, which sends faculty out to teach its students at an agency or institution. For nursing education to become a part of an educational institution which has control of faculty standards and finances is a goal which is becoming achieved more often each year.

New programs take into account the fact that education is a lifelong process which is not complete at the end of a particular program. They are geared to the stimulation of the thought process and not just to the learning of more and more facts. Educations should give a sense of direction to students, describe alternate goals from which to choose and assist them to learn to make wise choices for themselves and their patients.

This has implications for the refresher, who must not be lulled into a sense of false security by the mere learning of modern procedures. Nursing should be made as exciting as it really is before new methods are learned. The refresher may be employed at the same time as a graduate from any of the new programs. She will find that her adjustments and orientation needs will be different in some respects but similar in other respects. Today's student does not graduate thinking that she must know everything. She graduates with certain tools and she knows that she will continue to learn as she practices nursing. This holds true for the refresher also.

SUGGESTED READINGS

Hill, Richard J.: The Right to Fail. *Nursing Outlook,* April, 1965, p. 38.

Swafford, Elizabeth Hitt: A Diploma Program Graduate Goes to College. *Nursing Outlook,* January, 1965, p. 55.

REFERENCES

Aasterud, Margaret, and Guthrie, Katheryn: What can be Expected of the Graduate of an A.D.? *Nursing Outlook,* August, 1964, p. 52.

Anderson, Lois D.: Telecourse in Nursing. *American Journal of Nursing,* July, 1964, p. 79.

Boyle, Rena E.: Implications of Administrative Policies Regarding Transfer of Credits and the Granting of Advanced Standing for Nursing Education. A paper presented at the Preconvention Meeting of the Council of Schools, Georgia State League for Nursing, April 3, 1962.

Dineen, Mary A.: A Nursing Major Without Nursing. *Nursing Outlook,* April, 1965, p. 66.

Dustan, Laura C.: Is it the System? *Nursing Outlook,* May, 1964, p. 58.

Gray, James: *Education for Nursing.* Minneapolis, University of Minnesota Press, 1960.

Hansen, Margaret M.: Granting College Credit to Registered Nurse Students. *Nursing Outlook,* January, 1965, p. 53.

Lambertson, Eleanor: *Education for Nursing Leadership.* Philadelphia, J. B. Lippincott Co., 1958.

Let's Be Practical About a Nursing Career. Committee on Careers, National League for Nursing, 1964.

Levine, Myra E.: The Professional Nurse and Graduate Education. *Nursing Science,* June, 1965, p. 206.

MacDonald, Gwendoline: Baccalaureate Education for Graduates of Diploma and Associate Degree Programs. *Nursing Outlook,* June, 1964, p. 52.

Mechner, Francis: Learning by Doing Through Programmed Instruction. *American Journal of Nursing,* May, 1965, p. 98.

Montag, Mildred L., and Gotkin, Lassar G.: *Community College Education for Nursing.* New York, Blakiston Division, McGraw-Hill Book Co., Inc., 1959.

Monteiro, Lois: The Tape Recorder as a Teaching Machine. *Nursing Outlook,* October, 1964, p. 52.

Nursing Science, June, 1964, Vol. 2, No. 3:

DeChow, Georgeen H.: Preparing the College and Community for Associate Degree Education in Nursing: A Director's Point of View. p. 206.

Dunlap, Marjorie S.: Preparation of Nurse Faculty for Associate Degree Nursing Programs. p. 223.

McCandless, Mary R.: Preparing the Community for Associate Degree Education in Nursing and the Planning Year: A Consultant's Point of View. p. 199.

Montag, Mildred L.: The Logic of Associate Degree Programs in Nursing. p. 188.

Waters, Verle H.: Orienting Hospital Personnel to the Associate Degree Program. p. 240.

Ogden, Ruth P.: Nursing Education. *Hospitals,* April 1, 1965, p. 129.

Rogers, Martha E.: *Educational Revolution in Nursing.* New York, Macmillan Co., 1961.

Sandve, Wanyce C.: Diploma Programs Need Scrutiny. *American Journal of Nursing,* February, 1965, p. 103.

Scott, Eileen O., and Roche, Elizabeth J.: From a 3- to a 2-Year Diploma Program. *Nursing Outlook,* December, 1964, p. 24.

Saturday Review, December 19, 1964:

Boroff, David: Status Seeking in Academe. p. 45.

Dapper, Gloria: Spokesman for the Two-Year College. p. 55.

Merlo, Frank P.: The Burgeoning Community College Higher Education for All? p. 50.

Schwartz, Bert: Is it Really Higher Education? p. 52.

Stoppel, David A., and Cook, John B.: A Chemistry Course on Videotape. *Nursing Outlook,* April, 1965, p. 68.

Waters, Verle Hambleton: Distinctions Are Necessary. *American Journal of Nursing,* February, 1965, p. 101.

West, Margaret D., and Crowther, Beatrice: *Education for Practical Nursing.* 1960, Department of Practical Nursing Programs, National League for Nursing.

6

Responsibilities of Personnel Supervised by the Registered Nurse

It may seem unusual to examine the duties and responsibilities of persons at the lower level of the organizational chart first, but refreshers usually find it easier to understand their functions after they know the education, experience and background of those whom they supervise.

It is difficult to attempt to describe the responsibilities of personnel who work with the general staff R.N. because they vary so greatly among institutions and communities. Differences in assigned duties may be due to the composition of the labor market available to an area, dissimilar job specifications, priority goals of nursing leaders in a particular community or the subtle influence of current employees. It is impossible for the R.N. to perform the entire range of duties which have been assigned to her in recent years. As a result, she must delegate non-nursing tasks. What she has delegated has become the job responsibility of other workers. A few background comments will help you to understand some of the differences.

It is vital that the graduate nurse understand the purpose, function and background of her fellow workers. One of the greatest difficulties in nursing today is the overuse of personnel. Whenever we assign personnel to duties which they do not know or which we do not teach, the quality of our care diminishes.

A hospital needs to try to promote employment policies, in-service education, job descriptions and methods which will result in having the most skilled and best educated persons as close to the patient as possible. This is why it is so necessary to prepare and to utilize as many nurses available in a community as possible. Even when there is a fairly adequate supply of personnel, one often sees the nurse increasing the amount of time she spends at the desk rather than the amount of time she spends with the patient. At the present time, leaders in both nursing service and nursing education are trying to reverse this trend. Nonetheless, there are nurses who have coordinated activities at the desk and assisted doctors for so many years they feel most secure in this role and emphasize it. It takes education and a great deal of persuasion to make these changes possible. The next chapter will be concerned with functions of the R.N. in more detail.

In the meantime, I hope that the reader will also keep in mind that job descriptions, duties and functions of personnel which are described in this chapter are that of a particular group of hospitals in a particular part of the country. This area, a metropolitan center in the midwest, has a shortage of nurses, but this shortage is not as acute as it is in some other parts of the country. It should also be noted that all the causes of a nursing shortage are not fully understood. In one community there may be two hospitals without a nurse staffing shortage and other hospitals with an acute shortage. This may occur when salary scales are identical. A rapid turnover of personnel unfortunately perpetuates itself. If a nurse is employed at a hospital with a shortage of personnel, she may become frustrated, tired and sometimes discontented enough to resign. This again creates internal change and the vicious circle repeats itself. Few studies have been made of hospitals which do not have a high turnover rate. We are better acquainted with factors contributing to turnover rates than we are with factors contributing to stability of a nursing staff although there is some evidence to indicate that there is less turnover where nurses work closely with patients.

We do know that youth, marriage, pregnancy and a desire to travel contribute to turnover of staff. A nurse can find a job almost anywhere in the world. This is one of the advantages of becoming a nurse. Nonetheless, constant seeking of new positions may be a sign of dissatisfaction as well as a restless and adventurous spirit.

Eugene Levine has studied personnel turnover rates in hospitals. He reports that some positions must be filled two or three times during a year. In one study he states (referring to professional staff nurses), "Within the 12-month period covered by the study, resignations occurred in nearly half of all the staff nurse positions." In a work situation with this kind of constant fluctuation, some very odd things occur. An R.N. may be working with an L.P.N. with greater tenure. As a result the practical nurse may attempt to direct and instruct the registered nurse. Because a new R.N. does not recall which slip is required to order a new diet, the nurse aide may conclude that the nurse does not know what she is doing. What is often worse, the nurse herself may get the same idea. It is important to remember that the knowledge and effectiveness of the nurse should not be undermined by such unfamiliar details. Conversely, the R.N. may have the continual problem of having to teach new nonprofessional personnel.

Without going into these matters further, let us look at what the personnel on nursing stations are doing, the purpose of their jobs and the kind of persons who fill these positions. Many jobs once had a specific purpose; but they may lose or alter their purpose with time. A hospital finds it necessary to look at its job descriptions every two or three years to see if better use of personnel can be accomplished. A change in the labor market, new methods, new products, new arrangements of assignments or any number of possibilities may alter the utilization of a particular position. Nursing departments continuously try to be aware of such possibilities.

THE NURSE AIDE

The nurse aide's position gained prominence during World War II. This position was created to give nurses (who were few and far between because so many were in the armed forces) more time to perform the more highly skilled duties which were vital. Nurse aides cleaned bedside units, cleaned cupboards, changed linen for discharge units and ran errands. Their contact with the patient was minimal, and this was considered the proper way of doing things.

As time went on and the war was over, there was not only a continued shortage of nurses, but an increase in the number of patients. Most of the duties performed by nurse aides were reassigned to the housekeeping department. This was one of the first steps in taking away cleaning chores not only from the nurse, but from the nursing department.

Nurse aides were then used to take care of the "easy" patient. No one has ever adequately described an "easy" patient, but it is a term which continues to be used all too frequently. Unfortunately, it usually implies that the patient does not have any mechanical equipment attached to him, that he is not critically ill or that he does not require any treatments requiring technical skill. It may leave the patient who has emotional needs, educational needs, referral needs or any number of less obvious needs in the hands of our least educated personnel. As you work with patients, you will see this phenomenon occurring, and it will be something to guard against. See pp. 67–69 for A.N.A. Statement on Auxiliary Personnel in Nursing Service.

What Is the Nurse Aide's Background?

Although the background of the nurse aide depends upon the hiring policies of the hospital, she is often a person with no education beyond high school. Some hospitals accept persons who are not high school graduates. Once in a while, a girl who is working her way through college will be employed as a nurse aide. In any case the majority of nurse aides come to a hospital with no background in health education. Everything they do must be taught at the employing institution. The usual length of training time for an aide is one month. It must be remembered that on-the-job training emphasizes procedures. While a lecture on patient relations is usually included, it is vital that the R.N. remember that these persons do not have a background in any science, behavioral or otherwise. This is emphasized, not to diminish the importance of the nurse aide's work but to make sure that those who work with her give her adequate support and assistance.

What Does the Nurse Aide Do?

The nurse aide (male or female) should always work under the supervision of a registered nurse. She is taught to assist the staff in the care of patients. The key word is "assist." The aide should never be solely responsible for a patient.

Job descriptions will vary among hospitals. The following are common duties performed by persons working in this job classification under the supervision of a registered nurse:

1. Give morning and evening care to selected patients.
2. Give patients their food trays, nourishments and drinking water.
3. Feed selected patients.
4. Record and measure intake and output.
5. Position patients in bed.
6. Transport patients by wheel chair or litter.
7. Give and remove bedpans.
8. Give enemas to selected patients.
9. Apply hot water bottles, ice collars, etc.
10. Help patients with a tub bath, sitz bath or shower.
11. Take radial pulse, respirations and temperature (by mouth, rectum or axilla).
12. Weigh and measure height of patients.
13. Admit, discharge and transfer patients.
14. Collect urine, stool and sputum specimens.
15. Answer patients' lights.
16. Care for flowers, distribute mail and packages and run errands for patients.
17. Order linen and supplies as necessary.
18. Keep station neat and tidy.

In summary, the nurse aide comes to the hospital with no formal education. Preparation for her work consists of on-the-job training. Improved practice and further learning is accomplished through supervised experiences and inservice education.

THE ORDERLY

The orderly is used in many ways. He often becomes a jack-of-all-trades through on-the-job training. He may give care to patients, catheterize male patients, clean isolation units, transport patients, lift heavy or helpless patients, run the autoclave or deliver, clean and operate various pieces of equipment. The orderly is frequently in the difficult position of being under the direction of one department administratively and responsible to many persons in other departments throughout the hospital. When an orderly is "on call" to several departments, he often has many persons telling him what to do.

The alternative to this type of orderly utilization is to use him as a male nurse aide. If an institution is large enough and the community provides a large enough labor market, this is considered a better way to utilize orderlies. Their duties become similar to that of the nurse aide. They are particularly helpful in an area where there is a preponderance of orthopedic and urological patients.

This particular job is hard to fill, and there is often a great turnover. Clearer orderly job descriptions and closer supervision of orderlies are often necessary. Usually, a boy who is going to school functions well and learns quickly. However, his tenure is short which often means that as much as one third of his employment span may be spent in orientation and training. Most men want a position in which there is opportunity for advancement and this type of position does not provide it.

A.N.A. STATEMENT ON AUXILIARY PERSONNEL IN NURSING SERVICE*

Definition of Auxiliary Worker in Nursing

The term "auxiliary personnel" in nursing service is used in this statement to designate auxiliary personnel employed to assist the nurse in hospitals, nursing homes, and other agencies. These workers are employed and trained to perform tasks which involve specified services for patients as delegated by the professional nurses or licensed practical nurses.

Auxiliary workers in nursing service carry out tasks supportive and complementary to nursing practice. Although the performance of these tasks is essential to patient care, the auxiliary workers are neither professional nurses nor licensed practical nurses, nor do their activities constitute the practice of nursing. Furthermore, it is the belief of the American Nurses' Association that licensing of this group is not consistent with the supportive role of auxiliary personnel in nursing service.†

It is pointed out that this definition of auxiliary workers rules out all other trained and untrained personnel, of whom there are many. In this other con-

*Prepared by the A.N.A. Committee on Allied Nursing Personnel. *American Journal of Nursing*, July, 1962, p. 73.

†In some psychiatric facilities, for example, the worker who performs functions within the field of practical nursing is sometimes called a psychiatric aide or technician. Preservice preparation of workers performing these functions should be secured in a state-approved program leading to licensure as a practical nurse.

text are such employees as physical and occupational therapy aides and x-ray and laboratory technicians, as well as porters, diet maids, ward maids, messengers, receptionists, clerks. These are excluded because they relate either to the environmental care of the patient or may be assigned to more than one division of the agency. While in some measure they may be supportive to the nursing service, their employment, training, and supervision should not be the responsibility of the nursing service.

This statement is chiefly concerned with the group of auxiliary workers frequently referred to as "nurses' aides." The title of this group differs in various employment situations, where they are designated as nursing assistants, ward attendants, orderlies, nursing aides, et cetera. Because of this lack of uniformity in title, it was thought best, for the purposes of this statement to refer to this group as auxiliary workers in nursing service.

Selection

The ultimate responsibility for the selection of auxiliary workers in nursing service should rest with the department most closely associated with their work—that is, the nursing department. In the health agencies where there is a general personnel director responsible for employment, the staffing needs of the nursing service can be met adequately only if there is a close working relationship between the personnel director and the nursing service administrator.

Qualifications

The qualifications of auxiliary workers differ widely, but in general, preference should be given to those with at least a grammar school education and an interest in the care of the sick. The workers should be physically and emotionally healthy; mentally competent; maintain good grooming and appearance; speak correctly, quietly and audibly; exhibit a kind, courteous, and friendly manner; demonstrate willingness to work with others; and understand and practice ethical conduct. While the ages of auxiliary personnel show wide variation, ability to perform the expected tasks and to understand the nature of the supportive role in the care of the patient is more important than chronological age. The auxiliary worker should be employed only after a medical examination which includes appropriate physical and psychological tests.

Training

These auxiliary workers who render services which are supportive to the nursing care given by licensed nurses should be prepared for their duties by a planned program of on-the-job training in contrast to the preservice nursing. Subsequent training and evaluation of the auxiliary personnel in nursing should be an ongoing process, with responsibility for this specifically delegated to the nursing service administration of the institution or agency.

The extent and nature of the training program should be interpreted to all workers in the agency so that they will have an understanding of the role of the auxiliary workers in nursing service. There are two attitudes commonly held by professional personnel which need to be modified—one is that which tends to limit the tasks of auxiliary workers so that they cannot make the contribution to patient care which they should, and the other which allows them to take on more and more responsibility for nursing procedures so that eventually, with little or no preparation, they are actually assigned to nurse patients. It is obvious that the whole purpose of auxiliary workers in nursing service is put in jeopardy when either of these attitudes is present. It is also necessary to bear in mind that the practice of nursing by unlicensed persons is illegal and violators are subject to prosecution. The auxiliary worker should be taught to understand the nature of his personal responsibility and the danger to himself and patients should he attempt to practice nursing. Professional personnel must also realize that nurses have an obligation to protect the public by not delegating to a person less qualified any service which requires the competence of a nurse.

The aim of training of these auxiliary workers, therefore, should be to develop a program which is both safe for the patient and practical for the nursing service. In order to carry out effective on-the-job training for auxiliary workers in nursing service a qualified professional nurse instructor should be appointed. In large institutions where the number and turnover of personnel warrant it, this should be the sole responsibility; in other situations it may be joined with other duties, but it should never be secondary to them.

The training program should be well organized, including classroom instruction, demonstration, and supervised practice. Experience in a variety of situations has demonstrated that the length of time required for on-the-job training of the auxiliary workers varies widely, depending upon the ability of the worker and the characteristics of the nursing unit in which the workers are employed. No content, however, should be included in the training program which would purport to train the worker for more than simple, uncomplicated tasks to be performed under the direction of nurses.

Supervision

After the initial training period, the direct supervision of these auxiliary workers should be delegated to the nursing unit. These auxiliary workers should then be assigned to work under the immediate direction and supervision of a qualified nurse who selects and delegates the specific tasks to be performed by the worker. The vital point is to assure continuing supervision following the orientation period and that the supervision and evaluation of the auxiliary workers in nursing service should be the responsibility of a nurse so designated and prepared by the nursing service administration. The abilities and work performance of these auxiliary workers should be evaluated on a continuing basis, with written reports for the purpose of record and for indications for additional training and assignment.

THE PRACTICAL NURSE (L.P.N. OR L.V.N.)

The practical or vocational nurse (the term depends upon the state where the person is licensed) has increased in numbers at a fantastic rate. In 1930, there were 11 state approved schools of practical nursing and, in 1963, there were 829. The properly assigned practical nurse contributes immeasurably to good patient care. See pp. 71–73 for the ANA and NFLPN Statement of Functions of the Licensed Practical Nurse.

What Is the L.P.N.'s Background?

Most schools of practical nursing prefer that an applicant be a graduate of high school, although there are exceptions. Schools may accept students from 17 to 50 years of age. After the student has completed her practical nurse education, usually one year in length, she may then take an examination to qualify her for licensure. If anyone is interested in learning what schools are available in a specific area, she should write the National League for Nursing to obtain, *Let's Be Practical About a Nursing Career,* which lists the requirements of each state and contains a list of approved schools of practical nursing in each state.

Before 1948, a practical nurse was of questionable background because many were self-appointed. Some states did not have licensure laws. There were few standards with which to measure a practical nurse except by employing her and seeing what she could do. During World War II, nurse aides who had performed well were trained to do additional procedures and duties. Some of these women are still employed as unlicensed practical nurses.

What Does the Practical Nurse Do?

The practical nurse has gained an important place in the care of patients. Her work is done under the supervision of a registered nurse or a physician. She performs all the things done by a nurse aide in addition to the following duties:

1. Take blood pressure and apical pulse.
2. Assist physicians with physical examinations and selected treatments.
3. Prepare patients for surgery, treatment or diagnostic examination.
4. Apply compresses and packs to eye, ear, skin or to a wound.
5. Catheterize patients and insert an indwelling catheter.
6. Use selected hyperventilation and oxygen equipment.
7. Perform bladder and vaginal irrigations and give perineal care.
8. Assist with intravenous therapy. This usually means that she learns to watch fluid levels and injection sites and to observe the comfort of the patient.
9. Assist with gastric, chest and wound suction machines. She learns to read gauges and to observe the comfort of the patients.
10. Care for patients in isolation.
11. Chart in the patient's medical record.
12. Give selected medications.

Older nurses are sometimes threatened by the practical nurse. Her list of duties looks all too much like that of the registered nurse 20 years ago. The nurse must remember that total nursing care is far more encompassing than the accurate performance of procedures and techniques. This does not minimize the necessity of performing procedures correctly for the benefit of patient safety, comfort and privacy. Nonetheless, the practical nurse has a limited exposure to psychology, sociology, pharmacology, English and many other disciplines.

STATEMENT OF FUNCTIONS OF THE LICENSED PRACTICAL NURSE*

Education and Licensure

The LPN should be prepared and qualified for nursing practice by:

1. Education
   a. Preservice preparation in a program in practical nursing approved by the state board of nursing.
   b. Orientation and continuing inservice education.
   c. Instruction, within the scope of practical nursing, of the practitioner who qualifies for further training in specialized fields peculiar to the agency.
2. Licensure by state board of nursing

Personal Qualifications

Personal and vocational growth and development should be sustained by:

1. Maintenance of good health practices.
2. Active participation in and the promotion of nursing organizations; inservice education programs; workshops; institutes; other educational and community activities.

Role Description

The work of the LPN is an integral part of nursing. The licensed practical nurse gives nursing care under the supervision of the registered professional nurse or physician to patients in simple nursing situations. In more complex situations the licensed practical nurse functions as an assistant to the registered professional nurse.

A simple nursing situation is one that is relatively free of scientific complexity. In a simple nursing situation the clinical state of the patient is relatively stable and the measures of care offered by the physician require abilities based on a comparatively fixed and limited body of scientific facts and can be performed by following a defined procedure step by step. Measures of medical and personal care are not subject to continuously changing and complex modifications because of the clinical or behavioral state of the patient. The nursing that the patient requires is primarily of a physical character and not instructional.

In more complex situations, the licensed practical nurse facilitates patient care by meeting specific nursing requirements of patients as directed, such as preparing equipment, supplies and facilities for patient care, helping the professional nurse to perform nursing measures, and communicating significant observations to the registered professional nurse.

Legal Status

The legal responsibility of the LPN extends to two areas:

1. Licensure to practice practical nursing according to state law.

2. Performance limited to those acts for which he or she has been prepared. Although it is true that the LPN's responsibility extends to these two areas, bearing in mind the individual's personal responsibility under the law, it is equally true that the professional nurse has ultimate responsibility for nursing service, including the responsibility for assignment of all nursing personnel.

*This statement was approved by the Executive Board of the National Federation of Licensed Practical Nurses in October, 1963, and by the Board of Directors of the American Nurses Association in January, 1964. It appeared in *American Journal of Nursing*, March, 1964, p. 93.

Functions

The selection of the functions or the specific procedures to be performed by the LPN depends upon a realistic appraisal of the elements within the situations, such as the complexity of scientific principles underlying the procedure or function; the ability and skills the LPN has acquired and demonstrated; the amount and character of the supervision required by the LPN to perform the functions; and the patients' needs and the ability of the LPN to provide safe nursing care to meet those needs.

In this context, the LPN performs the following functions:

A. Participates in the planning, implementation, and evaluation of nursing care in complex situations, and in giving nursing care in simple nursing situations by:

1. Providing for the emotional and physical comfort and safety of patients through:
   a. Understanding of human relationships between and among patients, families and personnel.
   b. Recognizing and understanding cultural backgrounds, spiritual needs; respecting the religious beliefs of individual patients.
   c. Recognizing and understanding the effects of social and economic problems upon patients.
   d. Protecting patients from behavior that would damage their self-esteem or relationship with families, other patients or personnel.
   e. Participating in the development, revision, and implementation of policies and procedures designed to insure comfort and safety of patients and personnel.
   f. Assisting the patient with activities of daily living and encouraging appropriate self-care.
   g. Considering needs of the patient for an attractive, comfortable and safe environment.

For effective practice the LPN must know and utilize fundamental principles of human behavior and have an appreciation of the effects of stress upon individuals and groups.

A practical understanding of human growth and behavior makes it possible to note signs of change or disturbance in the patient's activity patterns. These may relate to illness, to individual responses to the institutional environment, and to personnel.

Representation and participation on committees and in conferences relevant to personnel and nursing care utilizes staff resources to develop a mutual understanding of the individual's role and responsibility in nursing service, e.g. a Committee on Infection Control.

2. Observing, recording and reporting to the appropriate person:
   a. General physical and mental condition of patients, signs and symptoms which may be indicative of change.
   b. Stresses in human relationships between patients and patient's families, visitors and personnel.
3. Performing nursing procedures for which the preparation of the LPN has provided the necessary degree of skill and judgment, such as:
   a. Administration of medications and treatments prescribed for the patient.
   b. Preparation and care of patients receiving specialized treatments.
   c. Performance of special nursing techniques in caring for patients with communicable diseases.
   d. Practice of first-aid measures.
   e. Preparation and after care of equipment for treatments, including sterilization and observation of aseptic techniques.
4. Assisting with the rehabilitation of patients according to the patient care plan through:

a. Awareness of and encouraging the interests and special aptitudes of patients.
b. Encouraging patients to help themselves within their own capabilities in performing activities of daily living.
c. Knowledge and application of the principles of prevention of deformities; the normal range of motion; body mechanics and body alignment.
d. Utilizing the community resources and facilities for continuing patient care.

B. Promoting effectiveness of the employing health service agency through:
1. Utilizing opportunities in contacts with patients' relatives to promote better understanding of policies pertaining to the health service.
2. Fostering cooperative effort through understanding the functions of all personnel involved in patient care.
3. Utilizing community resources and relationships for better understanding by the public of health services.

THE WARD SECRETARY

The ward secretary, sometimes called a ward clerk, is another position which has become increasingly common since World War II. The ward clerk has become a necessary part of the nursing station of any major size. She not only prevents hundreds of interruptions that take nurses away from patients, but she also learns to perform many clerical and receptionist functions which do not require a nursing education. Besides doing clerical work, a ward clerk functions as a receptionist. A great deal of general information can be given out by persons trained to do this job.

A station may have two shifts of clerical coverage (usually days and evenings). Night coverage is unusual. As patient turnover increased and the number of medications, examinations and treatments for each patient multiplied, the number of necessary records mounted and paper work became an eight hour a day job. Ward secretaries are lay persons who are trained on the job to do some of the following things:

1. See that a doctor receives his charts and locate a nurse to assist him if required.
2. Act as receptionist to visitors, relatives and even patients when they first come to the station.
3. Order nontreatment items for station and patients.
4. Answer the telephone and direct calls and messages to proper persons.
5. Answer the intercommunication system which is connected to patient rooms and dispatch the proper person to assist the patient.
6. Operate the addressograph.
7. Assemble forms for new charts, make out name tags, kardex cards, supply forms, etc.
8. Call doctors, interns, etc., and take messages for personnel who are paged over the loudspeaker system.

9. Chart certain items in the patient's chart, usually such things as temperature, pulse, respiration, height, weight, blood pressure, treatment and medications.
10. Transcribe physician's orders.

There is disagreement about whether ward clerks should perform certain of the latter tasks. The refresher will, therefore, find wide variations in specific duties.

THE STATION MANAGER

The station manager concept is another new idea being developed to relieve nurses of non-nursing responsibilities. This position serves as an excellent example of how imperative it is to see the actual job description of a position before one can discern its real responsibilities and requirements. A job title may be quite deceiving. A head nurse may be functioning as a nurse specialist, a supervisor, an assistant director of nursing or in any number of other ways. A station manager may function as a person who spends virtually all of her time transcribing physician's orders or she may be a man with a bachelor s degree in business administration. On-the-job training may be the only requirement beyond high school. The person may be a nurse or a non-nurse. The responsibilities may involve supervision of many persons from several departments or no supervision at all. In the latter case, coordination of activities may be the main responsibility. The station manager position is often misunderstood because of the needs and interpretations of the job by so many disparate types of institutions.

In one city the terms station manager and chart nurse basically describe the same job. In this particular case, both jobs involve responsibility for transcribing physician's orders. In another hospital the term ward secretary is used for a person who functions in the dual position of ward clerk and transcriber.

Some of these persons are responsible for supervision of non-nursing services to patients. In this case a station manager may be quite different. He or she may be asked to supervise the housekeeping personnel who clean the rooms, the dietary personnel who serve meals and nourishments on the station, the engineers who repair equipment on the station and other such personnel. When the job encompasses the supervision of personnel from such a variety of departments, it is usually administered under the department of hospital administration. In this case there are two supervisors on the nursing station, one for the nursing care (the head nurse) and the station manager who is responsible for all non-nursing services. Because all services culminate in patient service, clarification of responsibilities are required for such job differentiations. Such an arrangement usually accomplishes the removal of non-nursing duties from nursing personnel.

The need for these positions differs and their success varies according to many factors. Nonetheless, adaptations of this job may be found in many places.

THE VOLUNTEER

Volunteers, both male and female, serve in many areas of a hospital and perform a wide variety of services. They may function in occupational and diversional areas, they may make beds, serve customers in the coffee shop, make bandages or perform any of several other chores. They receive an orientation to the hospital as well as an orientation to their particular duties. It is important to remember that they always need the support and help of personnel employed in the area.

SUMMARY

When a nurse leaves one hospital and enters another, moves from one community to another or returns to nursing after an absence of several years, she will need to examine the job descriptions of those who work with her in order to clarify her own responsibilities. The nurse does not function alone. It is necessary that she know how her work is related to that of others who provide nursing care, either directly or indirectly, before she can begin to function in her new setting. With all these persons available to the patient, what are the responsibilities of the R.N.? The next chapter will describe some of the ways an institution utilizes the registered nurse.

REFERENCES

American Nurses Association Statement on Auxiliary Personnel in Nursing Service, April, 1962.

Chase, Elsa P.: Time-Tested Program of Aid Training. *American Journal of Nursing,* January, 1963, p. 90.

Fay, Audrey B.: Help is Where You Find It. *Nursing Outlook,* December, 1956, p. 673.

Henning, John F.: MDTA The Broad Program. *American Journal of Nursing,* June, 1964, p. 109.

Howe, Arlene: Supervisors Coordinate Patient Services. *Modern Hospital,* July, 1963, p. 77.

Lee, Anne Natalie: The Training of Nonprofessional Personnel. *Nursing Outlook,* April, 1958, p. 222.

Levine, Eugene: Turnover Among Nursing Personnel in Hospitals. *Hospitals,* September 1, 1957, p. 50.

Levine, Eugene, Siegel, Stanley, and DeLa Puente, Joseph: Diversity of Nurse Staffing Among General Hospitals. *Hospitals,* May 1, 1961, p. 42.

Licensed Practical Nurses in Nursing Services. National League for Nursing, 1965.

Orem, Dorothea E.: *Guides for Developing Curricula for the Education of Practical Nurses.* U.S. Department of Health, Education, and Welfare, OE-85004.

Randall, Margaret: *Ward Administration.* Philadelphia, W. B. Saunders Co., 1949.

Stevenson, Neva M.: The Better Utilization of Licensed Practical Nurses. *Nursing Outlook,* July, 1965, p. 34.

West, Margaret D. and Crowther, Beatrice, *Education for Practical Nursing, 1960,* Department of Practical Nursing Programs, National League for Nursing.

7

The Registered Nurse at Work in a Hospital

Any nurse who smokes, uses liquor in any form, gets her hair done at a beauty shop or frequents dance halls will give the director of nursing good reason to suspect her worth, intentions and integrity.

In addition to caring for your 50 patients, each bedside nurse will follow these regulations: Daily sweep and mop the floors of your ward, dust the patient's furniture and window sills.

Maintain an even temperature in your ward by bringing in a scuttle of coal for the day's business.

Light is important to observe the patient's condition. Therefore, each day fill the kerosene lamps, clean the chimneys, trim wicks. Wash the windows once a week.

The nurse's notes are important in aiding the physician's work. Make your pens carefully. You may whittle nibs to your individual taste.

Each nurse on day duty will report every day at 7 A.M. and leave at 8 P.M., except on the Sabbath when she will be off from noon until 2 P.M. Graduate nurses in good standing with the director of nurses will be given an evening off each week for courting purposes or two evenings a week if they go regularly to church.

Each nurse should lay aside from her pay a goodly sum of her earnings for her benefit during her declining years so that she will not become a burden. For example, if she earns $30 a month she should set aside $15.

And the nurse who performs her labors, serves her patients and doctors faithfully and without fault for five years will be given an increase by the hospital administration of 5 cents a day, providing there are no hospital debts outstanding.*

This frequently quoted job description of 1887 sharpens the contrast between yesterday and today. Salary range, authority status of the director, length of working hours, mid-Victorian influence, lack of technical tools as well as actual nursing duties are evident in this description. A moment of reflection will tell us that people with imagination

*Job description of 1887. *Canadian Nurse,* April, 1965, p. 307.

and dynamic ideas have led us and helped us to adapt to the many interdependent and interacting changes of every decade.

The present-day registered nurse can expect continually changing responsibilities. In order to participate in these changes, she must learn to utilize many available resources. One of the aims of this book is to help the refresher to prepare for her new role and to suggest some of the changes she might expect. In order to do this, you will need to learn what responsibilities are expected of the nurse employed in a hospital. Because responsibilities vary so greatly, you will find many places where they differ from what is herein described.

The term nurse does not have the definite meaning today that it did 20 years ago. The word may be used to describe a practical nurse, a diploma graduate or a woman with a bachelor's degree or more. Even the term registered nurse may be used to refer to persons with very different educational backgrounds. Although this may be a sign of transition and growth, it is no less confusing to the public and even to nurses.

A great deal has been written about nursing as a profession. There is much debate about whether nursing can be considered a true profession, although most authorities agree that it is at least a semiprofession. One characteristic of a profession is that there be a large amount of judgment and decision in the performance of the work. As this increases, that work then becomes more professional in its nature. Without arguing the pros and cons of nursing as a profession, it is necessary to understand that an increased amount of independent judgment and decision is required of the registered nurse.

Let us begin by saying that one of the most important functions of the R.N. is the management of direct bedside nursing care of the patient. This is different from management of a unit. While the nurse needs to know certain administrative principles, she needs them for a function which is quite different from what was traditionally known as nursing administration.

Another distinction, closely related to this, separates functions of the nurse based on medical care. The nurse will carry out physician's orders as she has in the past, but this is considered a dependent function because it is not initiated by the nurse. She will assist the physician whenever required. The nurse will also be giving care, which is her main responsibility. This is initiated by her and is a function independent of other disciplines.

The nurse is gradually coming to realize that she cannot be all things to all people. Through the years, this particular desire has caused her to dissipate her energies. She has taken over many doctor's tasks whenever he has not had the time. She has performed pharmacy duties, dietary functions and housekeeping tasks. It is flattering to think that such a variety of persons have such faith in our abilities, but nursing care has often suffered because of it. Future development and growth of nursing will rest upon what is selected, identified and ultimately accepted as nursing functions by the profession as a whole.

Before going into more detail about nursing, let us look briefly at our patient. We often overlook him because of our difficulty in understanding him.

WHAT WE EXPECT OF OUR PATIENTS

I recently sat in on a discussion with a class of refreshers about nurses' expectations of patients. The discussion started with a description of the ideal patient. The ideal patient was described as cooperative, independent when able to care for himself, passive when needing assistance, cheerful, friendly, outgoing, uncomplaining, brave, accepting of his care and thoughtful of personnel. He does not turn on his light very often and he has few visitors. One class member suggested that anyone with "ideal patient" qualities probably would receive little attention because "he needed so little." The group leader persisted until the list of pleasing patient qualities was almost ludicrous.

The discussion then circled around a description of the "difficult" patient. He was described as crotchety, demanding, uncooperative, inconsiderate of other patients as well as personnel. He turned his light on frequently and "made up excuses just to get the nurse in there."

It was apparent to everyone in the group that it is important to realize that we are prone to describe patients in terms that meet our needs rather than terms that indicate needs we might meet.

We tend to avoid the patient who upsets us and, as a result, that patient is likely to become more lonely and therefore more demanding rather than less. Our avoidance of such a patient prevents us from finding out what it is that is bothering him, bringing the patient and the nurse still farther apart. These patients give us a feeling that we have not been successful in our approach. This is true, but not in the sense that we think. Putting a label on a patient blocks problem solving. Calling a patient "irritable" is somewhat final. Asking what is bothering a patient who acts irritably opens the door to a possible solution of his problem.

It is therefore helpful to remember that our own response to a patient affects his behavior and our nursing care. When a patient is hostile, it is common to find the nursing staff developing hostility toward the patient. When these reactions occur, a nursing care plan made by a group of personnel can be very fruitful and prevent or at least reduce further tensions. This, then, returns us to the work of the R.N. in the hospital.

METHODS OF ASSIGNMENT

Team nursing has been developed in an attempt to permit the R.N. to use her knowledge and skills most effectively. As a method of assignment, it combines features of the case method of assignment with that of the functional method. As a result, the general duty R.N. has an expanded and somewhat different role. Review of the case method and the functional method helps to understand team nursing.

The Case Method

The case method, sometimes called the group method of assignment, was and perhaps is the ideal method. Several patients are assigned to a nurse who gives all the care to that group of patients. Nurses usually find increased satisfaction from giving total care to their patients and patients usually enjoy being able to identify with one person whom they can call their nurse. Because present-day personnel have such different educational backgrounds and are prepared to give such different levels of care, this method of assignment is rarely possible, although there are exceptions.

A nurse aide cannot provide the total care needed by a patient with emphysema because several medications, teaching and Bennett respirator treatments are required. An L.P.N. may or may not have been educated to give most of the technical care. In this case, the R.N. is the only person who is prepared to give this patient's total care; psychological, technical and educational. This is true of many patients. Because there are not enough R.N.'s, the case method is seldom used except for the purpose of student education.

The Functional System

The functional system is perhaps the most effective system for getting work done, but it is also the most impersonal method of assignment because it is so task-centered. Each person is assigned specific duties and work. One person may be assigned to the T.P.R.'s, p.r.n. enemas and weights of patients. Another person might be assigned to making all the beds of ambulatory patients and to help with semiambulatory patients. Another person might be assigned to the medications for the entire floor. The functional system leaves little provision for the nontechnical needs of patients because it is planned around routines and tasks rather than patients.

The Team System

Basically, the team system is a combination of the case method and the functional system. It attempts to utilize the differing skills of personnel according to patient requirements. A group of patients are cared for by several persons. Patients on a station are divided into two or three groups. A 40-bed station might be divided into two sections of 20 patients each or into three groups of 13 or 14 patients. Each group of patients is cared for by several persons (a team). The team of persons might be composed of an R.N., two L.P.N.'s and one nurse aide. Ideally, the distribution of the team changes with the needs of the patient group. In reality, this is only partially achieved.

The R.N. is the team leader, the L.P.N.'s and the nurse aide are the team members. The R.N. makes out the assignment of patients and is responsible for seeing that her group of patients receives optimum nursing care. For general care, she tries to match patient needs with the skills of her personnel. The nurse aide might be assigned to taking the T.P.R.'s, weights and serving extra nourishments if this is not done by the dietary department. The L.P.N. might be assigned to the medications. These are the functional aspects of team nursing. The R.N., as a team leader, is automatically assigned to make rounds of all 20 patients to ascertain their needs and make first-hand observations, to assist her team members to perform their work and to evaluate the care given to her patients. Each team member is also assigned to particular patients. This is the case method aspect of the team system.

In a larger sense, a team might include interdisciplinary personnel, such as the doctor, the physical therapist and the social worker. A description of this kind of team approach will be found in Chapter 14. For purposes of this discussion, we will limit ourselves to a brief description of the team system as a method of assignment and as it relates to the duties of the R.N. Figure 7–1 shows different combinations of patients and personnel of three teams.

THE TEAM LEADER

Team leadership cannot be learned quickly or superficially. Where a severe shortage of R.N.'s exists, L.P.N.'s and sometimes even nurse aides are asked to function as team leaders. Although they are assigned as team leaders, they cannot be expected to function as a person who has been educated for the job or as a person who has a background of psychology, sociology and physical sciences. "Both registered nurses and licensed practical nurses engage in the practice of nursing. The difference between the registered nurse and the licensed practical nurse is, therefore, not a difference in function but a difference in the degree of judgment which each possesses and utilizes."*

The next few pages might best be considered an orientation to team leading. There are four important functions of the team leader: delegation of care, teaching of personnel, appraisal of patient needs

Guide for Registered Nurses in the Assignment of Nursing Personnel. 1965, Minnesota Board of Nursing and Minnesota Nurses Association.

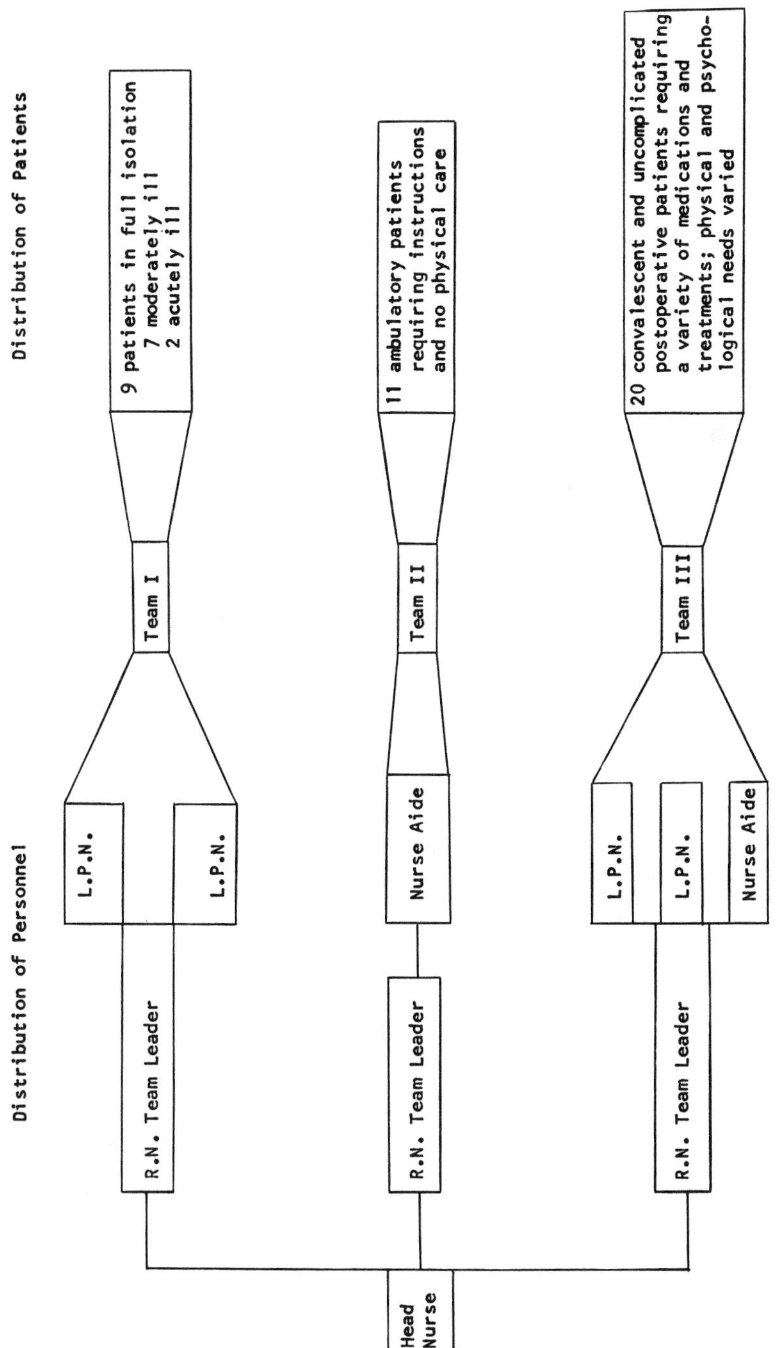

Figure 7–1. *Variations of the distribution of three teams on a 40-bed station.*

and planning of new goals of nursing care. Brief familiarization with these four functions will help you to better understand what the hospital R.N. does at work.

Delegation of Care

What care can be assigned and delegated to team members? Which patients require the R.N. background? Is a nurse aide able to give a bed bath to a patient with coronary thrombosis who seems to have accepted his physical restrictions? Could the nurse aide give a bath to the patient with coronary thrombosis who considers physical restrictions senseless? Both patients seem to require a bed bath. But would it be better for one of these patients to do without the fatiguing experience of a bed bath?

These are a few examples of what the R.N. must ask about her patients and her personnel. To match personnel with patients purely on the basis of duties and physical needs is a mistake. As a matter of fact, a nurse aide of some experience may well be able to care for a coronary by virtue of her personality. She could not give medical interpretation to the necessity of restrictions, nor would she have the tools to explore the reasons for his lack of compliance with medical instructions, but she might be able to help the patient to relax. In this way, she may contribute greatly to the care of such a patient.

Should the R.N. give physical care to patients? Yes. She may wish to learn more about a particular patient or she may wish to give special instructional care. There may be many reasons. Aside from caring for a few patients who are selected because of their special needs, the team leader should remain as free as possible in order to assist her team members with the care of the other patients. What better way to observe the interaction between personnel and patients? What better way to learn what might be helpful to team members? What better way to find out if the patient has further needs?

Major aspects of delegated duties should always be written clearly and legibly. A printed assignment form, such as the one on the opposite page, is always helpful. Oral review of the assignment and additional instructions are usually necessary also. The assignment sheet needs to be used in conjunction with information on a kardex or a nursing care plan.

It is also important for personnel to realize that the very nature of caring for a group of patients makes it inherently impossible to guarantee that some change may not be necessary during a shift. A patient may expire, a patient may require emergency resuscitation, or someone may require special observation. Unexpected contingencies should at least be anticipated.

One other element of delegation is the assignment of meal hours and coffee breaks. Both are pleasant breaks in the work day, and it is always more pleasant to eat with friends and colleagues of one's choice. This cannot be the only factor considered in these assignments. If a station has two teams, there are probably two R.N.'s on duty (aside from the head nurse). These two persons should not go to meals at the same time. Patients deserve to have at least a minimum number of the best prepared personnel available at all times. Socialization is no excuse for leaving a group of patients without this. Many nurses feel that because a shortage of personnel makes it sometimes necessary to leave patients without R.N. coverage, it is therefore all right. This merely

DAILY TEAM ASSIGNMENT

Station______ Team______ Date______

Care Conference on:________________

1. Check patients under the personnel to whom they are assigned.
2. Check special assignments at the top. If two persons work together, the names may be written in rather than a check mark.

PERSONNEL						
T.L.						
MEDS						
B.P.						
I & O						
T.P.R.						
OTHER						
COFFEE						
MEAL HOUR						
INSERVICE CL.						

ROOM	PATIENT NAME						

Figure 7–2. Sample daily team assignment. (St. Barnabas Hospital, Minneapolis, Minnesota.)

makes it a necessity on occasion, but does not justify it when it is not necessary.

In summary, the team leader must delegate both duties and patients to members of her team. That delegation must be based upon the needs of her patients and the education, experience and personality of her team members. In all reality, the team leader must realize that she is often faced with the task of trying to use the personnel she has in the best possible way. The skills of the team members at her disposal may not always match the needs of her patients, but she can give her patients the benefit of her best judgment in distributing their talents.

> The registered nurse determines, implements and evaluates the nursing care plan consonant with the physician's medical care plan. She must perform nursing functions or delegate them to other nursing personnel in accordance with agency policy and generally accepted nursing standards. She must direct and supervise all nursing activities performed by licensed practical nurses and all functions performed by auxiliary workers in support of nursing activities.*

Teaching Personnel

Although the burden of in-service education must not be placed on the team leader, she must learn a few simple techniques in order to teach team members when they are new to an area or have learned a procedure incorrectly or when a review is in order because something is infrequently used or performed. If a team member has never been exposed to a task or function, it is up to the head nurse or in-service instructor to prepare her. The team leader must first of all know how to do a procedure correctly herself. If she needs review, she has procedure books, a head nurse, supervisor or in-service instructor to call upon. Sometimes another R.N. may be the only person needed.

The team leader must be aware of what her team members know and whether they perform techniques safely and carefully. She often needs to give simple reviews or demonstrations of procedures at the bedside. The team leader can assist the in-service instructor by keeping her informed of learning needs that she identifies.

The team leader can improve her instruction by being aware of a few teaching guides. The teacher must be sure that the student can see what is being demonstrated. She must not only show the person what to do, but also explain what she is doing and why. After a verbal review of the steps, the learner should perform the procedure in the presence of the instructor soon after the demonstration. This gives the learner an opportunity to ask questions and find out whether she fully understood what was being taught. Personnel who receive on-the-job demonstrations are usually highly motivated because they are learning something immediately useful. For this reason, they are likely to be responsive and attentive.

***Guide for Registered Nurses in the Assignment of Nursing Personnel.* 1965, Minnesota Board of Nursing and Minnesota Nurses' Association.

Team leaders also teach by example. Their behavior and attitudes are imitated as often as their procedure skills. This is a more subtle but no less important kind of teaching performed by team leaders.

The team leader must further realize that teaching does not necessarily imply learning. If the teacher gives instructions that are not clear, if the learner is distracted or if she does not understand, learning did not occur. When this happens, it is helpful to know the reason in order to improve future instructions. The immediate concern of the team leader is that she be aware that no instruction is complete without at least one follow-up observation. It should be added that the team leader also has no way of knowing whether patient assignments are satisfactorily completed unless she follows up to find out. The same blocks to communication can occur with everyday written and verbal instructions.

Appraisal of Patient Needs

A great deal of attention is now being given to the nonphysical and nontechnical needs of patients. The reason for this is that we have often neglected them because of emphasis on procedures. An observant nurse of yesterday will notice that her patient's catheter is not running, but she is less likely to be attuned to her patient's nonverbal behavior. Is he lying rather rigidly in bed? Does he have an anxious expression? She needs to be reminded that her patient's verbal expressions should not be interpreted without some exploration. If he says he does not think he will ever get home, does he mean that he is worried about his bill, that he will be a burden to his wife, that he might have cancer or that he does not want to go home for some reason or other?

The nurse can learn to utilize more of her time to appraise her patient's needs, both physical and psychological. This does not make the nurse a psychotherapist. It simply means that she realizes that patients have psychological needs and that she will try to help her patients in all spheres. Physical and psychological comfort interact upon one another. A patient who lies on a wet draw sheet is both physically uncomfortable and embarrassed if it is due to urine. By the same token, a patient lying on a dry draw sheet can hardly be expected to have no worries.

The nurse must try to explore the meanings of her patients' comments by asking questions or trying to find out whether she understood them correctly. She cannot do this if she guides the conversation in an attempt to make herself comfortable. We all have a tendency to want to "cheer the patient up," to change the subject if we cannot think of an answer for the patient or to focus our attention on the hot pack or a new bouquet of roses.

The key to appraisal of patient needs is concentrated listening. None of us are as expert at this as we would like to be, but it is something which we can consciously practice. When we make rounds to our patients, we might sit down in a chair instead of standing near the door appearing anxious to hurry on to the next patient or to something more important.

It is strongly urged that every refresher read Ida Jean Orlando's book, *The Dynamic Nurse-Patient Relationship*, before returning to work. In order to better help patients, a knowledge of social data is important. Aside from information found on face sheets, the nurse may need to explore and utilize what she learns. We often find it interesting to know that someone was born in a log cabin and never went beyond the third grade, but we rarely base our nursing actions on this knowledge.

At some institutions, a so-called nursing history is obtained. Some utilize what is known as a structured interview. In either case the institution provides a sheet similar in appearance to a medical history and it is kept on the patient's chart. It may be helpful to know some of the items on such history and interview sheets, as we may wish to obtain similar information even if we do not have an opportunity to use a specific form.

Questions similar to the following are often asked. How long have you had this particular illness or symptoms? Do you have other illnesses? Have you been hospitalized before this admission? What kind of work do you do? How does this illness interfere with your job and income? Do you have difficulty sleeping? Is there anything which helps you to sleep? Do you wish to restrict visitors or telephone calls? Are you on any special diet? What are your special food likes and dislikes? How might we best help you during your stay? Other questions will occur to the nurse as she talks to her patients. It is vital that the nurse utilize this information when she plans patient care. This is an excellent way to involve the patient in planning his own care.

Observation, reporting and recording of both objective and subjective information is no less important than it was in the past. Environmental comfort, safety, physical appearance, mental condition, complaints, activity, vital signs, reaction to treatments and medications all must be noted and recorded. The chapters on nursing care will make this more apparent. The nurse must meet both the physical and the emotional needs of her patients. Nursing care is incomplete if either aspect is omitted.

Planning New Goals for Patient Care

Once we have delegated certain functions to our personnel, assisted them to carry out these functions and assessed the needs of our patients, we need to raise our sights and provide an up-to-date plan of care for each patient. A good, written plan of care provides the much needed communication between the patient and the many persons working different hours and different days of the week. Such a care plan is usually developed at a nursing care conference.

THE NURSING CARE CONFERENCE. The nursing care conference, the team conference or the patient care conference are terms used to describe a conference of team members where care of an individual patient is explored. It is not like a transfer report or a brief meeting to discuss work. The team leader is the discussion leader.

Certain efforts on the part of the leader contribute greatly to a successful conference. Make the group feel at ease so that everyone, nurse aide, orderly, L.P.N. and student feel encouraged to contribute their ideas. After a brief review of the patient's history and condition, begin to identify problems of the patient with the group and approaches which might help the patient, and decide upon goals for special concentration. Utilize any teaching opportunity which may arise as long as it pertains to the patient. Record the plan and close the conference after about ten or 20 minutes. If more time is needed, plan follow-up conferences for future days. End the conference with a summary of the plans to help the patient and prepare members for an evaluation of the plans in a few days.

THE NURSING CARE PLAN. The nursing care plan is usually written on a Kardex card for each patient. It usually specifies the problem, the plan of approach and nursing care goals. The amount of written detail depends somewhat upon the composition of the personnel on a nursing station. Writing down details prevents the results of many a false assumption. Because we know something, we often assume that everyone else also knows it. A blind patient might serve as an example. A notation that a patient is blind may not necessarily assure the patient that when personnel enter his room they will speak and identify themselves as they approach his bed. This is a courtesy to any patient who cannot see. If this is something which personnel forget or do not know, it is then necessary to record the reminder. A determination of a patient's nursing needs is often referred to as a nursing diagnosis.

Sample Nursing Care Plan

Nineteen-year-old girl admitted with acute back strain after an auto accident.

Aim—Help patient to express her needs.

Problems	Approaches
1. Lies in bed staring at ceiling, does not express self, is almost completely withdrawn.	1. Provide time and privacy to allow her an opportunity to talk. Sit down at bedside. 2. Explore some of her nonverbal expressions: twitching hands, watching nurse's facial expression.
2. Does nothing to occupy her time.	1. Inquire about possible hobbies. 2. Ask craft cart to visit to see whether she responds to any of their projects.
3. Unable to void (no physical explanation).	1. Give warm baths for back pain when she needs to void.

This particular patient was a challenge to the nursing staff. A certain amount of success was achieved each day. As a result, her nursing plan was altered and brought up to date as more information was known, as certain approaches were evaluated and as she improved both physically and psychologically.

OTHER RESPONSIBILITIES OF THE R.N.

Administrative Responsibilities of the Team Leader

Minimal administrative responsibilities are required in the sense that the team leader only delegates, plans, organizes and directs the work of two or three other persons. She has the assistance of her head nurse in these responsibilities. If she receives personnel who have been adequately oriented and come properly educated for their jobs, her administrative duties are narrow in scope although very important. She is not responsible for discipline of personnel, although she must know how to direct personnel without being "bossy" or autocratic. Personnel problems, administrative problems resulting from outside her team and major learning needs of personnel should be referred to the head nurse. She is the one who is ultimately responsible for the work of her personnel. It is the head nurse who is responsible for evaluation and guidance of those assigned to the station. If a team leader is thoughtful of her team members if she gives good nursing care herself and if she gives them adequate support, she will usually be able to function satisfactorily.

Keeping the Patient's Chart

The following is part of the A.N.A. *Statement of Guiding Principles on Reporting and Recording:**

Records should:

1. Be concise and meaningful, demanding a minimum of clerical time.
2. Be systematic and well organized.
3. Be accurate, eliminating needless repetition of remarks.
4. Portray physical, emotional, sociological and interpersonal reactions.
5. Be complete.
6. Be legible, containing only approved abbreviations.

A well-kept chart is an important guide for the doctor in making a diagnosis and prescribing treatment for the patient. The chart is an aid to nursing diagnosis and helps formulate a plan of nursing care, without which effective treatment and nursing care are really impossible.

*Prepared by General Duty Nurses Section Committee on Practice, American Nurses' Association, March, 1963.

The major changes in charting are to exclude superfluous notes and to make them more meaningful in order that they become more useful.

Evaluation

The R.N. is responsible for an informal type of evaluation of herself, personnel with whom she works and patient care for which she is responsible. At the end of the day, without undue self-criticism, the team leader may decide that she needs to study and practice better ways of assigning personnel. She may have decided that one L.P.N. needs a review class in isolation technique and refer this to the head nurse. She may decide that the nursing care of a particularly challenging patient has improved greatly as a result of some of her conferences. Evaluation does not need to have a negative connotation. It includes praise. Personnel should be exposed to this aspect of evaluation so that when suggestions are made for improvement, they know that strengths as well as weaknesses are recognized.

Charge Responsibilities of the R.N.

On the relief and night shifts, there is usually no head nurse or assistant head nurse. Some hospitals, however, put the assistant head nurse on the relief shift in order to provide uniform standards of supervision on the two most active tours of duty.

In most hospitals this is not true. Therefore, the R.N. may be responsible for all patients on the floor on the evening and the night shifts. The station may function as only one team, so to speak, regardless of how many teams exist at other times of day. In this case, the R.N. must make additional independent judgments about her patients. She also has a more direct responsibility to visitors and physicians. Her resource person on these shifts is the supervisor or someone with similar duties.

SUMMARY

At the present time, the general duty R.N. in a hospital is most likely to work as a team leader although other functions and assignments exist in many places. Even the duties of team leaders vary greatly among institutions.

Although there are many goals not yet achieved, the aims of today are to teach and encourage new approaches and new depths which will actually utilize the nurse as a therapeutic agent. The nurse of today is learning to let the patient participate in his care and plan his routine whenever possible. She will call upon the family if it seems appropriate. She is seeking to practice nursing based on sound principles while setting a consistent example of procedures so that she does not confuse nonprofessionals who do not have the knowledge to adapt procedures. On the other hand, she tries to be flexible so that her care can be adapted for a particular patient. She wishes to be well organized so that she is not inefficient, but she will not sacrifice individualized care for efficient routines. She is beginning to be able to combine the satisfactions of the practice of nursing with a life outside her work. She may not be with her patient as long as her sister of yesteryear, but her goal is to spend her time so that it will be of optimum value to her patient and not of a superficial nature.

SUGGESTED READINGS

Bermosk, Loretta S., and Mordan, Mary Jane: *Interviewing in Nursing.* New York, Macmillan Co., 1965.

Donovan, Helen M.: Making Rounds with a Purpose. *Nursing Outlook,* July, 1960, p. 394.

Henderson, Cynthia: Can Nursing Care Hasten Recovery? *American Journal of Nursing,* June, 1964, p. 80.

Interpretation of the Statements of the Code For Professional Nurses. Prepared by A.N.A. Committee on Ethical Standards, American Nurses' Association, 1964.

Kron, Thora: *Nursing Team Leadership.* Philadelphia, Ed. 2, W. B. Saunders Co., 1966.

Matheney, Ruth V., et al.: *Fundamentals of Patient-Centered Nursing,* St. Louis, C. V. Mosby Co., 1964, Chapters 1, 2, 3, 4, 6, 7 and 10.

Mercadante, Lucille T.: Leadership Development Seminars. *Nursing Outlook,* September, 1965, p. 59.

Orlando, Ida Jean: *The Dynamic Nurse-Patient Relationship.* New York, G. P. Putnam's Sons, 1961.

Pellegrino, E. D.: The Changing Role of the Professional Nurse in the Hospital. *Hospitals,* December 16, 1961, p. 24.

Prange, Arthur J., and Martin, Harry W.: Aids to Understanding Patients. *American Journal of Nursing,* July, 1962, p. 98.

REFERENCES

Abdellah, Faye G., Beland, I. L., Martin, A., and Matheney, Ruth V.: Patient-Centered Approaches to Nursing, New York, Macmillan Co., 1960.

Alfano, Genrose: Administration Means Working With Nurses. *American Journal of Nursing,* June, 1964, p. 83.

Bermosk, Loretta S., and Mordan, Mary Jane: *Interviewing in Nursing.* New York, Macmillan Co., 1965.

Bernardin, Estelle: Loeb Center—as the Staff Nurse Sees It. *American Journal of Nursing,* June, 1964, p. 85.

Criteria for Evaluating a Hospital Department of Nursing Service. National League for Nursing, 1965, No. 20–1168.

Donovan, Helen M.: Making Rounds with a Purpose. *Nursing Outlook* July, 1960, p. 394.

Fuerst, Elinor V., and Wolff, LuVerne: *Fundamentals of Nursing.* Ed. 3, Philadelphia, J. B. Lippincott Co., 1964, Units One & Two.

Guide for Registered Nurses in the Assignment of Nursing Personnel. Minnesota Board of Nursing and Minnesota Nurses' Association, 1965.

Henderson, Cynthia: Can Nursing Care Hasten Recovery? *American Journal of Nursing,* June, 1964, p. 80.
Hughes, E. C., Hughes, H., and Deutscher, I.: *Twenty Thousand Nurses Tell Their Story.* Philadelphia, J. B. Lippincott Co., 1958.
Interpretation of the Statements of the Code for Professional Nurses. Prepared by A.N.A. Committee on Ethical Standards, American Nurses' Association, 1964.
Kreuter, Francis Reiter: What is Good Nursing Care? *Nursing Outlook,* May, 1957, p. 302.
Kron, Thora: *Nursing Team Leadership.* Philadelphia, Ed. 2, W. B. Saunders Co., 1966.
Lambertsen, Eleanor C.: Challenges of the Sixties. Clarifying the Education and Role of Tomorrow's Nurse. *Hospitals,* January 1, 1960, p. 39.
Lambertsen, Eleanor C.: Toward a Clearer Definition of the Nurse's Function. *Hospitals,* July 16, 1961, p. 51.
1958, p. 88.
Matheney, Ruth V.: 1953–1963 Differentiating Nursing Levels. *Three Score Years and Ten 1893–1963,* National League for Nursing, 1963.
Matheney, Ruth V., et al.: *Fundamentals of Patient-Centered Nursing,* St. Louis, C. V. Mosby Co., 1964, Chapters 1, 2, 3, 4, 6, 7 and 10.
McManus, R. L.: Nurses Want a Chance to be Professional. *Modern Hospital,* October,
Mead, Margaret: Nursing—primitive and civilized. *American Journal of Nursing,* August, 1956, p. 1001.
Mercadante, Lucille T.: Leadership Development Seminars. *Nursing Outlook,* September, 1965, p. 59.
Merton, Robert K.: Status Orientations in Nursing. *American Journal of Nursing,* October, 1962, p. 70.
Orlando, Ida Jean: *The Dynamic Nurse-Patient Relationship,* New York, G. P. Putnam's Sons, 1961.
Pellegrino, E. D.: The Changing Role of the Professional Nurse in the Hospital. *Hospitals,* December 16, 1961, p. 24.
Prange, Arthur J., and Martin, Harry W.: Aids to Understanding Patients. *American Journal of Nursing,* July, 1962, p. 98.
Report of the Committee on Perspectives National League of Nursing, *Perspectives on Nursing,* National League for Nursing, 1965.
Ritvo, Miriam M.: Who Are "Good" and "Bad" Patients? *Medical Hospital,* June, 1963, p. 79.
Standards for Organized Nursing Services. American Nurses' Association, March, 1965, No. NS-1.
Statement of Guiding Principles on Reporting and Recording. Prepared by General Duty Nurses Section Committee on Practice, American Nurses' Association, March, 1963.
Tarnower, William: Psychological Needs of the Hospitalized Patient. *Nursing Outlook,* July, 1965, p. 28.
Ujhely, Gertrud B.: *The Nurse and Her Problem Patients.* New York, Springer Publishing Company, Inc., 1963.
Uris, Auren and Shapin, Betty: *Working With People.* New York, Macmillan Co., 1953.
Walker, Virginia H., and Hawkins, James L.: Management: A Factor in Clinical Nursing. *Nursing Outlook,* February, 1965, p. 57.

8

Teaching Today's Patient

TODAY'S PATIENT

Today's patient basically is not different from yesterday's patient. He still needs his physical needs taken care of when he is unable to do so for himself. He still needs attention to his worries, and he still requires a safe pleasant environment where personnel are not indifferent to him. His knowledge and experience, however, greatly modify his expectations.

Yesterday's patient was more submissive. When he came to the hospital, he put himself in the hands of personnel with few questions and great trust. He was confined to bed for a long time, and personnel had an opportunity to get to know him. By the same token, he learned to know them. There was more time and the general pace of the hospital was slower.

Today's patient knows that hospital care and treatment is complex and expensive. He has read our popular magazines, and he may well have had a friend or relative who considered his hospital care less than perfect. His stay is usually brief and he rarely is cared for by the same person for any length of time. These things conspire to make him anxious whenever he enters a hospital.

Many of our patients are elderly. Therefore, they will have more illnesses in their lifetimes, and they will have chronic diseases which may be controlled with varying degrees of success. As a result, they have more experience with illness and with hospitals. A patient might be kept alive by a nylon blood vessel or a transistor battery or treated with the bone of an unborn calf or the organ of another person. The very newness of such procedures contributes to uneasiness and requires more knowledge and understanding of care and treatment received. As a result, the nurse has a greater responsibility in the area of patient teaching.

OBJECTIVES OF PATIENT TEACHING

Objectives of patient teaching can be thought of as extensions of immediate care. By this I mean that the nurse should remain one or more steps ahead of the patient's present state of illness. This is the responsibility of the professional nurse who must lead her staff in providing a truly comprehensive type of nursing care.

One objective of patient teaching is to prevent further complications of a present illness as well as to prevent a recurrence of the illness. Neither can be accomplished without the participation and understanding of the patient. A woman who is hospitalized for coronary heart disease will serve as an example. The success of her treatment is partially dependent upon her ability to follow instructions which are aimed at preventing further strain on the heart at the present time. Additional knowledge will be required when she goes home to help prevent a recurrence of the disease later on.

A second objective of patient teaching is to help the patient to know what his treatments and diagnostic examinations entail. When a patient returns to the x-ray department three times for an intravenous duogram, he should know that this is a necessary part of the examination and that it does not mean that some particularly startling abnormality has been found on his x-ray. Because this type of teaching is mainly information-giving, we sometimes forget to ask the patient if he has any questions about such procedures.

A third objective of patient teaching is to promote general health, whether it be within the limitations of a disease or not. The nurse will want to promote good health and hygienic habits both for the patient and his family.

The attainment of these objectives helps the patient and his family to develop a positive attitude toward his care. This is not achieved by the nurse alone. It comes about through her work with her patient, who must actively participate in the attainment of these objectives. We all too often forget the truism: Education can be considered successful only when learning has taken place.

MAJOR AREAS OF PATIENT TEACHING

In the past, the patient was not supposed to know very much about his care and treatment. What he knew came from only one source, the physician. The nurse was not supposed to divulge any information. The stock answer to a patient's question was, "Your doctor will have to tell you that." Today a prime responsibility of the nurse is to answer her patient's questions. Some information definitely remains within the province of the doctor. The nurse does not give out diagnosis or interpret medical findings, but she does help the patient to understand his

(Text continued on page 99.)

INTRODUCTION TO YOUR MEDICAL TEAM

YOUR DOCTOR is a member of the medical staff at The Charles T. Miller Hospital which gives him the privilege of admitting you and using the facilities and services of the hospital.

Assisting your doctor:

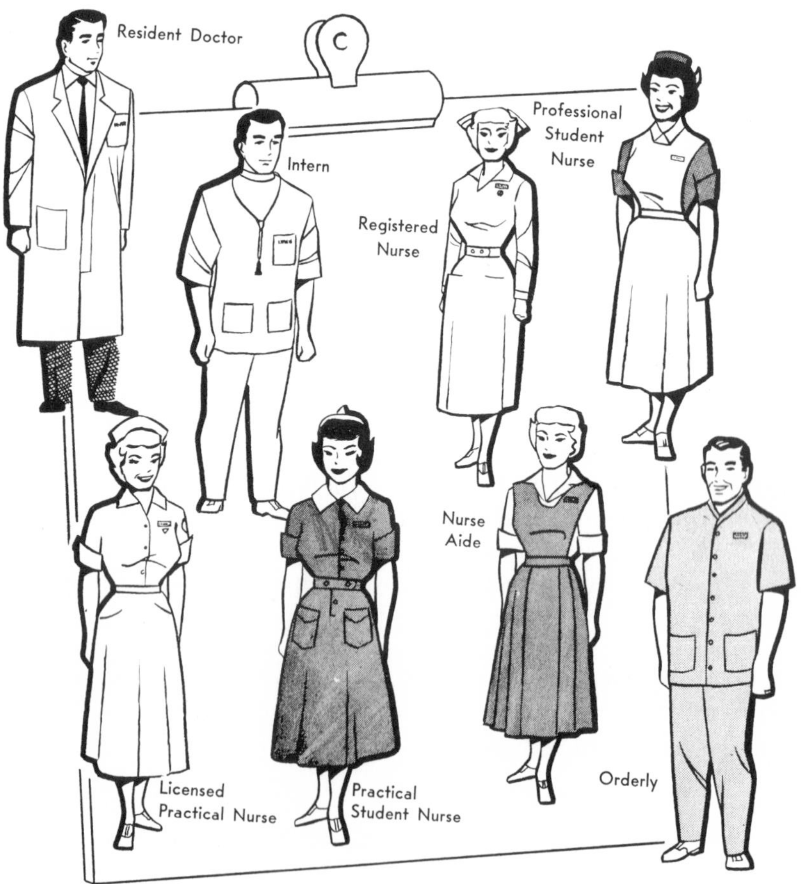

OTHER WORKERS IN WHITE who will be visiting you for tests, treatments, or other services are the medical technologists, laboratory and X-ray technicians, and members of the departments of inhalation therapy, physical medicine, and dietary.

Figure 8–1. *Sample information for a patient hospital brochure. (Courtesy Charles T. Miller Hospital.)*

PHYSICAL MEDICINE offers a program which assists patients in reaching the maximum of their physical and vocational needs through **PHYSICAL** and **OCCUPATIONAL THERAPY.**

In the **PHYSICAL THERAPY DEPARTMENT**, physical measures, such as heat, electricity, massage, exercise, and other rehabilitation methods are employed. Treatments may be continued on an out-patient basis after discharge from the hospital.

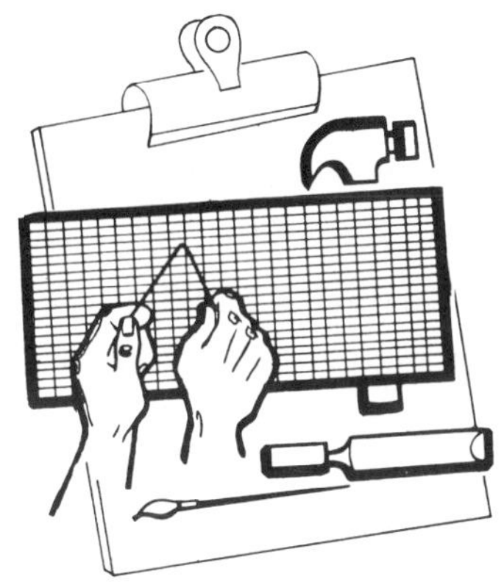

OCCUPATIONAL THERAPY offers a program of arts, crafts, recreation, and other selected activities for the patient's rehabilitation.

The **INHALATION THERAPY DEPARTMENT** works toward the improvement of conditions and abnormalties of the respiratory system by administration of oxygen and other therapeutic gases.

Figure 8–1. *(Continued)*

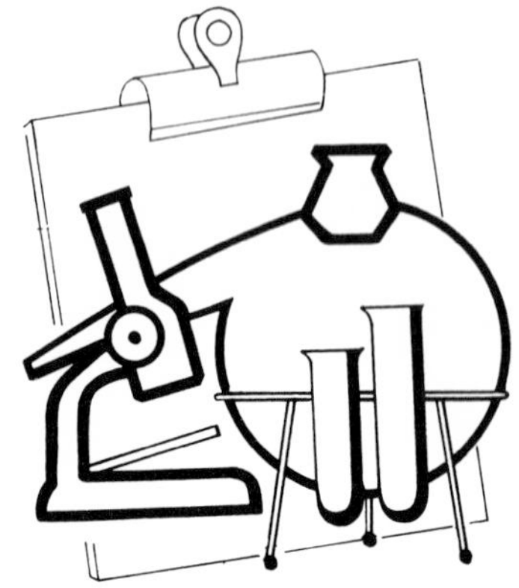

During your hospital stay your physician may use the services of the **RADIOLOGY DEPARTMENT, LABORATORY,** and **BLOOD BANK.** In these areas, physicians who have specialized in the fields of X-ray and laboratory medicine (radiologists and pathologists) direct the work of trained experts who perform the countless scientific tests and examinations so important in the diagnosis and treatment of your illness or injury. These departments are also equipped to render such specialized services as radio-active isotope studies, radiation therapy, electroencephalograms, and pulmonary function studies.

Chest X-rays and certain routine laboratory tests are a requirement for every new patient on admission. All other examinations are ordered only by your doctor. X-ray films are the property of the hospital as a part of your medical record.

The Red Cross furnishes blood to the Miller Hospital Blood Bank. In times of emergency, this is supplemented by blood drawn in the Hospital Blood Bank. To insure an adequate supply at all times, patients receiving transfusions are urged to send donors to the Red Cross or Hospital Blood Bank for prompt replacement.

If additional information is desired, ask your nurse for the pamphlets describing these units.

Figure 8–1. *(Continued)*

You have had an introduction to the people who are directly concerned with your care and treatment. BEHIND THE SCENES many other employees also contribute to your welfare.

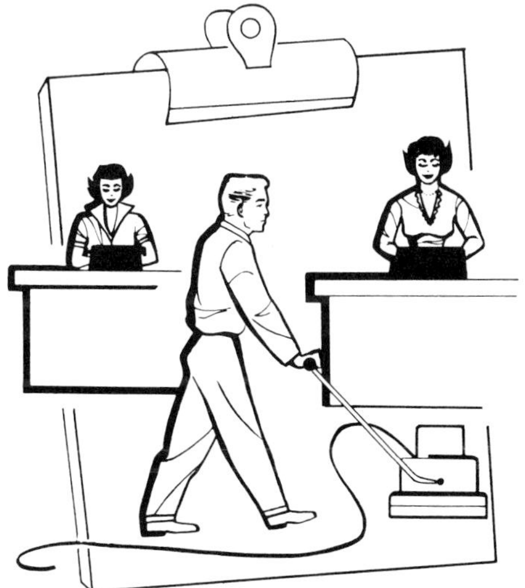

The Miller Hospital maintains a commercial-size laundry which provides the enormous daily requirements of clean linen. A large housekeeping staff has the important task of keeping our hospital clean.

Repairing the equipment and the general over-all maintenance of the hospital are the responsibilities of our Engineering and Maintenance Departments. Licensed engineers operate our boiler plant twenty-four hours a day.

The daily business functions of the hospital are carried on by workers in the Business Office, Purchasing Department, Personnel Office, Medical Records, Switchboard, and Admitting Office.

These departments, along with those previously described, are all coordinated by the Administrator and together comprise today's most complex, essential form of organization.

Figure 8–1. *(Continued)*

THE CHARLES T. MILLER HOSPITAL

ACCREDITATIONS AND MEMBERSHIPS

Approved by:

The Joint Commission on Accreditation of Hospitals

Representing:

American Hospital Association
American Medical Association
American College of Surgeons
American College of Physicians

Licensed by:

Minnesota State Board of Health
City of Saint Paul

Member of:

American Hospital Association
Upper Midwest Hospital Conference
Minnesota Hospital Association
Twin City Hospital Association
Metropolitan Saint Paul Hospital Planning Council

EDUCATIONAL PROGRAMS

Postgraduate Medical Training Program for Interns and Residents

Residency in Administration

Affiliating Professional Student Nurse Program

Miller Hospital Vocational School of Practical Nursing

Training Course for Surgical Licensed Practical Nurses

Supplemental Training in Surgery for Registered Nurses

Laboratory Course in Medical Technology

X-ray Technology Course

Figure 8-1. *(continued)*

care and treatment. In general, there are five areas of teaching responsibility which belong to nursing personnel.

Orientation to the Immediate Surroundings

When a patient is admitted to a hospital, he first needs to know several things about his immediate environment. He must know how to call a nurse. He should learn how to operate his bed if it has controls that he can operate. He will need to know how to operate his radio and television and how to adjust his reading lights. Where should he hang his clothes? Where is the bathroom?

He will feel comfortable sooner if he knows who is in his environment. If he is in a multiple-bed room, introduction to the other patients will make him more at ease. It will also help him to learn who the personnel are and if not their names, at least ways of identifying job categories.

Patients especially need to identify with one or two persons among the personnel. The person who will give him his direct care is very important to him. It is also important for him to know who is in charge of the area. If the head nurse or team leader has not seen him or if she has seen him but not identified herself, the patient may be left with a feeling that there is indifference on the part of those responsible for his care.

Information About the General Routine

It will also help the patient to know what time to expect his meals, when his doctor is likely to come, when the newspaper boy comes to the station and other details which will lessen the strangeness of his new surroundings.

Will an intern examine him? What are the visiting hours? Where is the nearest telephone? All the things which become routine to hospital personnel are new and important to both the patient and his family.

Most hospitals have prepared brochures to give much of this information to the newly admitted patient. Such brochures relieve the nurse of explaining repetitious material to each patient, but written materials need to be reviewed with each patient to assure understanding of information and awareness of services available. The initial patient and family contacts are important as they set the stage for individualized care in the future.

Review of Treatments and Special Examinations

Each patient will have specific orders which pertain only to him.

He will need to know what they are, their purpose and when and how they will be carried out.

The patient who knows some of the following facts about his care will be far better satisfied than the one who does not. A sleeping pill is ordered if I need one. It can be repeated if it does not work. I will have castor oil this afternoon in preparation for a colon x-ray tomorrow. I will be able to take my sleeping pill at about 10:30 P.M. when the effects of the castor oil are over. I will not be able to have anything but water between midnight and 6:00 A.M. Then I will not be able to have anything to eat or drink until after my x-ray, which will be done in the x-ray department at about 9:00 A.M. I can have breakfast afterwards (about 10:00 A.M.), and my doctor will probably not know the results of my x-ray until the following morning. I need not take a bath or shower until after lunch so that I will have had time to take a little rest. All these things sound very commonplace, but they make a patient far more relaxed. If he does not know these things, he is likely to lie in bed anxiously wondering what is going to happen to him next and when.

Many hospitals have developed printed pamphlets about common procedures and diagnostic tests. They usually describe the purpose of the test or procedure along with a description of the principal things which the patient will experience. One hospital has 15 such individual pamphlets. They include such subjects as the B.M.R. test, the EKG. examination, the stomach x-ray, care in an isolation room and care in the intensive care unit, as well as others which help a patient and his family to understand his care and treatments.

Written material needs to be supplemented with verbal review by the nurse. This gives the nurse a chance to evaluate further needs of her patient, and it gives her patient an opportunity to ask questions and to describe any special difficulties he might have with a particular procedure.

Information Regarding the Particular Disease

Every patient will need to have instructions which are related to his condition and to him in particular. If a patient has diabetes, he will need to know about urine testing, proper foot care, how to measure insulin, etc. Even if he has had diabetes for a long time, he may need help in one specific aspect of his care. Reading material might be a beneficial adjunct to verbal instruction. Suggested readings at the end of this chapter include only a small sampling of literature available to patients.

If a patient goes home with a dressing on a wound, he must know whether he can take a bath and change the dressing. If he is to change it, he needs to have proper dressings available and he should know how to handle the soiled ones, especially if the wound has been infected.

He also needs to know how to handle clean dressings properly in order to prevent infection.

If the patient has had a stroke, he will need to know many things. His family will need to be included in the instructions. Knowledge of his home is required to make sure that the instructions being given can be carried out. It is essential that the patient have an opportunity to practice procedures in the hospital before he is discharged.

Information After Discharge

If a hospital has a social worker or public health nurse who visits patients after discharge, the patient has an excellent opportunity to apply and adapt any learning he received at the hospital under supervision. Such a person will know what the physician ordered and what nursing instructions were given. She will also be able to keep hospital personnel informed about the effectiveness of their teaching.

If a hospital does not have such a person, personnel must be cognizant of community agencies available to help patients, and they must take the initiative to refer those who could benefit from a particular service. Planning for follow-up home care needs to be done with the guidance of the patient's physician. It is vital that the hospital pass on adequate information so that patients receive optimum benefit from referrals.

In either case, how the patient will manage at home must be considered while he is still in the hospital. If he is likely to need assistance, even if it is merely someone to cook meals, it should be planned ahead of time.

WHAT DOES THE PATIENT KNOW WHEN HE ENTERS A HOSPITAL?

When a patient enters a hospital today, he has undoubtedly read about his disease. In addition, his physician has discussed his condition with him. Some of his information may be reliable, but some may not be accurate. Misinformation is often difficult to refute. If the patient is convinced that his source of information is authentic, he will be equally convinced that his information is correct. Most popular magazines have health reports or health columns. A report in such a magazine may be accurate, but it may give a false impression. A patient may expect a treatment which is available only for research or which was successful only in a small sample of patients. As a result, he sometimes has impossible expectations from his care and treatment. Readily available medical information has still another effect. It keeps the public informed about new treatments and medications. Thus, patients can realistically have greater expectations from their medical care.

A physician tells his patient more than he used to. He usually knows what his treatments are and why he is receiving them. If a patient was upset at the time his physician talked to him, it is necessary for the nurse to be aware that her patient might have misunderstood the information. This is why it is so important for the nurse to assess her patient's knowledge and understandings at the time of admission. She can clarify questions and report any apparent needs for further medical interpretation to the doctor.

WAYS OF IMPROVING OUR TEACHING

What we teach is often less important than when and how we teach it. A patient may have been given accurate information, but it may have been presented somewhat condescendingly so that irritation or feelings of insecurity interfered with his learning. It may have been taught at a level which was not comprehensible to him because it assumed learning which he did not have. It may have been discussed at a time when he was distracted by worry or when another problem was more important to him. The patient may have seen no useful purpose for having the information when it was given. Such blocks to learning, as opposed to methods of teaching, re-emphasize the necessity of observing our patients carefully.

Planning Teaching Activities

The nurse's teaching activities will be most effective when she consciously plans it into her work. This is especially essential when teaching major matters. She needs to know what she will teach and how she will teach her material. She can then go to her patient to plan when she will show him how to irrigate his colostomy, measure his insulin, walk with crutches or whatever his particular need happens to be. The patient should be informed of her intentions in advance in order to give him time to gather his thoughts and questions.

Besides setting a time for teaching, the nurse must plan her approach. It needs to be geared to the patient's age, education, cultural beliefs, apparent intelligence, visual or hearing difficulties and his general health. Recent sedation may inhibit his ability to learn. If a patient has either intellectual or sensory limitations, it is wise to give small amounts of information at more frequent intervals. Repetitive teaching is sometimes necessary.

Remember that one of the most active things that a patient might do is to listen. We must be sure, however, that he is listening and that he does not just appear to be listening.

What aids will augment our teaching? There are many. Various reading materials are available. Sometimes printed materials are written with professional consultation such as the pamphlet, *Strokes (a guide for the family)*, published by the American Heart Association. Nontechnical books written by patients who describe their experiences with a particular disease are also helpful. An example is *Episode* written by Eric Hodgins, who describes his experience with a stroke.

Besides written material, there are diagrams, slides and actual equipment which the patient might learn to use. Some patients have Bennett respirators in their homes. Some use sterile disposable syringes, some rent hospital beds, some require wheel chairs, some use crutches, some will need ileostomy sets. The list of possibilities is endless. In many cases, reading material can be combined with technical instructions for the operation of a specific device or piece of equipment.

Planned teaching is important but it has one limitation. If a nurse decides that all her teaching should be on a planned basis, she will miss some very important openings for incidental teaching. If we do not seize certain moments, we may miss some of our most significant teaching opportunities. When the patient asks a spontaneous question, motivation for learning is certainly present. Answering such a question carefully along with providing an opportunity for further questions often leads to some of the best health education received by the patient.

Teaching by Example

The patient may not be so convinced that cleanliness is an aid to prevention of infection if he notices that our shoes are dirty and our uniforms are telltale gray. The adolescent will not believe that we are convinced of what we say when we talk about clean hair and our own is greasy.

The obese nurse talking about low calorie diets and the importance of weight reduction is far less persuasive than the nurse who has managed to control her own weight. The patient is more likely to be influenced by the nurse who seems convinced that her information is significant enough to follow herself.

Assessing the Patient's Needs

By asking the patient questions and exploring his present knowledge, you can assess what teaching is necessary. Besides asking questions about what is known, it may be helpful to learn how he feels about what he knows.

The latter is important, as it may indicate how he will participate in his care and his attitudes toward future treatment. His feelings about his condition, his care and his prognosis may reveal fears which the nurse might help to alleviate. This, in turn, may further ease other adjustments.

Too much information as well as too little can be inappropriate. Each patient will have moments of saturation which need to be considered. Some patients will only want to know pertinent information immediately affecting them. These patients are likely to dismiss additional information as being useless. Whenever a patient seems to have reached his saturation point or is disinterested because the information does not have immediate application, further discussion should be postponed until later.

If a patient receives too little information, he may feel anxious and remain curious about various aspects of his treatment or condition. People often incorrectly fill in gaps in their knowledge, thereby coming to false conclusions. We often blame the patient for such misinformation when it may be due to some omission in our teaching. This makes assessing of the patient's understanding doubly important.

Anyone who has ever taught a class—formal or informal—and followed it by a test of the salient points has experienced some degree of depression. Such a test invariably reveals that far less "clearly presented" material was absorbed than the teacher would like to think. Once the nurse learns that much of what she says is either not heard or not understood, she will no longer assume that everything she teaches is learned.

After the main points of a particular procedure have been described, the patient should be given an opportunity not only to ask questions but to review the material with the nurse to make sure it was clearly understood. The nurse can ask the patient a few key questions about a concept, a procedure or a principle behind a procedure. In this way, she can discover whether further knowledge is required by her patient.

SUMMARY

In summary, we might approach patient teaching with four questions: (1) What does the patient already know? (2) Is he anxious to learn or does he need motivation and better insight into the help such information can be to him? (3) What is the best way to teach this material? (4) Did he understand what was taught him? The patient needs an opportunity to observe and imitate the nurse, to practice and become familiar with a new skill and to study written materials. This, in conjunction with patient interviews and nursing care plans, contributes to making the care of each patient distinctly individual.

SUGGESTED READINGS FOR PATIENTS

(See also references for Chapters 10 and 14).

Brams, William A.: *Managing Your Coronary*. Philadelphia, J. B. Lippincott Co., 1960.
Do It Yourself Again. American Heart Association.
Facts About Strokes. American Heart Association, 1960.

The Heart of the Home. American Heart Association.
Help Yourself to Recovery After Mastectomy. American Cancer Society.
Home Nursing Handbook. Metropolitan Life Insurance Co., 1959.
Ray, Marie B.: *How to Conquer Your Handicaps.* New York, Bobbs-Merrill Co., 1948.
Rosenthal, H., and Rosenthal, J.: *Diabetic Care in Pictures.* Ed. 3, Philadelphia, J. B. Lippincott Co., 1960.
Strokes (a guide for the family), American Heart Association, 44 E. 23rd St., New York 10, 1958.

SUGGESTED READINGS FOR NURSES

Bowe, Agnes B.: Beyond Procedures—Incidental Teaching. *Nursing Outlook,* November, 1958, p. 628.
Brown, Esther Lucile: *Newer Dimensions of Patient Care, Part 3, Patients as People.* New York, Russell Sage Foundation, 1964.
A Cancer Source Book for Nurses. American Cancer Society, New York, 1963.
Facts About Diabetes. American Diabetes Association, 1956.
Fuerst, Elinor V., and Wolff, LuVerne: *Fundamentals of Nursing.* Philadelphia, J. B. Lippincott Co., Ed. 3, 1964, Unit 8.
Hewitt, Helon E., and Pesznecker, Betty L.: Blocks to Communicating With Patients. *American Journal of Nursing,* July, 1964, p. 101.
Russell, Robert B.: View From the Pillow. *American Journal of Nursing,* December, 1961, p. 88.
Sheldon, Nola S.: Bathing the Patient. *American Journal of Nursing,* December, 1953, p. 1451.
Wandelt, Mabel A.: Teaching is More Than Telling. *American Journal of Nursing,* May, 1957, p. 625.

REFERENCES

Bowe, Agnes B.: Beyond Procedures—Incidental Teaching. *Nursing Outlook,* November, 1958, p. 628.
Brown, Esther Lucile: *Newer Dimensions of Patient Care, Part I, The Use of the Physical and Social Environment of the General Hospital for Therapeutic Purposes.* New York, Russell Sage Foundation, 1961.
Brown, Esther Lucile: *Newer Dimensions of Patient Care. Part 3, Patients as People.* New York, Russell Sage Foundation, 1964.
A Cancer Source Book for Nurses. American Cancer Society, New York, 1963.
Facts About Diabetes. American Diabetes Association, 1956.
Fuerst, Elinor V., and Wolff, LuVerne: *Fundamentals of Nursing.* Philadelphia, J. B. Lippincott Co., Ed. 3, 1964, Unit 8.
Garrett, Annette: *Interviewing: Its Principles and Methods.* Family Service Association of America, 192 Lexington Ave, New York, 1942.
Hershey, Nathan: Informed Consent. *American Journal of Nursing,* July, 1965, p. 101.
Hewitt, Helon E., and Pesznecker, Betty L.: Blocks to Communicating With Patients. *American Journal of Nursing,* July, 1964, p. 101.
Hodgins, Eric: *Episode.* New York, Atheneum, 1964 (Fortune editor who had C.V.A.).
The Institute of Physical Medicine and Rehabilitation, New York University Medical Center, 400 E. 34th St., New York 16: Publication 1—*Primer for Paraplegics and Quadriplegics.* June, 1961.
Publication 2—*Understanding Aphasia.* July, 1958.
Publication 3—*Functional Fashions for the Physically Handicapped.* January, 1961.
Publication 4—*Essentials of Living with Pulmonary Emphysema.* January, 1963.
Reik, Theodor: *Listening With the Third Ear.* London, Garden City Books, 1948.
Report of the Committee on Perspectives National League for Nursing. *Perspectives For Nursing,* National League for Nursing, 1965.

Russell, Robert B.: View From the Pillow. *American Journal of Nursing,* December, 1961, p. 88.

Schmidt, Ruth: Life at Home. *Nursing Outlook,* June, 1958, p. 330.

Sheldon, Nola S.: Bathing the Patient. *American Journal of Nursing,* December, 1953, p. 1451.

Skinner, Geraldine, Bateman, Evelyn, and Nichols, Kathleen: To Nurse is to Teach. *American Journal of Nursing,* January, 1958, p. 92.

Tollefsrud, Valborg E.: We're For Educating Our Patients. *American Journal of Nursing,* August, 1956, p. 1009.

Wandelt, Mabel A.: Teaching is More Than Telling. *American Journal of Nursing,* May, 1957, p. 625.

9

Diagnostic Laboratory and X-ray Examinations

Depending upon the size of the institution, the departmental organization and departmental responsibilities, the nurse will perform varying tasks related to the patient who requires diagnostic examination by the laboratory and/or the x-ray department. This chapter will only review the most common examinations.

One important aspect of all such examinations is that the patient know what is going to happen to him. Will he leave his room for the examination? Will the technologist come to him for the examination? Must he actively participate in providing a specimen for the test? The nurse is responsible for explaining this kind of detail to the patient. She is usually expected to describe at least minimum details of an examination, as discussed in the last chapter.

Aside from the explanation of a diagnostic study, the nurse may have other areas of responsibility. First of all, the nurse or a member of her department may be assigned the task of ordering the particular test after the physician has requested it on the order sheet in the chart. In such a case, the nurse must know which slip is to be used for the requisition of the order, what information is required by the department which is to perform the study and what preparation of the patient is needed for the examination. If a hospital has ward managers or some type of secretarial help on its nursing stations, the nurse will not need to perform the clerical details. In any case there are other vital things of which the nurse must be cognizant.

LABORATORY EXAMINATIONS

Samples of urine, feces, sputum, spinal fluid, blood, wound drainage, bone marrow and other body fluids can be studied. Tissues are examined for cell type. Fluids are examined for drug level, electrolyte content, bacterial invasion, function of a specific organ and many other factors which are vital to diagnosis and treatment. The nurse lays the groundwork for many of these tests and participates in the collection of specimens in varying degrees.

The Order

The order originates from the physician and is requested by him on the patient's chart. It is then transcribed or set in motion. A proper slip must be prepared for a hematology, tissue, urine, bacteriology or chemistry study. These are common types of examinations performed by a laboratory. Some laboratories perform all of their examinations in one laboratory. Some hospitals have separate laboratories for each of these functions, and some merely have separate sections within one laboratory for the performance of these different studies.

A necessary part of some tests is an appointment time, and so a telephone call to the department may be required. An example might be the metabolism test. It is important for the person who is to perform this test to know how many such tests she will have for the next day in order that she might give the best possible patient service.

The Preparation

Once a test is ordered by the physician and requested of a particular department, it is then necessary to tell the patient about the examination. Some tests are as simple as a finger prick for a hemoglobin count, and some are more lengthy and complex such as the five-hour glucose tolerance examination.

Most hospitals have written procedures and/or patient brochures for examinations requiring patient preparation. Each station may have general reference material, such as a paperback edition of Garb's *Laboratory Tests in Common Use*. This and similar books briefly describe many tests, giving the nurse pertinent information. In the absence of such materials, she must ask the laboratory about details of any examination which is unfamiliar to her.

Regardless of how simple or complex a test is, some degree of written and/or verbal review must be given the patient. He must know where, when and how the examination is to be performed. The more technical aspects of a test should be explained and interpreted by the physician.

The following is an example of the kind of information which is required by nursing personnel who are responsible for collecting specimens. The patient needs to be informed of items 2 and 3. This was written to expedite the collection of a 24-hour urine specimen for urobilinogen.

1. Obtain gallon container with preservative from the urine laboratory.

2. When the patient voids, discard the specimen and record the date and time. This is the beginning of the 24-hour specimen period.

3. Place all urine voided during the next 24 hours in the container.

4. Send the container to the laboratory at the end of the 24 hours with the proper identification slip attached to it.

Specimen Collection

The collection of specimens for laboratory examination is done by many persons. The physician may obtain a tissue specimen from a biopsy, the nurse may obtain a nose and throat culture, or the laboratory technologist may collect a blood sample.

There are certain "musts" for specimen collection regardless of who collects it. The name on the request slip must be checked against the patient's name. Mrs. Smith's slip must not go with Mrs. Smythe's urine specimen. The use of identification bracelets worn by patients is one safeguard against such incidents. Regardless of whether the patient wears a bracelet or not, some check must be made before a specimen is collected and sent to the laboratory.

A second "must" is that a specimen must be collected in the proper type of container. If a specimen is collected in a container without a preservative when a preservative is necessary, this adds delay, cost and frustration to the patient's hospitalization. If a urine sample must be kept on ice, the charge nurse must make sure that everyone involved knows it must be kept on ice so that the specimen does not spoil.

A third "must" is that the patient be instructed about the collection of any specimens which he might directly influence. He needs to know if a feces, urine or sputum specimen is needed. He needs to know if he is to fast, force fluids, rest or participate in some other way.

A fourth "must" is that once collected, the specimen be carefully and properly handled. Specimens should be taken directly to the laboratory as soon as they are collected. Whether or not the hospital provides a messenger service, has a dummy service or uses some other method of delivery, specimens should go to the laboratory immediately. A urine specimen forgotten in a patient's bathroom, a nose and throat culture left to dry before it can be placed on a slide or agar plate or a spinal fluid specimen left to deteriorate are all examples of improper handling of specimens. Tubes which might roll or break should be held upright in a glass or some other kind of holder to prevent breakage, spilling or absorption by a cotton stopper resulting from tipping of a tube. Careful aseptic techniques must be used for the collection of cultures. Nothing should touch the inside of the tube except the specimen, and contamination of the outside of the tube must be prevented.

The refresher might be asked to obtain a clean voided specimen of urine. This is sometimes ordered rather than a "cathed" urine specimen in order to eliminate the possibility of introducing infection by the insertion of a catheter. In this case, the genitalia are cleansed and the patient voids into a sterile container.

Specimen collection is often the direct responsibility of the nurse. She must remain aware of the necessity of accurate identification of patient and specimen, the use of the proper collection container, the need for patient instruction and participation in many cases, as well as the necessity of prompt delivery of the specimen to the area where examination and analysis will take place.

Report of the Results

Nursing personnel are frequently the first persons to see the report of an examination, because it is usually sent directly to the nursing station. Should there be something unusual about the results of an examination, there may be occasion for the nurse to telephone the report to the physician, rather than to wait until he comes on his next routine visit. Results of examinations are reported to the patient by his physician.

There are many methods of reporting abnormal test results, and it is up to the institution to explain its system to newly employed personnel. Some hospitals expect laboratory personnel to report abnormal findings to the physician. Some expect the nurse to report such findings either upon the request of the physician regarding a specific patient whom he may be watching particularly closely, or the nurse may be expected to do this on her own initiative. Some laboratories stamp "Call M.D.—this finding is not within normal limits" on the report which is returned to the station to be placed on the chart. In this case, the nurse is notified when to call the physician and is not expected to know the normal range of countless tests.

How does the nurse know whether a test result is within normal limits if the laboratory does not tell her? Some laboratory records have the norm of each test for that particular hospital printed on them. Some places provide each nursing station with a book of norms which is kept readily available. Many drug companies print free booklets which list normal ranges for many examinations. It is important to know that lab norms vary with laboratory techniques and other factors, so they are not as interchangeable among institutions as many people suppose.

In all cases the report of the examination is placed on the patient's chart, whether it is a typewritten description of a biopsy examination by a pathologist, a white blood cell count recorded on a small slip which is glued onto a page of the chart or a report that is copied on the chart by a lab or clerical assistant.

There are countless numbers of laboratory tests. Many are performed by the average hospital laboratory and some are performed by specialty laboratories equipped to do only certain tests. In the latter case, specimens must be mailed for analysis. This may mean that findings are not known for several weeks. At the opposite extreme, ten different tests may be performed on one blood sample using an automated system which coordinates an auto-analyzer with a computer. In this case, results may be reported within one hour after the specimen has been drawn. Such extremes combined with variable techniques and norms point out the impracticality of memorizing details of anything other than common tests. Laboratory technologists must be consulted whenever available reference material is not adequate. Regardless of who collects a specimen, its source, its purpose or the method used, the nurse will participate to some degree.

X-RAY EXAMINATIONS

The modern x-ray department serves two functions: diagnosis and treatment. Deep x-ray therapy, cobalt and radioisotope therapy are performed in x-ray departments. Only diagnostic studies will be discussed here, as radiation therapy requires nursing care which can best be described in a medical-surgical textbook.

The Order

Like the laboratory test order, the x-ray order originates from the physician who requests it on the patient's chart. The order is then transmitted to the x-ray department in writing and by telephone if it is the type of examination which requires an appointment time. X-ray request forms often ask for the diagnosis and general condition of the patient so that these things can be considered at the time of the x-ray and when the x-ray is read by the radiologist and the patient's physician.

The Preparation

Also like the laboratory test, the next step is to tell the patient about the examination, give him a pamphlet describing the examination, if there is one, and allow him an opportunity to ask questions.

Many x-rays do not require any physical preparation. If a patient is to have an x-ray of an arm or a leg, he merely needs to be informed of it in most cases. If he is to have an examination of certain internal

ABOUT YOUR COLON X-RAY

The colon x-ray examination is a picture of the large intestine made visible by a special opaque solution. It is an important part of your diagnostic study. In order that it be successful, we need your assistance in following a few instructions.

TONIGHT:

Before being settled for sleep, you will be given a cathartic and an enema to cleanse the intestinal tract in preparation for the X-rays.

You will not have anything to eat or drink between midnight and the next morning.

IN THE MORNING:

You may wash and brush your teeth, and you will be given a light breakfast of tea and toast if no other X-rays are to be taken. So that you will have time to comb your hair and to put on your robe before you are taken to X-ray, you will be notified approximately ten minutes in advance.

IN THE X-RAY DEPARTMENT:

You will be taken into a room and be prepared for an enema with a special contrast medium which is visible by X-ray. The room will be darkened so that the doctor can use the fluoroscope machine to examine the large intestine as the fluid flows into it.

Following this, the bathroom in the X-ray Department will be available to you to expel the solution before returning to the X-ray room for completion of the examination.

AFTER THE X-RAY EXAMINATION:

After you have been escorted to your room, you may have your meal and drink fluids as usual, unless otherwise directed.

THANK YOU FOR YOUR ASSISTANCE. PLEASE FEEL FREE TO ASK YOUR NURSE ANY FURTHER QUESTIONS.

Figure 9–1. *Instructions given to patients at St. Barnabas Hospital who are to have a colon x-ray examination.*

organs such as the kidney, colon, gallbladder or stomach, he will require other preparation as well. An example of the kind of instructions needed for such an examination is the following guide for a barium enema (colon x-ray):

1. Telephone the x-ray department for an appointment.
2. Write the patient's diagnosis and surgical history on the request slip.
3. Give the patient a barium enema pamphlet and review it with him.
4. Use the following routine unless the patient is elderly or very young, or the physician orders otherwise:
   Castor oil 2 oz. at 2 P.M. the day before the x-ray examination.
   Enema at 8 P.M. the evening before the x-ray examination.
5. Patient may have nothing by mouth except for sips of water after midnight.
6. Breakfast of tea and toast at 7:00 A.M.—nothing by mouth after this until the x-ray examination is completed.
7. After the x-rays are taken, the patient may eat as usual.
8. Give 2 oz. milk of magnesia at 8 P.M. the evening of the x-ray examination.
9. Offer patient soothing rectal ointment for any discomfort after the x-ray examination.

Transportation to the X-ray Department

Depending upon the number of x-rays performed each day, nursing personnel may or may not be asked to bring patients to and from the x-ray department. If a great number of x-rays are performed, either the x-ray department provides transportation service to the department or a transportation pool for all departments of the hospital may be available for this task. Such a pool is often referred to as an escort service.

Some patients do not require assistance to get to and from the x-ray department. A few can walk to the department by themselves if their condition warrants it and if they are given clear instructions on how to find the department. It is important that personnel who are responsible for transportation service do not abuse this. Many patients are expected to go to and from x-ray for a colon x-ray examination, for instance. If the patient feels weak or is elderly, he should go by wheel chair. After all, it is exhausting to have enemas and castor oil. Some patients may be able to go to x-ray by themselves, but are too weak to return by themselves after the examination. The type of examination and the age and condition of the patient should determine whether the patient requires a wheel chair, a litter or merely directions for getting to the department.

When a patient goes to another department a few precautions will prevent loss or soiling of his personal belongings. Patients should wear a hospital gown whenever the examination involves barium or any dye which will affect his bowels. He should be provided with slippers if he has none, he should wear a bathrobe, and he will need to have his lap covered with a blanket to prevent exposure and to keep him warm and comfortable. If a patient is to have an examination which requires sedation, dentures and eye glasses should be left at the bedside where they can be placed in appropriate containers to prevent breakage or loss.

Report of Results

X-ray results are usually reported to the physician the next day unless there is some urgency in the findings. X-ray reports are also typewritten and eventually placed on the patient's chart.

Interpretation of the findings are made by the physician and reported to the patient by him. The nurse will read the report in order to keep herself apprised of the patient's medical condition. The physician will be able to clarify her questions. In any case she may gear some of her nursing care to the report if it is indicated.

Common X-ray Examinations

Without attempting to review all types of x-ray examinations or any one x-ray in detail, the following have been selected for review and up-dating purposes, based on questions asked by many refreshers.

STOMACH OR UPPER G.I. The patient drinks barium. The stomach and small intestine are then viewed under fluoroscopy and films are also taken. The patient returns at intervals for follow-up studies of the small bowel.

COLON X-RAY OR BARIUM ENEMA. Barium is instilled into the colon which is viewed under fluoroscopy. Films are also taken.

GALLBLADDER X-RAY. The patient may be given tablets containing an opaque dye the evening before the x-ray or he may be given an intravenous opaque dye to make the gallbladder visible. If the material is to be given in the x-ray department by vein, it is called an I.V. cholangiogram. If the patient takes the tablets, it is called a cholecystogram.

I.V.P. (INTRAVENOUS PYELOGRAM) OR UROGRAM. In the x-ray department, intravenous dye is injected to make the kidneys, ureters and bladder visible on x-ray.

DUOGRAM. A duogram is a combined I.V.P. and I.V. cholangiogram.

BRONCHOGRAM. Iodized contrast material is injected in the

bronchial tubes to make the bronchial tree visible in order to see foreign bodies, tumors or bronchial dilation.

PNEUMOENCEPHALOGRAM. A small amount of spinal fluid is removed. This is followed by air injection which permits x-ray viewing of the ventricular and subarachnoid spaces.

VENTRICULOGRAM. Ventricular fluid is withdrawn through holes made by a trephine in the skull and replaced by air for visualization of the ventricles. This x-ray procedure is performed in the operating room.

MYELOGRAM AND SPINOGRAMS. By injection of a contrast medium, the subarachnoid spaces of the spinal canal can be visualized for the diagnosis of various types of spinal cord tumors, cysts and intervertebral disks.

VASCULAR RADIOGRAPHY. An opaque medium is introduced into the vascular system in order to view the arteries and veins. This has been made possible by cineradiography which literally takes movies of circulating blood. When it is done in order to visualize the blood vessels in the head, the dye is injected into the carotid artery and is called cerebral angiography. It is called angiocardiography when it is performed to view the cardiac chambers and larger thoracic blood vessels for diagnosis of congenital and acquired heart defects. When the dye is injected for diagnosis of blood vessels of the extremities, it is called femoral angiography.

Written permits are required for many of these x-ray examinations. Hospital policy will dictate which ones require this.

The nurse must know the site of injection for the angiogram, and she must be aware that possible bleeding might occur after the examination. She, therefore, must check the site at intervals, apply pressure if there is any sign of bleeding, and call the physician if there is more than a small amount of bleeding or temporary oozing.

MAMMOGRAMS. This is an x-ray of the mammary glands which aids in the diagnosis of breast tumors and diseases. This relatively new type of x-ray has been made possible by the development of an especially sensitive type of film which makes it possible to visualize soft tissue.

OTHERS. Chest x-rays and x-rays of various bones of the body are done much like they were in the past except that they are done more frequently, and newer techniques make all x-ray examinations a more accurate aid to diagnosis.

Nuclear Medicine

Nuclear energy can be used to treat and diagnose disease. When a radioactive drug is administered for diagnostic purposes, the concentration of this material is determined for the particular organ being studied. This is accomplished by the use of radiation detection machines which ascertain the radioactivity of the thyroid, brain and other organs.

Ultrasonography

The use of high-frequency sound equipment has been developed as another aid in diagnosis. In ultrasonography, a high-frequency inaudible sound pulse is sent to a tissue. An echo is then received. The strength of the echo from abnormal tissue differs from that received by normal tissue. This has been used to detect brain lesions, renal calculi and breast tumors, and is presently being studied for the diagnosis of disease in other organs.

SUMMARY

The role of the laboratory and x-ray departments will continue to grow in the area of accurate diagnostic procedures. Expanded knowledge from medical research, automation and technological inventions

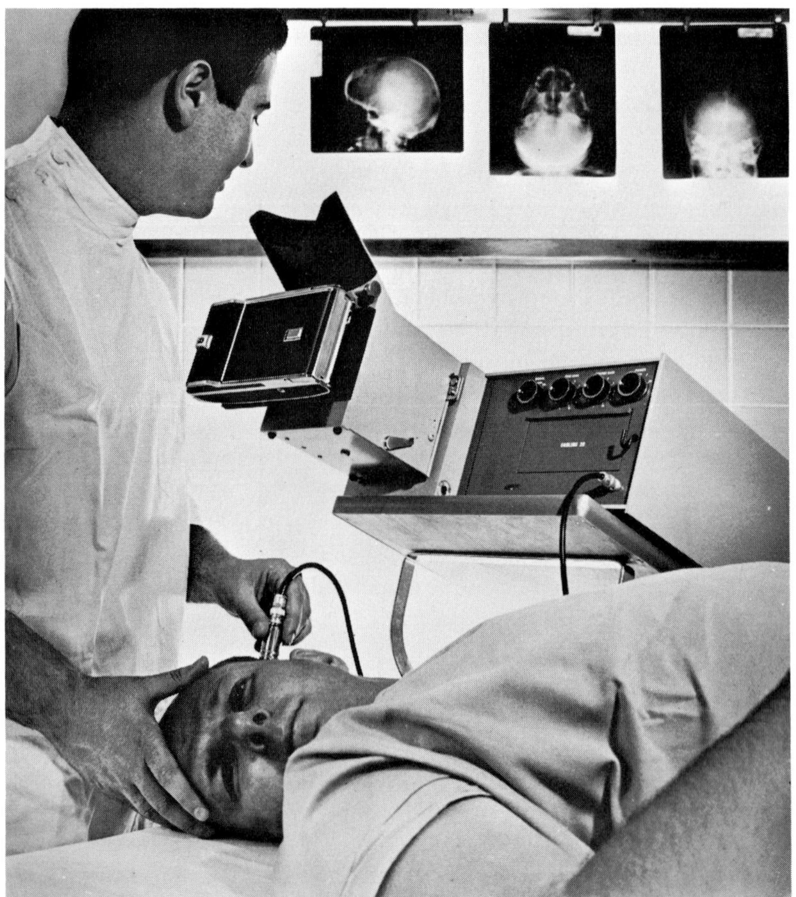

Figure 9–2. *Ultrasonoscope is used to detect intracranial lesions. (Smith, Kline & French.)*

will continue to increase effectiveness and accuracy. The nurse may want to spend a half day in the x-ray department to observe x-ray procedures so that she may better prepare her patients. Once a nurse is employed, she will be kept informed of newer methods used at her employing institution.

SUGGESTED READINGS

It is recommended that you study x-ray and laboratory tests in relation to your patients so that you can relate them as they are related in the textbook of your choice and as they are related in Sutton's *Bedside Nursing Techniques.*

REFERENCES

Blaivas, Murray A.: Computerized System Speeds Blood Test, Cuts Costs. *Modern Hospital,* April, 1965, p. 117.

French, Ruth M.: *Nurses' Guide to Diagnostic Procedures.* New York, Blakiston Division, McGraw-Hill Book Co., 1962.

Garb, Solomon: *Laboratory Tests in Common Use.* Ed. 3, New York, Springer Publishing Co., 1959.

Garnett, Theodosia V., and Barbata, Jean C.: *Collection of Laboratory Specimens and Diagnostic Procedures.* Paterson, New Jersey, Littlefield, Adams & Co., 1964.

Radioactive Medicine. A pamphlet for the patient, Squibb, November, 1964.

Robbins, L. L.: Future Trends in Radiology. *Hospitals,* March 1, 1964, p. 68,

Sutton, Audrey L.: *Bedside Nursing Techniques.* Philadelphia, W. B. Saunders Co., 1964.

Vennes, Carol Hocking, and Watson, John C.: *Patient Care and Special Procedures in X-ray Technology.* St. Louis, C. V. Mosby Co., 1959.

10

Major Changes in Dietary Service

Four major areas of dietary service will be of particular interest to the refresher. First, the responsibility of the nurse in this area has changed greatly. If a hospital employs a dietitian, her work in this area may have diminished. If it does not, her work may have increased. Second, technology has greatly contributed to change in the preparation and service of food. Third, nutritional divisions have made the "basic 7" passé and, fourth, certain special diets have been developed and modified as a result of expanded knowledge in biochemistry. Without attempting to review nutrition or expecting the refresher to do so in her spare time, it is hoped that the description of the highlights of these four areas will be of assistance. The suggested readings will help those who require or desire more knowledge of this field.

NURSING RESPONSIBILITIES FOR FOOD SERVICE

It is not possible for a refresher to review nutrition in detail. If you are employed in a hospital in which considerable dietary responsibility is connected with your job, a review of special diets is especially recommended. Nurses are gradually taking less responsibilty for non-nursing services in order to gain more time for patients. Present-day student experience in the dietary department has greatly changed in most schools of nursing. The student no longer spends weeks preparing special diets and writing out menus. She has observation periods in the dietary department in order to gain insight into the complexity of food preparation. She then has instruction from a dietitian, who correlates her teaching with individual patients and the general curriculum. As a result, diet therapy is better understood as part of total therapy of the patient.

Some institutions have various kinds of decentralized dietary service. This may mean that one person is assigned to each station to provide dietary service to that area. Such a person may not be a dietitian; she may be a food aide, someone similar to the nurse aide in terms of her function as related to the dietitian. This person visits patients, discusses their meals, their likes, their dislikes, etc., and sees that the patient receives his preferences within the confines of the diet which is prescribed by the physician. She may also distribute and collect patient trays, record food intake, and in some cases, she is even responsible for feeding patients. Feeding patients, however, is still the job of the nurse in most instances. Decentralized dietary service may also be found in a hospital without a traditional kitchen. In this case, the kitchen, as well as the service, is decentralized.

The nurse may be employed in such situations, or she may be employed in situations in which she is still responsible for serving food and even for interpreting special diets. Most likely she will find herself in a situation in which some food service responsibility has been removed but not all of it. A rather common practice is to have someone from the dietary department come to the station to distribute trays and to collect trays. The nurse is then responsible for positioning the patient, observing and recording his food intake and feeding patients.

If a hospital is large enough to employ a dietitian, the nurse is rarely responsible for giving the patient all his dietary instructions. Nonetheless, the nurse should be aware of the basic principles of a special diet and be able to interpret it somewhat generally. Because nurses have frequent contacts with patients, they will have an awareness of some of the learning needs of patients which must be conveyed to the dietitian. In this way, the dietitian and the nurse do not overlap in their duties; they complement one another.

TODAY'S FOOD SERVICE

Selective Menus

The selective menu has become very common. Although the range of food possibilities does not resemble that of a restaurant, it gives the patient an opportunity to omit foods which he dislikes. A selective menu can be used for special diets as well as general diets.

When a selective menu is used, it is usually divided into three parts (see Figure 10–1): one for breakfast, one for lunch and one for dinner. The patient circles his selections on the menu, which is distributed a day in advance.

In conjunction with the selective menu, a food aide or food technician (comparable with our practical nurse) usually visits patients to collect the menus. This gives dietary personnel an opportunity to eval-

SOFT DIET Sat. 10-23-65	SOFT DIET Sat. 10-23-65	SOFT DIET Sat. 10-23-65
Breakfast (circle what you desire)	**Lunch** (circle what you desire)	**Dinner** (circle what you desire)
Orange juice or Apple juice	Grape juice or Pineapple juice	Strained soup, crackers or Grapefruit juice or Orange juice
Cheerios, cream or Cream of wheat, cream	Baked salmon & cream-ettes or Cottage cheese & fruit plate	Baked haddock fillet, lemon or Soft salisbury steak
Soft cooked egg or Grilled bacon	Vanilla ice cream or Orange junket	Mashed potatoes Buttered green beans
Jelly Toast—white or dark Toast slices, one or two	Bread—½ slice or 1 slice Butter Jelly	Royal Anne cherries or Banana & cream
Coffee (black or with cream) Tea Milk	Coffee (black or with cream) Tea Milk	Bread—½ slice or 1 slice Butter Jelly
		Coffee (black or with cream) Tea Milk

Figure 10–1. *Sample Selective Menu.*

uate their services. It also gives dietary personnel a chance to discuss dietary problems with patients who need special help. The more technical assistance is given by a dietitian.

Hot Food Hot and Cold Food Cold

Modern equipment has been developed to eliminate the age-old problem of hot food cooling off and cold food warming up during its transfer from the kitchen to the patient. There are several types of equipment which can prevent this.

One method of keeping food hot is a specially designed plate holder. A hot lead pellet is placed under the regular plate of hot food. This will stay hot for about 45 minutes, ample time to transport the food. Another piece of equipment is a food cart which has a refrigerated area and a heated area. Such a cart is usually prepared in the dietary department where hot foods are placed in the heated section and cold foods are placed in the refrigerated section. The electric cord is disconnected when the cart leaves the kitchen and is immediately connected again when it arrives in the patient area. Thus, foods remain at the proper temperature until the tray is actually removed from the cart and taken to the patient's room.

Food Preparation

Food preparation has become more of a science and less of an art just as it has in our homes. Frozen foods, dehydrated foods and prepared foods also contribute to the ease of hospital cooking. There are fewer artisans of pastry and specialty dishes in the hospital kitchen than there used to be. Sometimes even the hospital administrator is unaware of these changes, as exemplified by the following incident. After the Board of Governors had finished an excellent dinner ending with a superb cheese cake, the administrator told the dietitian that the pastry cook had done an especially fine job on the dessert. The dietitian replied that the pastry cook was ill and that the dessert had been a defrosted product which any of us could purchase from our corner grocer. This episode would certainly shatter the image of a fine pastry cook and warm the heart of any frozen-food manufacturer. In any case good cooks are getting harder to find, and good prepared foods are becoming easier to find.

New Equipment

Electronic ovens are available for cooking. Special high pressure, frozen-food cookers are manufactured. Such devices will prepare a five-pound frozen-food package in a matter of minutes. Large open broilers are made. Some even simulate outdoor charcoal broilers. Ovens are better insulated, as is dish washing equipment. Such machines combined with general air conditioning may not make a kitchen a cool place during summer months, but it is far more comfortable than it used to be.

Other equipment enables a kitchen staff to serve hundreds of meals in the same amount of space that used to accommodate the preparation of only 75 meals. Conveyor belts for dirty dishes save countless steps. When dirty dishes arrive in the kitchen they are moved to the washing area via a conveyor belt. From the cafeteria dirty dishes also arrive on the belt. Dishes are often plastic. Some dishes are even disposable.

Some food cabinets have doors in the back and in the front. Foods

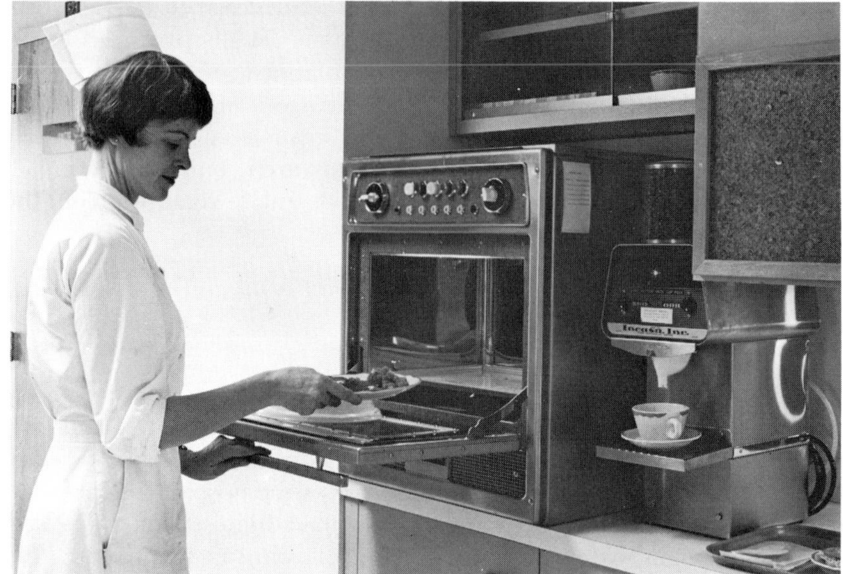

Figure 10–2. *In a tradition-breaking food service system, patients' trays are delivered to nurses' stations in refrigerated carts. Trays are assembled in a "noncooking kitchen" from prepared foods. (From McCune, Elizabeth: Food Service and Dietetics.* Hospitals, *April 1, 1965, p. 62.*

are placed inside from the back door, which opens onto the kitchen where foods are prepared. The front door opens onto the cafeteria where the food is removed for service to the diners. Some are made to hold hot foods, some to hold cold items.

Prepared packets of seasoning may replace the sugar dispenser, the salt and pepper shakers and similar items. Trays are often provided with prepackaged condiments similar to that used on airplanes and in restaurants.

Technological developments will continue to provide better food service through better use of space, provision of new tools and equipment and more efficient methods. Computers can be used to write menus, to compute meal nutrients, to order foods and to regulate costs. Future food service may be so influenced by our space age that the modern up-to-date kitchen of today's hospital may be obsolete in the next decade.

Vending Machines

Although a hospital usually has to provide some kind of individualized food service for patients, it now has the option of installing food vending machines for its employees and visitors. This is becoming a big business, and the varieties of foods are rather surprising. Hot soups, sandwiches, ice cream and soft drinks are the commonest items available. Some institutions install these machines mainly for the purpose of providing round-the-clock food service. They provide food service for personnel and for patients and families at odd hours. Without them many hospitals are unable to provide food at a moment's notice for 24 hours, seven days a week. The vending machine can be a real service to the family who must keep a night vigil. Instead of machines, some institutions utilize a local catering service for certain types of meals.

Snack Carts

Another important innovation to food service is the snack cart, sometimes called a nourishment cart. Most hospitals provide meals at hours which do not correspond to what we are used to in our daily lives. Breakfast is served at about the right hour for the average working man (although a little early); lunch is early or late according to the individual's habits; and dinner is always an hour or two before the average person eats at home. Aside from meals, every American has become accustomed to the "coffee break" in both the morning and the afternoon. Some of us are also used to a night snack. While this is less common, it is particularly needed when supper is so early. In addition, food consultants recommend that we should not go without food for more than 14 hours.

Taking these things into consideration, some institutions send a cart to each patient at about 10:00 A.M., 2:00 P.M. and 8:00 P.M. This cart carries coffee, tea, juices and milk. For the patient who needs extra calories, malted milks, sandwiches and ice cream may also be available. Where this service is not provided, the nurse is often found in the kitchen making coffee or tea for patients who request it.

Experiment With Meal Hours

One hospital has tried what, at first glance, seems like a somewhat revolutionary idea. The changed eating habits of Americans are considered in the plan. De Paul Hospital, in St. Louis, provides only two main meals a day. A kind of continental breakfast (a roll and coffee) is served about 7:30 A.M. A brunch is then served at about 10:30 A.M. This eliminates most of the HOLD trays in the morning. At about 2:00 P.M., a snack is made available. Dinner is then served at about 5:30 P.M., and an evening snack is offered before bedtime. This particular regimen more closely resembles the eating habits of many persons. It also takes into consideration that patients are inactive, have smaller appetites and in most instances would prefer not to gain weight during hospitalization.

In order to make such a drastic change from a traditional three-meal a day schedule, patients, physicians and personnel were thoroughly oriented about the reasons for this schedule, and it has been considered a success.

FOOD GROUPS

The hard-to-remember "basic 7" food groups have been reduced to four in number. For those who would like to recall the basic 7, they were leafy green and yellow vegetables, fruits, potatoes, milk and cheese, meat and eggs, cereal and butter. Careful counting by the novice reveals that there are nine items in the basic 7. Let bygones be bygones. The new easy-to-remember food groups are: (1) dairy foods, (2) meat, (3) vegetables and fruits and (4) breads and cereals.

Dairy foods include cheese, ice cream, butter and other milk products. The meat group includes meats, fish, poultry, eggs and a few vegetables, such as dried beans. All vegetables and fruits are included in the third group, and all breads and cereals are included in the fourth group. Figure 10–3 shows a guide to an adequate daily nutritional intake according to current knowledge.

GENERAL CATEGORIES OF HOSPITAL DIETS

Clear Liquid Diet

The purpose of a clear liquid diet is primarily to replace water, salts and carbohydrates. It is used for postoperative patients who require non-gas-forming fluids for a short period of time. Clear broths, plain flavored gelatins, clear tea, coffee and carbonated beverages are used.

Full Liquid Diet

The full liquid diet may be ordered to give the patient a little more nourishment before he is given solid foods. Strained cream soups, thin refined cooked cereals, strained fruit juices, plain ice cream, sherbet, junket, custard and milk may be added to the items on the clear liquid diet.

Soft Diet

The soft diet is low in cellulose and connective tissue. It is used where mechanical ease of chewing and/or digestion is desired. If a patient has had oral surgery, it is vital that all foods be soft in consistency so that no tissue damage occurs. Toast would not be included. If the diet is ordered for digestive reasons, toast would be included. Puréed foods are not commonly used because they are so rarely eaten. Meats are sometimes omitted as well as high fiber vegetables and fruits with skins and seeds. No fried foods and little or no spices are used.

Light Diet

This diet is very similar to a regular diet and is sometimes used just before a patient is placed on a general diet. The major difference between the light and the general diet is that fried foods, course foods and rich desserts are omitted. The diet is complete nutritionally.

General Diet

There are no restrictions on the general diet, also known as the full, house or regular diet. In order to prevent digestive disturbances, fried foods and rich desserts are given sparingly.

Patients advance in their diets more rapidly than they used to. Light and soft diets are considered transitional diets between liquid and general diets. Some institutions may provide a soft or a light diet, but not both. In any case the patient progresses from a liquid diet to a general diet with great speed compared with that of the past.

THERAPEUTIC DIETS

Every day new knowledge in the field of biochemistry becomes available through research. As a result, nutritional therapy becomes more important to more persons. This section will review the highlights of only four modified special diets. They were selected because they are becoming more common or because changes have occured in recent years.

Weight-Reducing Diets

There are few of us who do not have at least one theory on how to lose weight. Our conclusions are influenced by wishful thinking, scientific information, current food fads and a great deal of in-between meal snacking.

Popular magazines are chock full of recipes and gourmet food ideas. These are usually found alongside articles on how to diet. The two ob-

(Text continued on page 128.)

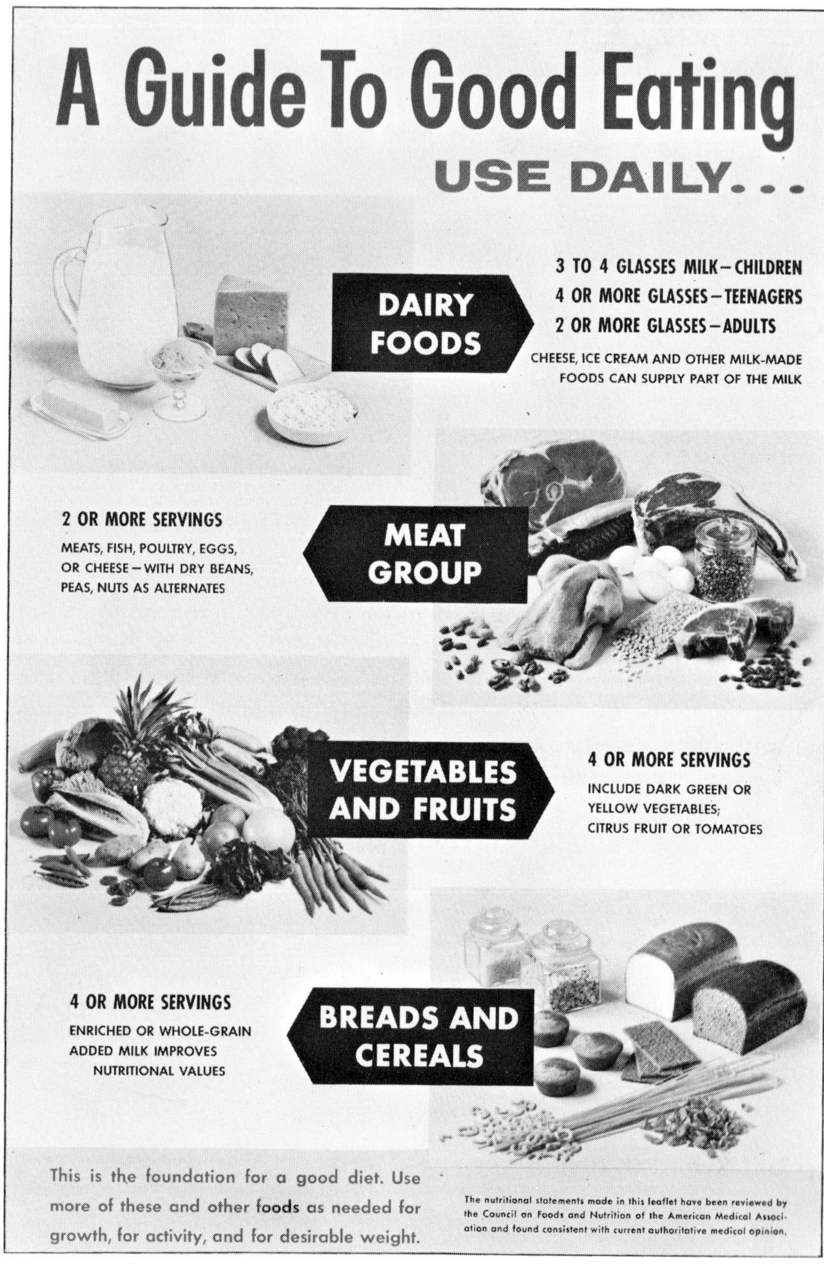

Figure 10–3. *A guide to good eating. (Courtesy National Dairy Council, Chicago, Illinois 60606.)*

A Guide to Good Eating helps you plan or choose pleasing and satisfying meals that provide good nutrition. It suggests minimum amounts of food from each of 4 food groups which should be included in each day's meals. This menu plan shows one way to include the 4 important food groups in a day's meals:

Breakfast

Fruit
Cereal or Egg or Both
Toast or Roll and Butter
Milk Coffee

Dinner

Main Protein Dish
Vegetable Potato
Bread or Roll and Butter
Milk Dessert

Lunch or Supper

Main Protein Dish Vegetable Bread and Butter
Milk Fruit

Vary your menus to suit your taste. In using the dairy foods for their important calcium . . .

1 glass milk = 8 ounces or ¼ quart
1 slice American cheese (1 oz.) = ⅔ glass milk
½ cup creamed cottage cheese = ⅓ glass milk
½ cup (¼ pint) ice cream = ¼ glass milk

In the meat group, 2 servings should give at least as much protein as 4 ounces cooked lean meat (⅓ pound raw). About equal amounts of protein come from . . .

1 ounce cooked lean meat, poultry, or fish
1 egg
1 slice cheese, American or Swiss (1 ounce)
2 tablespoons creamed cottage cheese (1 ounce)
2 tablespoons peanut butter (1 ounce)
½ cup cooked dried beans or peas

An average serving of vegetables or fruits is ½ cup; of bread, 1 slice; of cereal, ½ to ¾ cup.

The nutritional statements made on this leaflet have been reviewed by the Council on Foods and Nutrition of the American Medical Association and found consistent with current authoritative medical opinion.

Figure 10-3. *(continued)*

viously belong together, but few view it in this manner. People look at losing weight as a temporary project. "If I could just get rid of ten pounds, then I'd be all right." Crash diets are often followed by crash eating. Types of diets are endless in number. You can choose to starve for 48 hours, eat all you want of certain items or live on food substitutes for a certain period.

Statistics tell us that overweight is a predisposing factor to many diseases. As a result, physicians may prescribe diets, but the majority of diets are self-initiated. Most authorities will agree that reducing the size of our portions is superior to drastic rules which completely omit certain foods. A rapid temporary loss of weight is temporarily rewarding but rarely lasting. It is generally agreed that only altered eating habits will maintain a weight loss.

A great deal more is known about calories, fat metabolism and carbohydrate and protein utilization. Experimental diets attempt to see whether body chemistry can safely and successfully be altered for the purpose of weight reduction. This knowledge may alter the balance of what we eat, but it is probable that it will not allow us to eat and be anyting but fat. In any case, if dieting consists of anything other than reducing the quantity of food to a little below maintenance requirements, a physician should be consulted.

Low Sodium Diets

In the past, salt free (sodium chloride free) or low salt diets were common. It is more usual today to find low sodium diets, as it is the sodium which causes retention of fluids. Low sodium diets may be mild, moderate or severe in the amount of sodium restriction. There are many salt substitutes available on the market, but they should never be used unless the physician so orders. Some of these products have potassium, which may be contraindicated if a patient has kidney disease. Some have ammonium, which is contraindicated if liver disease is present. Therefore, reducing sodium intake by a salt substitute should be carefully checked before use. Generally speaking, protein foods are particularly high in sodium.

Mild Sodium Restricted Diet. The use of table salt and cooking salt is restricted. Salt preserved foods, such as bacon, dried beef, salted fish and ham should be avoided, as well as things like salted nuts, potato chips and crackers.

Moderate Sodium Restricted Diet. In addition to the above, prepared cereals, ordinary bread, anything cooked with soda or baking powder are avoided. Frozen peas, fish and canned vegetables and meat and soups are eliminated unless specially prepared without salt. Salt free butter and margarine are used.

Severe Sodium Restricted Diet. This diet is very limited and requires the advice and guidance of a dietitian. Special instructions are required by any patient who is asked to follow this regimen, as their foods are particularly circumscribed. *Food for Your Heart,* published by the American Heart Association may be helpful to patients on a low sodium diet.

Low Cholesterol Diets

The amount of research into the relationship of fat in the diet, blood cholesterol and atherosclerosis is immense. In atherosclerosis, fatty substances are found on the inside lining of arteries. This can lead to strokes or certain kinds of heart attacks. These fatty substances interfere with the flow of blood to whatever organs the particular artery serves. One theory is that a high level of fatty substance (measured by the cholesterol in the blood) may result in fatty deposits in the arteries and that this can be reduced by a diet low in saturated fats. Dr. Ancel Keys of the University of Minnesota has performed major research in this field, and he is a proponent of this theory. Other researchers have other ideas. In spite of this, present evidence weighs in favor of this possibility, especially in certain individuals. This is why patients may be asked to lower their fat intake and to substitute a substantial amount of vegetable oil for solid animal fat.

Foods high in saturated fat are animal fats, such as whole milk, cream, cheese, butter and meat. These foods are reduced in the low cholesterol diet. Foods high in polyunsaturated fat are fish and vegetable oils, such as corn oil. These foods can be substituted for some of the animal fat foods. Reduction of saturated fat and addition of polyunsaturated fat usually reduces the serum cholesterol.

Low cholesterol diets should never be used except under the direction of a physician. Most current nutrition books will be of help in the details of such a diet.

Diabetic Exchange System

Diabetic diets have been greatly simplified by the development of food exchanges. They permit measuring of foods rather than weighing foods. They also permit the exchange of foods according to desire without long involved calculations.

There are seven lists of exchanges (see Figure 10–4). List 1 contains foods that do not need to be measured. List 2 contains vegetables; List 3, fruits; List 4, breads; List 5, meats; List 6, fats; and List 7, milks. Each numbered list contains portions of foods of comparable calories and nutrients. For example, 1 cup of strawberries yields 10 grams of

(Text continued on page 132.)

LIST 1 FOODS THAT NEED NOT BE MEASURED (Insignificant carbohydrate or calories)

Coffee	Gelatin (unsweetened)	Saccharin and other noncaloric sweeteners
Tea	Rennet Tablets	Pepper and other Spices
Clear Broth	Cranberries (unsweetened)	Vinegar
Bouillon (fat free)	Mustard (dry)	Seasonings
Lemon	Pickle (unsweetened)	

LIST 2 VEGETABLE EXCHANGES

Group A—Raw vegetables may be eaten in any quantity desired. If cooked a single cupful is permitted. If desired an additional cup may be taken in exchange for a group B vegetable.

Asparagus	Cucumber	Dandelion	Mushrooms	Rhubarb (without sugar)
*Broccoli	Eggplant	Kale	Okra	Sauerkraut
*Brussels Sprouts	*Escarole	Mustard	*Parsley	String Beans, young
Cabbage	*Greens	Poke	*Peppers, green or red	Squash, Summer
Cauliflower	Beet Greens	Spinach	Radishes	*Tomatoes
Celery	Chard	Turnip, Greens	Romaine	*Water Cress
*Chicory	Collards	Lettuce		

Group B—One serving equals ½ cup, or 100 Gm. Carbohydrate, 7 Gm.; Protein, 2 Gm.; Calories, 36

Beets	Onions	Pumpkin	*Squash, Winter
*Carrots	Peas, green	Rutabagas	Turnips

*These vegetables have a high vitamin A content; at least one serving a day should be used.

LIST 3 FRUIT EXCHANGES Carbohydrate, 10 Gm.; Calories, 40

Use only unsweetened fruits—fresh, cooked, canned or frozen.

Fruit	Amount	Fruit	Amount
Apple, 1 small (2″ diam.)	80 Gm.	Grape juice, ¼ cup	60 Gm.
Applesauce, ½ cup	100 Gm.	Honeydew melon, ⅛ (7″ diam.)	150 Gm.
Apricots, fresh, 2 med.	100 Gm.	Mango, ½ small	70 Gm.
Apricots, dried, 4 halves	20 Gm.	*Orange, 1 small	100 Gm.
Banana, ½ small	50 Gm.	*Orange juice, ½ cup	100 Gm.
Berries (blackberries, raspberries, *strawberries), 1 cup	150 Gm.	Papaya, ⅓ med.	100 Gm.
Blueberries, ⅔ cup	100 Gm.	Peach, 1 med.	100 Gm.
*Cantaloupe, ¼ (6″ diam.)	200 Gm.	Pear, 1 small	100 Gm.
Cherries, 10 large	75 Gm.	Pineapple, ½ cup	80 Gm.
Dates, 2	15 Gm.	Pineapple juice, ⅓ cup	80 Gm.
Figs, fresh, 1 large	40 Gm.	Plums, 2 med.	100 Gm.
Figs, dried, 1 large	20 Gm.	Prunes, dried, 2	25 Gm.
*Grapefruit, ½ small	125 Gm.	Raisins, 2 tbsp.	15 Gm.
*Grapefruit juice, ½ cup	100 Gm.	*Tangerine, 1 large	100 Gm.
Grapes, 12	75 Gm.	Watermelon, 1 cup	175 Gm.

*These fruits are rich sources of vitamin C; one serving a day should be used.

Figure 10–4. *The seven lists of foods for the diabetic exchange system. (From The American Dietetic Association, Chicago, Illinois.)*

LIST 4

BREAD EXCHANGES Carbohydrate, 15 Gm.; Protein, 2 Gm.; Calories, 68

Bread 1 slice	25 Gm.
Biscuit, roll 1 (2" diam.)	35 Gm.
Muffin 1 (2" diam.)	35 Gm.
Cornbread 1½" cube	35 Gm.
Flour 2½ tbsp.	20 Gm.
Cereal, cooked ½ cup	100 Gm.
Cereal, dry (flakes, or puffed), ¾ cup	20 Gm.
Rice or grits, cooked ½ cup	100 Gm.
Spaghetti, noodles, etc. ½ cup	80 Gm.
Crackers, Graham (2)	20 Gm.
Crackers, Oyster 20 (½ cup)	20 Gm.
Crackers, Saltine (5)	20 Gm.
Crackers, Soda (3)	20 Gm.
Crackers, round, thin (6-8)	20 Gm.
Vegetables	
Beans (Lima, navy, etc.) dry, cooked ½ cup	90 Gm.
Peas (split peas, etc.) dry, cooked ½ cup	90 Gm.
Baked beans, no pork ¼ cup	50 Gm.
Corn, ⅓ cup	80 Gm.
Parsnips, ⅔ cup	125 Gm.
Potatoes, sweet, or yams ¼ cup	50 Gm.
Potatoes, white, baked or boiled 1 (2" diam.)	100 Gm.
Potatoes, white, mashed ½ cup	100 Gm.
Sponge cake, plain 1½" cube	25 Gm.
Ice Cream (omit 2 fat exchanges) ½ cup	70 Gm.

LIST 5

MEAT EXCHANGES Protein, 7 Gm.; Fat, 5 Gm.; Calories, 73

Meat, and poultry (beef, lamb, pork, liver, chicken. etc.) 1 slice (3" x 2" x ⅛")	30 Gm.
Cold cuts, 1 slice (4½" sq. ⅛" thick)	45 Gm.
Frankfurter, 1 (8-9 per lb.)	50 Gm.
Codfish, halibut, etc. 1 slice (2" x 2" x 1")	30 Gm.
Salmon, tuna, crab, lobster ¼ cup	30 Gm.
Oysters, shrimp, clams 5 med.	45 Gm.
Sardines, 3 med.	30 Gm.
Cheese, cheddar, American 1 slice (3½" x 1½" x ¼")	30 Gm.
Cheese, cottage, ¼ cup	45 Gm.
Egg, 1	50 Gm.
Peanut butter, 1 tbsp.	15 Gm.

Limit peanut butter to one exchange per day unless carbohydrate is allowed for in diet plan.

LIST 6

FAT EXCHANGES Fat 5 Gm.; Calories, 45

Butter or margarine, 1 tsp.	5 Gm.
Bacon, crisp, 1 slice	10 Gm.
Cream, light, sweet or sour, 2 tbsp.	30 Gm.
Cream, heavy, 1 tbsp.	15 Gm.
Cream cheese, 1 tbsp.	15 Gm.
French dressing, 1 tbsp.	15 Gm.
Mayonnaise, 1 tsp.	5 Gm.
Oil, or cooking fat, 1 tsp.	5 Gm.
Nuts, 6 small	10 Gm.
Olives, 5 small	50 Gm.
Avocado, ⅛ (4" diam.)	25 Gm.

LIST 7

MILK EXCHANGES Carbohydrate, 12 Gm.; Protein, 8 Gm.; Fat, 10 Gm.; Calories, 170

Milk, whole 1 cup	240 Gm.
Milk, evaporated ½ cup	120 Gm.
Milk, powdered ¼ cup	35 Gm.
*Milk, skim, 1 cup	240 Gm.
*Buttermilk, 1 cup	240 Gm.

*Add 2 fat exchanges if milk is fat free.

Figure 10-4. *(continued)*

carbohydrate. One fourth cup of grape juice can be substituted for this, as it also yields 10 grams of carbohydrate. The patient's prescribed diet tells him how many items from each list he may have at each meal. This also provides balanced vitamin and mineral intake and is determined by the nutrient composition of food, according to fat, protein and carbohydrate.

Looking at List 4, my physician might say that I can have one item from this list at each meal. I might decide to have a slice of toast one morning, a muffin the next and dry cereal flakes the next. In most cases this system allows latitude in the diabetic diet and permits the eating of foods on an ordinary menu. Candies, jams, cakes and sugar, etc., are still foods which must be avoided. The basic content of the diabetic diet is not as changed as the method of calculating it.

DIETS FOR INBORN METABOLIC DISORDERS

Inborn errors of metabolism occur as a result of mutant genes transmitted to offspring. Some of these errors cause mental retardation. This is an important area of nutritional research. Many future advances will be in the area of controlling the effects of inborn disorders of metabolism, names of which will not always be familiar to us.

In January of 1965, the American Academy of Pediatrics recommended that all newborn infants be tested for P.K.U. (phenylketonuria). The care and prevention of this disease exemplifies the results of research into biological values of food and relationships between hormones, calories, vitamins, enzymes and amino acids.

This particular disease is responsible for 1 per cent of the mentally retarded and can be prevented by dietary care if the disease is recognized in time.

Phenylalanine (an amino acid) is not oxidized due to an enzyme deficiency. By reducing phenylalanine in the diet, retardation can be prevented. This particular type of retardation cannot be reversed so that it is imperative that it be prevented. Therefore, diagnostic tests are being performed on newborns before they are discharged from the hospital. Legislation varies. Some states require a test, some permit testing, and others have no legislation regarding the condition. The Guthrie test, a diagnostic blood test, is usually performed after the infant has been on milk for 24 hours, upon discharge from the hospital and again when the infant is four to six weeks of age. The latter check picks up borderline cases of the disease. Urine tests for galactose and fructose utilization, other causes of physical and mental retardation, can also be performed, and tests for maple syrup disease and cystic fibrosis are being perfected.

SUMMARY

Food service has been greatly affected by technology. Research into the cause, diagnosis and treatment of disease makes therapeutic diets a growing field. If a patient's diet is viewed as a part of his total therapy, it does not get lost in the cooking and providing of trays. Nurses are assuming less responsibility in food service which has been greatly affected by technological advances, but they continue to assist in patient teaching.

SUGGESTED READINGS

American Heart Association booklets, 44 E. 23rd St., New York 10, N.Y.:
Your Mild Sodium-Restricted Diet
Your 1000 Milligram Sodium Diet
Your 500 Milligram Sodium Diet
Planning Fat-Controlled Meals for Unrestricted Calories
Planning Fat-Controlled Meals for 1200 and 1800 Calories

Behrman, Deaconess Maude: *Cookbook for Diabetics.* New York, American Diabetes Association, 1959.

Deutsch, Ronald M.: *The Nuts Among the Berries.* Ballantine Books, Inc., 101-5th Avenue, New York, 1961.

Mayo Clinic Diet Manual. Committee on Dietetics of the Mayo Clinic, Ed. 3, Philadelphia, W. B. Saunders Co., 1961.
Note: This would be helpful as a reference for many different kinds of special diets.

Meal Planning With Exchange Lists. Chicago, Illinois, American Diabetes Association and American Dietetic Association, 1956.

Morris, Ena: How Does a Nurse Teach Nutrition to Patients? *American Journal of Nursing,* January, 1960, p. 67.

Shafer, Kathleen, et al.: *Medical-Surgical Nursing.* St. Louis, C. V. Mosby Co., 1964, Chapter 5.

REFERENCES

Deutsch, Ronald M.: *The Nuts Among the Berries.* Ballantine Books, Inc., 101-5th Avenue, New York, 1961.

Doughday, Wm. H.: Dietary Treatment of Adults with Diabetes Mellitus. *Journal of the American Medical Association,* June 14, 1958, p. 859.

Fincke, Margaret L.: Inborn Errors of Metabolism. *Journal of the American Dietetic Association,* April, 1965, p. 280.

Hartman, Jane: Dietary Advances Will Affect Renovation. *Modern Hospital,* March, 1965, p. 148.

Kelly, Cordelia: Nurses, Nutrition, and the General Public. *American Journal of Nursing,* February, 1958, p. 217.

Keys, Ancel, and Margaret: *Eat and Stay Well.* New York, Doubleday & Co., Inc., 1963.

Kornblueh, Margaret: How Does Your Diet Rate? *Nursing Outlook,* July, 1965, p. 61.

Krause, Marie V.: *Food, Nutrition and Diet Therapy.* Ed. 4, Philadelphia, W. B. Saunders Co., 1966.

Kruse, Frank K.: Physical Medicine Versus Dieting for Obesity. *American Journal of Nursing,* April, 1954, p. 451.

McCune, Elizabeth: Food Service and Diabetics. *Hospitals,* April 1, 1965, p. 61.

Mayer, Jean: Obesity Control. *American Journal of Nursing*, June, 1965, p. 112.
Morris, Ena: How Does a Nurse Teach Nutrition to Patients? *American Journal of Nursing*, January, 1960, p. 67.
Parente, Barbara P., et al.: Adaptations of Exchange Lists—Use in Planning Metabolic Ward Diets. *Journal of the American Dietetic Association*, April, 1965, p. 267.
Russell, Pat: Vending Snack Bar Conserves This Hospital's Dietary Staff. *Modern Hospital*, March, 1965, p. 144.
Shafer, Kathleen, et al: *Medical-Surgical Nursing*, St. Louis, C. V. Mosby Co., 1964, Chapter 5.
Stare, Fredrick J.: Good Nutrition from Food Not Pills. *American Journal of Nursing*, February, 1965, p. 86.
Turner, Dorothea: *Handbook of Diet Therapy*. Chicago, University of Chicago Press, 1959, Chapter 7.

11

Care of the Patient's Skin

In the next three chapters an attempt will be made to illustrate a non-disease-centered approach to nursing care. It is similar to that used in some of today's nursing schools and textbooks. This approach reduces repetitive teaching, which used to be required when each disease entity was covered separately. It reduces the number of hours necessary to teach certain areas of nursing and brings important concepts into sharper focus so that they may be better applied. It decreases the number of facts to be memorized. As a result, the nurse is ultimately better able to use judgment based on general concepts instead of finding it necessary to recall many points which were related to specific conditions.

It is hoped that the next three chapters will combine a review of old learning with a description of newer material so that you will be able to apply it to a majority of your patients when you go back to nursing.

The objective of this particular chapter is to help you to realize how important the skin is as a defense against injury and disease and to provide you with information which will be helpful in preventing and minimizing skin problems. There will be no attempt to review diseases of the skin. For those who will be dealing with skin diseases, assistance can be found in your medical-surgical textbook.

BRIEF REVIEW OF ANATOMY AND FUNCTION OF THE SKIN

Anatomy

The skin has two layers which are supported by subcutaneous tissue. The outler layer, the epidermis or epithelium, is stratified. This layer prevents dehydration of deeper tissues and contains nerve endings for reception of the sense of touch.

The second layer is the dermis, which consists of blood vessels, nerves, sebaceous glands and ducts of the sweat glands. It also contains smooth muscular tissue as well as fibrous and elastic tissue which gives the skin its strength and elasticity.

Functions

The skin has several vital functions. As a sense organ, it helps us to interpret our environment by touch. This was Helen Keller's way of learning about the world. We forget how frequently it is used. When we buy clothing, we feel and touch the material. When we buy a melon, we squeeze it to see how ripe it is. Little children want to feel and touch everything. It is one of the ways we explore and learn about our environment.

A second function of the skin is to protect us from injury from the outside. It acts as a buffer against physical injury and as a defense against invasion of foreign substances and organisms. More than local irritation can occur when the skin is injured and no longer intact. Septicemia from a paper cut, and tetanus from a penetrating wound are but two examples of what can happen when the skin is broken.

The skin is concerned with metabolism. It excretes salts in perspiration and acts as a container for body fluids. This can be seen in a burn or a decubitus ulcer when there is wound drainage. In the case of a third degree burn, a serious disturbance in fluid and electrolyte balance can occur if the size of the area is of any consequence.

A fourth function of the skin is to regulate body temperature. When the body becomes warm, the skin cools the body by evaporation of perspiration. The skin tries to retain heat when the body becomes cold by acting as an insulator. "Goose pimples" are formed by the contraction of muscular tissue in the dermis for the purpose of retaining body heat.

Nursing care is closely related to the functions of the skin, the patient's condition and general preventive measures.

GENERAL PURPOSE OF NURSING CARE OF THE PATIENT'S SKIN

The patient's skin will need the attention of the nurse whether the diagnosis is cancer, heart disease, stroke, hip fracture, brain injury, cholecystitis or eczema. The nurse must realize that her observations of a patient's skin may be important in the possible detection of some systemic disease. Color change of the skin may indicate a vital change in the patient's general condition. In pediatrics, observations of a child's bruises and cuts may be important in the detection of a child beating or merely evidence of the extent of injuries from a fall or accident. Daily observations of the skin of a long-term patient should lead to action aimed at preventing decubitus ulcers. Descriptions of scales, redness, pustules, etc., are vital in the care of patients with a skin disease. In the case of actual skin disease, a review of the specific disease should be added to the nurse's general knowledge about skin care.

The aim of nursing care should always be to attempt to maintain a healthy skin which is unbroken, clean, dry and comfortable to the patient. Nursing care will vary with the age and activity of the patient as well as his diagnosis and general condition. It may also vary according to the climate and whether or not a hospital or home has air conditioning. In any case care of the patient's skin is an important part of general physical care.

BATHING THE PATIENT

Most hospitals provide a soap which contains hexachlorophene, not only for personnel but also for patient bathing. These soaps are sometimes a little more irritating than others, although manufactures are learning to counteract this effect to a considerable degree. The purpose of using a soap with this ingredient is to lessen the bacterial count on the skin.

A daily bath is a hospital ritual which few hospitals have eliminated unless there is a shortage of personnel. As students we gave baths to patients every other day because there were not enough hands to go around. Some hospitals have what is called "week-end" care. This means that a patient only gets his face, hands and back washed on week-ends when there are fewer persons on duty. I know of only a few institutions in which the daily bath has been eliminated in order to improve patient care. Where this has been done, personnel believe that it is better for the patient's skin to have a bath only two or three times a week. Patients usually agree. It should be added, however, that this is often done on an individual basis and not as a routine.

There are many reasons why it is hard for a nurse to omit the daily bath without feeling guilty. She feels that the patient expects this service as part of his room rate. She feels that her employer expects this of her. In some cases these things are true. In spite of this, the daily bath is often related to the nurse's comfort rather than that of the patient. I will belabor this point somewhat, in the hope that the refresher might think about this as an example of a traditional routine that needs examination, when it is applied to every patient.

Patient's Comments

I recently visited a friend who was dying of cancer. He was exhausted from discomfort and intermittent sleep. He had a complete bed bath every day. He was somewhat jaundiced and had pruritus. Every day he asked if he might have a bath only two or three times a week. He said the bath exhausted him, that it made his skin dry and uncomfortable and that he would appreciate it so much if the nurse would spend this time sitting and talking to him.

Another patient at a different hospital told the nurse that she had washed her face and hands before breakfast, had taken a shower prior to her admission the afternoon before and felt no need for a bath or shower. The nurse said a bath might relax her, handed her a towel and showed her to the tub room. The patient acquiesced but later told a friend how foolish she had felt because she had been made to feel that she were not quite competent enough to understand her hygienic needs. She was also a little irritated because she felt perfectly capable of making this decision herself.

Another patient found it especially irritating to have to take his bath in the morning when he preferred to have a bath at night. Still another patient was bathed before his barium x-ray and as he put it, "That was not when I needed it."

Nurses' Comments

"I am afraid to omit a bath because one patient told me this was the most important part of her day." "I once saw a patient get very angry because an aide had not given her a bath." "I think my head nurse expects this for all of her patients." "I feel more comfortable talking to a patient if I am doing something for him."

All these comments have some justification. If the nurse knows that her head nurse is adamant about a bath a day for every patient, she certainly is not in a very good position to start a one man crusade. Nonetheless, it might behoove her to discuss the matter with her head nurse in order to find out if this is really true. It is also true that once in awhile a patient thinks that a daily bath is part of his room rate and demands it. If there is a patient, however, who would benefit from having a bath less frequently, the reasons should be discussed with him. We should not let possible exceptions perpetuate a routine which needs re-examination in terms of the individual patient.

When to Bathe and When Not to Bathe

There are a few common-sense guides for intervals between patient baths, but these guides must be related to each patient. Such guides may or may not be related to the patient's diagnosis.

As we become older, our skins become thinner and less elastic. Subcutaneous fat disappears, wrinkles occur, and our glands become less active. Therefore, we wish to preserve some of the natural body oils rather than wash them away continually, creating a dry and sometimes irritated skin. This is an opportunity for teaching care of the skin.

Even in climate-controlled atmospheres in modern buildings, the air becomes somewhat drier during the winter. Daily bathing of older patients can create dry skin. As a consequence, the nurse must institute additional measures to combat the dry skin. She applies lotions and elbow covers, and uses other methods to prevent the skin from becoming uncomfortable.

Aside from cleanliness, the purpose of bathing is esthetic. Prevention of odors can be accomplished by cleansing selected parts of the body and by using deodorants, making total bathing unnecessary in many cases. When a bath is not given, daily care should include care of the face, hands and back, and cleansing of the underarms and perineum.

The adolescent patient who has overactive sebaceous glands and a tendency toward acne needs a daily bath to cleanse his skin of oils and waste products. He might need two baths a day if the nurse feels it would be beneficial. This is an opportunity for health teaching about care of the skin for this age group. It should be emphasized that care of the skin of an adolescent must not be the same as that of an older person.

A patient who has an elevated temperature and perspires profusely is in need of a daily bath or perhaps a bath b.i.d. The nurse should incorporate this into the written plan of care, not leaving it up to someone on another shift. Our daily bath routine rises to haunt us many times. We not only insist on bathing patients every morning, but it rarely occurs to us to do it more often just as it never occurs to us to do it less often.

Patients who have drainage need particular attention. If a patient is incontinent, thorough cleansing is required to prevent skin breakdown due to reaction of the excreta on the skin. This is also necessary for any patient who has wound drainage. Skin breakdown can occur rapidly from the irritation of such secretions. Thorough cleansing is required at frequent intervals. Some type of skin protection in the form of an ointment or paste may be necessary if the skin is constantly exposed to drainage, as in the case of a new colostomy.

One of the advantages of giving a bed bath is that the nurse is provided with an opportunity to observe the patient's skin. In the case of the patient who is up ad lib., taking a tub bath or a shower, we often forget that it is important to inspect the skin. This can be done when the patient is given a back rub. Observations of the skin of ambulatory patients are too often minimized.

REDUCING SKIN PROBLEMS

Dry Skin

Dry skin occurs in the aged, in the dehydrated patient, in the long-term patient, following the removal of a cast and with inactivity, and it is more likely to occur in blondes and redheads than in brunettes. It is also more likely to occur in patients with underactive glands such as the hypothyroid patient.

When patients have dry skin, the skin needs to be kept clean, but complete bathing should be done with discretion as already discussed. An adequate dietary and fluid intake is essential. Use of lotion or oil on the skin is recommended if there is nothing to contraindicate it. Powder can have a drying effect on the skin so that it should be used sparingly or not at all.

Sensitive Skin

Some patients have a hypersensitive skin. They may have severe allergies or merely have certain minor sensitivities. They may have a soap intolerance or merely have a fair complexion. These patients may require a special soap if they get a rash from regular soap. For the same reason lotions, oils, powder, make-up and deodorants should be carefully selected. In order to provide care which will not increase skin irritation, the patient will need to be consulted.

Some institutions have what is called "special" or "nonallergic" linen for such patients. This linen is usually rinsed two or three extra times after the regular laundry process in order to make sure that there is maximum removal of bleaches, dyes, soaps and other chemicals.

Pruritus

Pruritus may occur as a result of jaundice, allergies or venous stasis. It is hoped that the nurse can help to minimize the discomfort of this symptom.

The patient needs to refrain from scratching irritated areas. Nails should be kept short, clean and filed smoothly. Special care in bathing should be taken. Anything that might increase skin irritation should be avoided. Light-weight bedding should be used and cotton rather than wool blankets may be helpful. The nurse should suggest clothing which does not rub or retain body heat and moisture. If the patient has venous stasis it is sometimes helpful for him to lie down and elevate his feet for about five minutes of every two hours. If these measures fail to make the patient more comfortable, notify the physician, who will order medication to help relieve the patient's distress.

Areas Receiving Heat and Cold Treatment

The nurse applies heat and cold to the patient in the form of a soak, a compress, a special pad or blanket, a pack and several other ways. She must perform these treatments without injury to the skin. Consideration of the many factors already discussed is essential during the application of hot packs, heating units, cooling blankets, ice collars, hot water bottles, etc. Written procedures should be consulted as guides to good nursing practice. The nurse will need to implement these procedures in relation to her knowledge about the skin. Frequent observations will help her to apply such treatments to her particular patient.

Wound Areas

It is important that wound healing is not retarded by the type of dressing used. When gauze is applied to a draining wound, it usually sticks to the area. As a result, healing tissue is often pulled away when the dressing is removed. Telfa type dressings will prevent this. Gauze can be used to cover dry lesions.

Many nonallergic and nonirritating tapes are available. Tape should be removed from draining wounds by pulling toward the lesion from each side in order to prevent injury to new tissue on the edge where healing is taking place.

Whenever regular adhesive is used, the skin should be inspected daily. When it is taken off, tape marks should be removed with a solvent. The area should then be washed with soap and water to prevent skin irritation.

The Skin of a Patient Having Deep X-ray Therapy

Whenever a patient is receiving deep x-ray therapy, his skin is likely to have great sensitivity. The radiated part of the body should be treated like a sunburn. No soap should be used in all cases, and no water should be used when the skin is blistered. The physician will recommend oils which can be applied to the skin during the time that the skin is especially irritated.

Skin Breakdown

Causes. Skin may break down due to intrinsic causes, such as circulatory collapse or neurological disease. Paralysis, loss of sensation, lack of adequate circulation, inadequate nutrition or secondary infection are examples. Skin may break down due to extrinsic causes, i.e., pressure on certain areas which deprives the tissue of adequate circulation, such as excessive application of heat, cold or friction, wrinkles in the sheet, bed crumbs, casts, braces, lack of air circulation from lying on a heating pad, or pressure from an arm board.

These causes point to many measures which can be prevented by good nursing care. A great deal of research into the care and treatment of decubitus ulcers has been done at Walter Reed Hospital. They have found that these sores can be due to poor nursing care when skin is healthy and when the general condition of the body is good. They have also discovered that there are causes of decubitus ulcers which are not related to poor nursing care, such as devitalized skin and a negative nitrogen balance due to disease.

The nurse is charged with making every effort to prevent decubitus ulcers in all of her patients. She must also give general care and topical treatments in a manner that will minimize the likelihood of skin damage.

POTENTIAL AREAS OF DECUBITUS ULCERS. When a patient is in the prone position, pressure points include the knee, the iliac crest, the clavicle, the chin, the forehead and the sternum. Pressure points of a patient who lies on his side are the ear, the shoulder, the wrist and the ankle. Potential pressure points of a patient lying on his back include the scapula, the coccyx, the sacrum, the ischial tuberosities, the heel, the elbow and the occiput.

STAGES OF A PRESSURE SORE. The first stage of a potential pressure sore is redness which disappears soon after pressure to an area is removed. This is a warning signal which nurses often ignore because the symptom of redness disappears so readily.

The second stage of a pressure sore produces redness which does not disappear when pressure is removed. Superficial damage or loss of epithelium occurs, and a blister may form. This means that a pressure sore has begun.

The final stage of a lesion shows necrosis of surrounding skin, underlying tissue and muscle. It is surprising to learn that only about 12 per cent of such a lesion is visible. The rest of it is beneath the visible necrosis. A sore can develop to the final stage within 24 hours, reminding us of how important it is to pay attention to any pressure on the patient's skin.

TURNING. One of the most important things the nurse can do is to plan a turning schedule for each patient which can be followed around the clock by all personnel. The frequency of the turning schedule can be geared to the condition of the patient's skin. If redness does not occur in two or three hours, the turning schedule is appropriate. If the skin becomes red, the interval between position changes should be shortened. Turning also needs to be geared to the patient's daily schedule. He should not be prone at meal hours or at an hour when he is likely to need the bedpan.

When he is turned, pressure points should be gently massaged. Lotion may be used if the areas seem particularly dry. A draw sheet should be used to turn and lift patients in order to prevent burning of the skin caused by friction from being moved about in bed. Effort must also be made to support but not to touch a sore in order to prevent further injury when the patient is turned or moved.

Bedding should be checked whenever the patient is turned. Bottom sheets should be free of crumbs and tucked in tightly to avoid wrinkles. Too much bottom linen can cause wrinkles and lumps which often exist from overprotection of the mattress. Linen should also be dry and free of patches.

Diet. Patients need an adequate fluid intake. Selecting fluids which the patient especially enjoys can help immeasurably. The physician may order supplementary vitamins. A high protein diet is ordered for patients who have decubitus ulcers, because a large amount of protein is lost from these lesions. Thin patients are encouraged to gain weight and obese patients are encouraged to lose weight, as both extremes increase the susceptibility to pressure sores.

Nursing Accessories. The use of sheepskin, 4-inch foam rubber and many synthetic products are now available to place under areas particularly prone to pressure sores. They are considered quite successful in the prevention of decubitus ulcers. The use of an alternating pressure pad may be helpful. The principal thing for the nurse to remember is that such measures should be initiated BEFORE a sore has begun.

The air mattress, described in Chapter 18, is used for patients who can only be in one or two positions over a long period of time such as a patient with a cervical fracture. The Foster frame or the Stryker frame also needs to be considered in these cases. The physician, however, must make the final decision in the use of such devices.

Stockinet over the elbows is often successful in relieving skin irritation of a patient who reads a great deal and wears short-sleeved gowns or pajamas.

Exposure to a regular light bulb can be given without a doctor's order in some places. This varies with the hospital and even with the area within a hospital sometimes. An infant with a diaper rash is often greatly benefited by simple exposure to air for 20 minutes three times a day. Air is also beneficial to adults. When a light is used, it should not exceed 60 watts, or 20 minute exposure periods, or be less than 18 to 24 inches from the patient. Even if hospital policy does not require a physician's order for use of a light bulb, the nurse should always secure permission from the physician whenever it is to be used on a patient with a sensory loss.

The use of doughnuts and rubber rings are no longer recommended nursing measures. These devices surround a lesion and restrict the flow of blood. A particularly effective method of relieving pressure is to place a foam rubber pad (about 4 inches thick) on each side of a pressure point. This prevents contact with the bed and still permits flow of blood to the area.

The nurse should make sure that any bandage, appliance, cast, brace, etc., does not chafe or press on the skin. If a patient is ambulatory and has circulatory or neurological impairment, the nurse must make sure to check him carefully. Shoes need to be well fitting.

Socks need to be of proper size and without holes or darns which might cause pressure. Because these patients cannot feel discomfort, the nurse must be especially vigilant.

TREATMENT OF DECUBITUS ULCERS. The patient's physician should be kept informed of any suspicious areas of potential breakdown, and he will need to be kept informed of the condition of any sores. The patient must not lie on the affected area. He may need to use certain medications to protect the skin, to toughen the skin, to combat infection or to heal a wound. The number and kinds of medications are too numerous to mention. If a pressure sore becomes large and does not respond to medication and nursing care, excision of the lesion and skin graft may be necessary to obtain healing.

SUMMARY

Caring for the patient's skin provides the nurse with a unique opportunity to utilize her skills and observation powers. Nursing procedures can best be executed with knowledge about the skin. The nurse may be able to prevent potential discomfort and complications such as decubitus ulcers by instituting measures which are hers to initiate and to carry out. This is an area which clearly demonstrates what nursing intervention can do.

SUGGESTED READINGS

Hickey, Mary Catherine: Hypothermia. *American Journal of Nursing*, January, 1965, p. 116.

Hicks, Mary L.: Decubitus Ulcers 1. Alternating Pressure Pad. *American Journal of Nursing,* July, 1958, p. 1008.

Matheney, Ruth V., et al.: *Fundamentals of Nursing*. St. Louis, C. V. Mosby Co., 1964, Chapters 12 and 13.

Shafer, Kathleen Newton, et al.: *Medical-Surgical Nursing,* St. Louis, C. V. Mosby Co., 1964, Chapters 2, 8 and 9.

Sutton, Audrey Latshaw: *Bedside Nursing Techniques.* Philadelphia, W. B. Saunders Co., 1964, Chapters 2 and 16.

REFERENCES

Basic Nursing Care. Telecourse Study Guide for Nursing Students, Kenny Rehabilitation Institute, 1964-65.

Cannell, Ina June: 2. Plastic Spray. *American Journal of Nursing*, July, 1958, p. 1009.

Fuerst, Elinor V., and Wolff, LuVerne: *Fundamentals of Nursing.* Ed. 3, Philadelphia, J. B. Lippincott Co., 1964, Unit 14.

Hickey, Mary Catherine: Hypothermia. *American Journal of Nursing*, January, 1965, p. 116.

Hicks, Mary L.: Decubitus Ulcers 1. Alternating Pressure Pad. *American Journal of Nursing,* July, 1958, p. 1008.

Keane, Claire Brackman: *Essentials of Nursing*. Philadelphia, W. B. Saunders Co., 1964, Chapter 9.

Matheney, Ruth V., et al.: *Fundamentals of Nursing*. St. Louis, C. V. Mosby Co., 1964, Chapters 12 and 13.

Shafer, Kathleen Newton et al.: *Medical-Surgical Nursing*. St. Louis, C. V. Mosby Co., 1964, Chapters 2, 8 and 9.

Sutton, Audrey Latshaw: *Bedside Nursing Techniques*. Philadelphia, W. B. Saunders Co., 1964, Chapters 2 and 16.

Taylor, John C.: Decubitus Ulcers. *Nursing Science*, August, 1964, p. 293.

Verhonick, P. J.: Decubitus Ulcer Care. *American Journal of Nursing*, August, 1961, p. 68.

Verhonick, P. J.: Decubitus Ulcer Observations Measured Objectively. *Nursing Research*, Fall, 1961, p. 211.

12

Care of the Patient With Anoxia

Hypoxia and anoxia, terms often used interchangeably, mean oxygen deficiency in the body tissues. Patients manifest this phenomenon by such symptoms as dyspnea, cyanosis, irregular respirations, altered respiratory rate, etc. Nurses need to review certain information before giving care to patients having these symptoms.

THUMBNAIL REVIEW OF AIR EXCHANGE

Approximately 20 per cent of ordinary air contains oxygen. In a normal state of health and in an atmosphere containing this concentration, breathing is unlabored and regular, and occurs at a rate of about 18 times per minute. Skin tone, nail beds and lips are usually described in terms of the color pink as opposed to the color blue (cyanosis) in white-skinned persons. When a patient has had cyanosis, one sometimes hears the expression, "He has pinked up."

Oxygen is carried to body tissue via hemoglobin, the protein in our red blood cells. Air is first breathed into the lungs. When it reaches the air sacs (alveoli) of the lungs, the oxygen content of the air crosses the alveolar wall, enters the capillaries and is then carried throughout the body by the red blood cells. At the same time and place, returning blood unloads carbon dioxide which is exhaled into the air.

TYPES OF ANOXIA

It is obvious from this brief review of anatomy and physiology that there are various types of anoxia which stem from many different diseases. Medical treatment, therefore, is geared to the cause and manifestation of the condition.

Anemic Anoxia

In anemic anoxia, oxygen is decreased in the blood due to an insufficient amount of red blood cells and/or hemoglobin carrying the oxygen. This is associated with conditions such as hemorrhage, anemia and carbon monoxide poisoning. Transfusion of whole blood or packed cells (whole blood with 200 to 300 cc. plasma removed) is a common treatment. Oxygen is ordered in some cases.

Anoxic Anoxia

In anoxic anoxia, the blood does not become 100 per cent oxygenated in the lungs. Such interference of oxygen exchange in the alveoli occurs in cancer of the lung, pneumonia, asthma and tuberculosis. An obstruction in the respiratory passage can also cause this. Treatments are as varied as the diseases which are related to this kind of hypoxia.

Histotoxic Anoxia

In histotoxic anoxia, the oxygen supply to the tissues is not diminished, but the ability of the tissue to utilize oxygen is curtailed. This occurs in poisoning by cyanide. It can also be due to toxic effects of narcotics and anesthetics on the enzyme systems of cells.

Stagnant Anoxia

In stagnant anoxia, circulatory insufficiency causes low blood oxygen. Low blood pressure, circulatory collapse or shock may result in this condition, which is usually treated with a stimulant drug and a blood transfusion.

MANIFESTATIONS OF ANOXIA

Anoxia is manifested in many different ways. Dyspnea, labored or difficult breathing, is one of them. It is a tiring and unpleasant symptom which usually creates apprehensiveness on the part of the patient and may or may not be accompanied by pain. It is very frightening to be unable to catch one's breath, and it is very exhausting to have to strain consciously for each inspiration. Patients may say they are "breathless," have a "shortness of breath sensation," or complain of "lack of air."

Anoxia may also be manifested by headache, depression or general apathy. The patient might become weak and slow in his reactions. Sleepiness or wakefulness may occur.

The nurse will observe many symptoms. Breathing may be labored, as evidenced by an anxious look on the patient's face or retraction at the clavicle, sternum or diaphragm. Pupils may be dilated, cyanosis or extreme pallor may be evident. The mouth may be held open, and the tongue and lips may be dry. Respirations may be regular or irregular, shallow or deep, rapid or slow. The patient may have a cough—dry, "wheezy" or productive.

Although the severity of symptoms will vary, the patient will complain of some and the nurse will see others. It is, therefore, up to the nurse to take certain nursing measures to aid the patient and to keep the physician informed of symptoms so that he can make medical decisions at the appropriate time.

NURSING MEASURES IN THE CARE OF A PATIENT WITH DYSPNEA

Acute Care

If a patient is admitted to the hospital with severe dyspnea, there are certain things which the nurse can do immediately. Patients find it easier to breathe in a sitting position. Therefore, the head of the patient's bed should be raised. When the patient's thorax is in a vertical position, he is said to be in the orthopneic position.

The nurse must see that someone is asked to call the doctor, intern or resident, as the case may be. This task should be done by the nurse only when there is no one else to do it. The nurse will need to give instructions to the person who calls the physician, but her services are primarily needed by her patient when he is in acute distress. If he cannot be attended for a few minutes, he needs to be made as comfortable as possible and be protected with side rails.

Oxygen equipment should be brought to the room and made ready for immediate use, along with intravenous equipment and emergency drugs. Most hospitals have an emergency tray, cart or box which is available for such times.

The patient needs reassurance. The nurse will best be able to maintain a calm and helpful demeanor if she has planned in advance what she will need and do if a patient with dyspnea is admitted. The physician's orders should be carried out as soon as possible. Some will undoubtedly be Stat. orders.

As time passes and the immediate discomfort of the patient is relieved and immediate care is provided, the patient may be undressed and have his vital signs taken. This, along with questioning the patient about anything other than his most immediate needs, should be postponed until the more urgent things are taken care of.

Daily Care

Day-to-day care of the patient with dyspnea or a tendency toward this symptom chiefly consists of proper positioning of the patient, provision of physical and mental relaxation, rest, patient teaching and carrying out medical orders in a safe effective manner. If the patient is receiving oxygen continuously, his temperature is usually taken rectally.

POSITION. The patient should be kept in a position which makes it easiest for him to breathe. A Fowler's or semi-Fowler's position, with knees bent (if there is no contraindication), is usually comfortable. No one position should be used continuously, since contractures, pressure sores and fatigue need to be prevented. A footboard should be used if the patient will be on bed rest for any length of time. Some patients need to spend periods of time resting forward on an overbed table on which a pillow is placed.

PHYSICAL REST. Physical rest can be increased by many nursing measures. If the patient requires cardiac rest, the nurse should always get help when turning or lifting the patient so that the patient is not asked to exert himself unduly. A draw sheet can be used for raising the patient up in bed when he slides downward. His bed can be made from the top to the bottom if he becomes particularly uncomfortable while in a supine position. He will also need help with his personal hygiene and may need to be fed if he is acutely ill, exceptionally weak or required to be on complete bed rest over a period of time.

MENTAL REST. The nurse can also contribute greatly to the patient's mental comfort by giving him explanations about his care and treatment, listening to expressions of his needs and reassuring him when he becomes anxious. The nurse can save him much anxiety by anticipating his needs, keeping necessary equipment near him and informing him when she expects to return to his room. The signal cord should be within reach at all times so that the patient can be spared any anxiety about not being able to call the nurse. Frequent visits to the patient, getting to know him, and overall interest help to reduce anxiety about his symptoms and restrictions. The nurse can truly help her patient through a difficult period.

Patient teaching should begin when the patient is first confined to bed. A patient with asthma, tuberculosis or cardiovascular disease has many teaching needs. He needs to know why he is not permitted to smoke, why bed rest or limited activity is needed for eventual recovery and how to reduce strain, both physical and mental. Patient teaching must always prepare for the next stage. This gives the patient an understanding of the next step and a new goal to look forward to. There are many excellent materials which patients can read. See the list of suggested readings for patients at the end of Chapter 8.

MEDICAL ORDERS. Medical orders will give the nurse many tools which will contribute to the well-being and eventual improvement of the patient. It is vital that medications for pain be given so that the patient does not find himself in acute distress. It is up to the nurse to keep the physician informed about the effectiveness of the ordered pain medication. Cough depressants should be given generously to prevent strain from coughing and to loosen secretions when they exist. Respiratory stimulants also need to be given on time and before distress becomes acute. Humidity, steam and oxygen should be given properly and safely. Bowel activity needs to be known so that constipation or impaction is prevented by whatever measures are ordered.

METHODS OF ADMINISTERING OXYGEN

There are several pieces of equipment which may be operated with or without oxygen. The Croupette, a plastic tent which is principally designed to provide humidity to an infant or child, can be operated with a small motor or with oxygen. Attached to the Croupette is a pint-sized jar which is filled with distilled water. This water is forced into a fine spray into the tent to provide humidity for the infant or child. The physician will decide whether a compressor motor or oxygen is to be used.

Various types of incubators are on the market. It has been found that premature infants may develop blindness (retrolental fibroplasia) which is thought to be caused by too high an oxygen concentration during early life. Because of these findings, these machines are made so that they can be operated by compressed air or oxygen. When oxygen is used, physicians expect the nurse to make sure that no more than a 40 per cent oxygen concentration is administered to the premature infant.

The Bennett respirator and the Bird respirator are commonly used to give aerosol treatments to patients. They may also be used to assist patients who cannot breathe by themselves. Such pieces of machinery are not difficult to operate, but the nurse must know why they are used. You will need to review how to operate the particular model owned or rented by your employer. This is a good example of why a nurse should not learn procedures until returning to work. You might learn how to operate one piece of machinery only to find that your employing institution uses another brand, type or model which provides a similar type of assistance to the patient. Written procedures should always be available to employees, as a procedure might well have been learned but not used for six or eight months. Details of operation are usually forgotten when so much time elapses.

Oxygen, when administered by itself, may be administered to patients by four principal methods: the tent, the mask, the cannula or the nasal catheter. There are advantages to each, and it will be up to the physician to select the method. The mask is usually considered the best method for emergency therapy and for patients who need a high concentration of oxygen over short periods of time. The tent is used when the patient needs continuous therapy along with a cool atmosphere with controlled humidity. The cannula and catheter are used for patients who require moderate concentrations of oxygen.

THE INHALATION THERAPIST

In larger hospitals and in hospitals where lung and heart surgery is performed, the inhalation therapist may be part of the team of persons available to help the patient.

The inhalation therapist is usually responsible for the technical and clerical aspects of the operation of inhalation therapy equipment. Such a person or department is frequently under the supervision of the anesthesiology department.

Inhalation therapy personnel set up and supervise the operation of oxygen equipment. They are familiar with the operation, care and maintenance of equipment. They will see that adequate records are kept so that patient records, charges and inventory location lists are maintained.

Inhalation therapists are responsible for assisting the nurse in the care of patients receiving oxygen. They conduct formal and/or informal classes in the proper use of this equipment in areas where it is used. They make sure that safety rules are maintained.

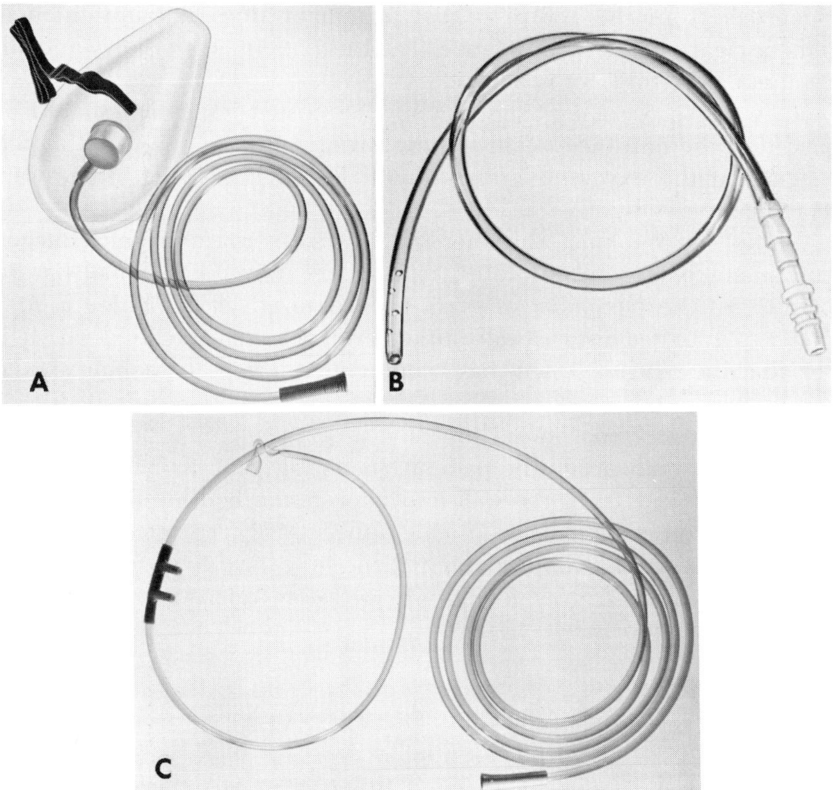

Figure 12—1. *Oxygen mask with connecting tubing (A) nasal catheter (B) and nasal cannula with connecting tubing (C). (Courtesy Pharmaseal Company.)*

Inhalation therapy is a new field and standards and guidelines are being established. The American Association of Inhalation Therapists is a nonprofit organization sponsored by the American Society of Anesthesiologists and the American College of Chest Physicians. One of its chief objectives is to develop educational programs in this field.

PRECAUTIONS DURING THE ADMINISTRATION OF OXYGEN

Oxygen supports combustion. It is for this reason that all precautionary measures rest with eliminating likelihood of any spark which might start a flame.

No Smoking

The "No Smoking" rule must be adhered to no matter how oxygen is administered. It is a good idea to remove ash trays, matches and cigarettes from the room so that a smoker does not unthinkingly light a cigarette. It is imperative that the patient, his visitors and his roommates be told not to smoke.

Two "No Smoking" signs should be posted. One sign should be placed at the entrance to the patient's room and the other one should be put on the oxygen cylinder or on the oxygen outlet at the wall, as the case may be.

The "No Smoking" rule should apply to any room in which oxygen equipment is stored or located, as there is always a potential hazard because of the possibility of small unrecognized leaks. Where a flowmeter is plugged into a wall outlet, even when it is closed off, it is felt that the oxygen system has been opened and that smoking should not be permitted.

In multiple-bed rooms, this may cause problems which the nurse will have to manage. If the patient has only a "standby" flowmeter, it can be removed from the wall and kept at the bedside in readiness. In this way other patients will not be unnecessarily restricted. If oxygen is being used in the room, other patients will have to go elsewhere to smoke or refrain from smoking. On occasion, relocation of some patients may be necessary.

Handling Oxygen Cylinders

Because oxygen cylinders are heavy, they need to be handled carefully in order to avoid accidents. When a cylinder is not in use, both the flowmeter valve and the cylinder valve should be turned off. Should a tank be accidentally tipped over with the cylinder valve on, it might spin on the floor rapidly and become very difficult to control. On the other hand, when oxygen is being used, a valve should be turned all the way on. Valves of an oxygen tank should always be all the way on or all the way off.

Cylinders should be stored in a cool, well-ventilated area which is not near flammable gases. Hands with grease and oil should always be washed thoroughly before handling oxygen equipment of any kind, as the combination of oxygen and petroleum products can be dangerous.

Safety When a Tent Is Used

Because of the combustible nature of oxygen, no electrical apparatus can be utilized inside the tent. Bed lamp switches, electric razors, hearing aids, telephones, T.V. or radio controls, signal cords, transistor or battery operated gadgets may not be used inside an oxygen tent. In some hospitals, signal cords are approved for use inside a tent because the actual switch is not located inside the tent. The nurse will

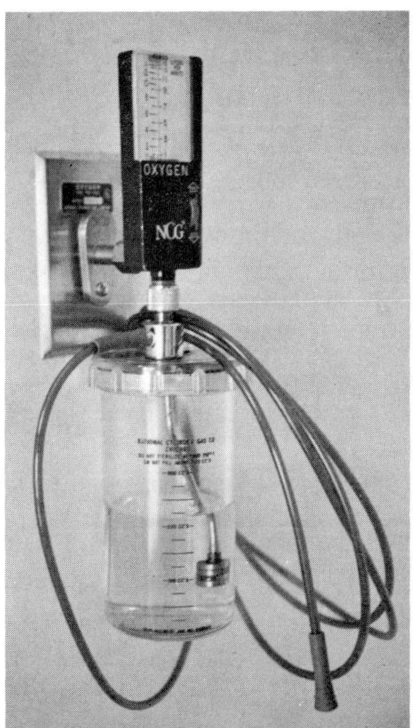

Figure 12–2. *Wall outlet with oxygen gauge, humidity bottle and connecting tube which can be attached to a nasal cannula, a nasal catheter or a mask. (Courtesy National Cylinder Co.)*

need to know if this is true where she works. In pediatrics, wind-up toys cannot be used inside a humidity tent if it is run by oxygen.

The nurse must give back rubs with powder, water or approved noncombustible substances as oily lotions and alcohol are not to be used inside tents. When an EKG. or x-ray machine is used, the oxygen tent must be turned off and the canopy opened during the procedure. If the patient is not able to tolerate this, an oxygen mask may be substituted during the examination.

Ten liters per minute is a recommended minimum flow for an oxygen tent. This prevents carbon dioxide build-up inside the tent. The canopy should always be tucked in around the mattress and top covers to prevent leakage of oxygen into the room and to make sure that the patient is receiving the maximum effect from his therapy.

Electric beds are approved for use with oxygen tents if no part of the motor is inside the tent. Fabrics which create static electricity should be avoided. The National Fire Protection Association no longer restricts the use of wool blankets inside a tent.

Safety When a Catheter, Mask or Cannula Is Used

General oxygen safety rules apply to these methods of oxygen administration also. However, electrical equipment may be used with somewhat less rigid precautions. T.V. controls, call lights and radios may be operated if they are not near the patient's head where the oxygen apparatus is working. Electrical equipment, such as the alternating pressure mattress and some types of heating pads, can be used if they are positioned at the foot of the bed. It is vital that operating instructions for such equipment be read, as many of these machines come with the precaution that oxygen may be used if it is at least 3 feet away.

Other Precautions

Oxygen is frequently discussed in terms of percentage rather than liters. Normal air contains about 20 per cent oxygen. This figure is important to know in relation to therapeutic percentages. A cannula and catheter produce about 35 per cent oxygen when run at about 4 to 6 liters, which is considered a usual rate. A tent provides about 45 per cent oxygen when run at 10 to 12 liters. When it is vital that the percentage be known, as in the case of a premature infant, the percentage of oxygen being administered can be measured by an oxygen analyzer, a device designed for this task.

It is also important that humidity be given with oxygen as it is very drying to mucous membranes if administered alone. This is why one will not see oxygen being given without humidity except in an emergency.

Certain machines, such as the Bennett respirator or the Isolette, have a knob or lever which regulates the percentage of oxygen. Usually there are three settings: 40, 60 and 100 per cent. Such machines should always be run at the 40 per cent setting unless the physician orders otherwise. Should a physician order 100 per cent oxygen, the nurse should receive a new order every six to eight hours.

The nurse will want to observe her patients frequently and see that they are receiving benefit from therapy. She must see that there are no leaks or kinks in the oxygen tubing. She must see that the mask is tight and without leaks, that the catheter is at the back of the throat or that the cannula is inserted in the nares, as the case may be. If the patient has a mask, the nurse will want to remove the mask and cleanse and dry the face, as the patient may become very warm and uncomfortable. Nasal catheters and cannulas should be cleansed and reinserted as necessary and at eight-hour intervals.

If the patient is in a tent, the canopy must be tucked in well, and the nurse must plan her work so that she opens and closes the tent as seldom as possible in order to prevent frequent dilution of the oxygen concentration. The patient will need special attention to warmth, because a tent is usually about 68° F. and there is a rather rapid circulation of air which creates a draft. Flannel gowns and pajamas as well as blankets are necessary to keep the patient warm. One special precaution about tents is needed. They are not soundproof. Patients can hear perfectly well through a tent, so that it is imperative that personnel be reminded of this to prevent any conversation which might cause anxiety in the patient.

NURSING PRECAUTIONS IN TRANSFUSIONS

Because two types of anoxia may be treated with blood transfusion, it is fitting that we review nursing precautions during transfusion in this chapter.

Before Transfusion

The nursing department is usually responsible for ordering the type and cross-match preceding a transfusion. The nurse must be aware that it is imperative to communicate the number of pints of blood which the physician deems necessary to the laboratory so that the proper amount of blood be prepared.

Once the blood is ordered, both the nursing and laboratory departments are responsible for the proper identification of the blood when it leaves the laboratory. Blood should not be obtained from the laboratory until it is time for it to be administered to the patient. If there is any delay, the blood should be returned to the laboratory within about 45 minutes, so that it may be placed under refrigeration of the proper temperature.

During Transfusion

Once the blood is brought to the patient's bedside, blood transfusion tubing (which contains a filtered drip chamber) is usually connected to a small bottle of normal saline or 5 per cent dextrose in 0.2 per cent saline. The name of the patient should be compared with that on the bottle of blood. Once the fluid is running properly into the patient's vein, the solution is clamped off and the blood is allowed to run in.

There are certain untoward effects to which the nurse must be alert during a transfusion. Blood should be started slowly and speeded up only slightly after the first five minutes. A patient should be checked every five minutes for the next ten minutes of a transfusion and every 15 or 20 minutes after that. The patient must be observed for hives or rash, chill or fever, headache, nausea or vomiting, dyspnea or change in color. In the case of possible blood incompatibility, the patient may also complain of fullness in the head, chest pain and back pain. It is imperative that the nurse clamp off the blood whenever any of these symptoms occurs. Both the physician and the laboratory should be notified so that the symptoms can be evaluated and the cause determined.

After Transfusion

Once the transfusion is completed, the necessary records should be made out. Some laboratories ask that blood tubing and blood bottle be kept for 24 hours after the transfusion so that both tubing and blood bottle can be checked in case of a delayed blood reaction.

EMERGENCY CARE IN THE EVENT OF CARDIOPULMONARY ARREST

Whenever a patient has a cardiac arrest or cessation of respirations, resuscitation is successful only if it is done immediately. Emergency equipment such as an emergency drug tray, a cardiac massage board, a throat suction machine and a tracheotomy tray are available at most hospitals, along with a defibrillator and a heart monitor. Each nurse will be responsible for knowing the policies and procedures regarding cardiopulmonary resuscitation at her particular institution.

When a patient is in need of resuscitation, the nurse must remain with the patient and do four things. She will summon help by using the patient signal cord, the patient telephone or calling out. She must then clear the patient's airway, begin mouth-to-mouth breathing and start external heart massage if the first two measures fail to revive the patient.

Mouth-to-Mouth Resuscitation

Initially, the patient's mouth can be quickly inspected for any possible obstruction to the airway. Foreign bodies can usually be removed with the finger if they are lodged in the larynx.

If the larynx is apparently clear, the patient should be placed on his back. Grasp the patient's chin with one hand and place the other hand on his forehead. Extend his head so that his tongue does not rest on the back of the throat. If this is not done, air from mouth-to-mouth or mouth-to-nose breathing cannot reach the lungs.

The nurse then places her mouth over the patient's mouth and blows into the patient until his chest rises. While she does this, she either pinches the patient's nose or rests her cheek on the patient's nose to stop any air leakage. She then removes her mouth to allow the lungs to deflate. This should be done in a steady rhythm about 12 to 15 times a minute. This method of artificial respiration is presently recommended instead of other methods.

Closed-Chest Cardiac Resuscitation

The American Heart Association, Inc., the American National Red Cross, the Industrial Medical Association, and the United States Public Health Service have made the following statement, "External cardiac resuscitation is a proved and accepted life-saving technique and should be applied as an emergency procedure by properly trained individuals of the medical, dental, nursing and allied health professions and of rescue squads."*

Drowning, electric shock, asphyxiation and heart attack are conditions which might necessitate the implementation of closed-chest resuscitation. Persons should be trained in this procedure before attempting it.

(Text continued on page 160.)

*American Heart Association, The Closed Chest Method of Cardio-Pulmonary Resuscitation–Revised Statement (Editorial). *Circulation*, May, 1965, p. 641.

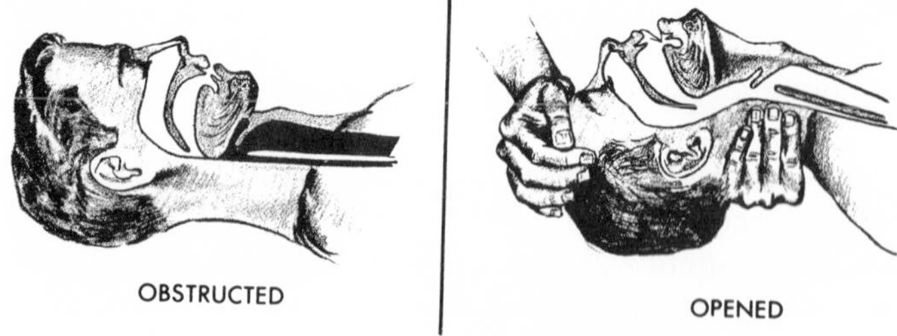

AIRWAY

The tongue is attached to the lower jaw and floor of the mouth. In an unconscious patient, the head flexes, the jaw relaxes and the tongue drops back to obstruct the air passage. To restore breathing, the first thing to do is to open the airway. The simplest and quickest method is:—(1) Lift the neck with one hand; and (2) Tilt the head backward into maximum extension with the other hand. This draws the tongue forward and opens the airway. This should always be the first maneuver performed. Sometimes, this alone will allow the patient to resume spontaneous breathing.

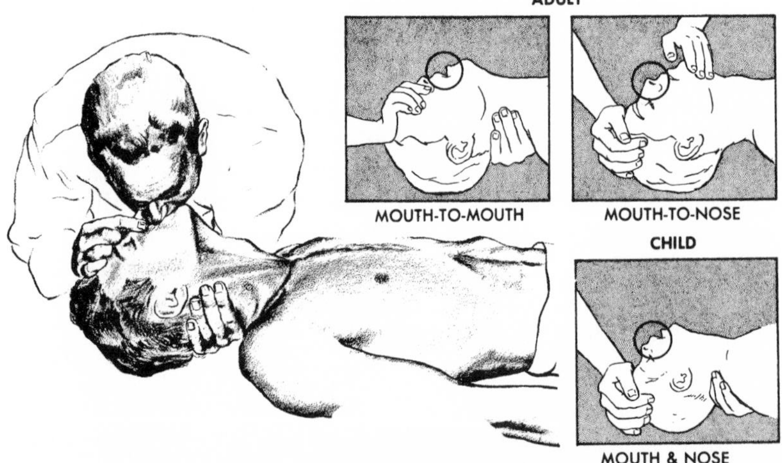

BREATHING

If the patient does not resume spontaneous breathing, start mouth-to-mouth resuscitation. First, pinch the nose shut with your thumb and index finger to prevent the escape of air. The rescuer's cheek can also be used to seal the patient's nose. Then open your mouth widely, take a deep breath, place your mouth over the patient's mouth to get a good seal, and inflate his lungs with about twice the amount of a normal breath. Remove your mouth and allow him to exhale. Repeat the cycle 12 times per minute. For mouth-to-nose resuscitation, you can prevent the escape of air by pushing the patient's chin upward to close his lips. Then open your mouth widely and get a good seal around the nose before inflating. In small children, place your mouth over their mouth and nose, use smaller amounts of air, and increase the rate to approximately 20 times per minute. Babies may require a faster rate and only small puffs of air from your cheeks. You will know that you are inflating the lungs with every breath by:—(1) Seeing the chest rise and fall; (2) Feeling the lungs expand; and (3) Hearing the air escape from the lungs during exhalation.

Figure 12–3. *Principles of Cardiopulmonary Resuscitation—opening the airway, mouth-to-mouth breathing, and external heart massage. (Medical Supply Company, Rockland, Illinois.)*

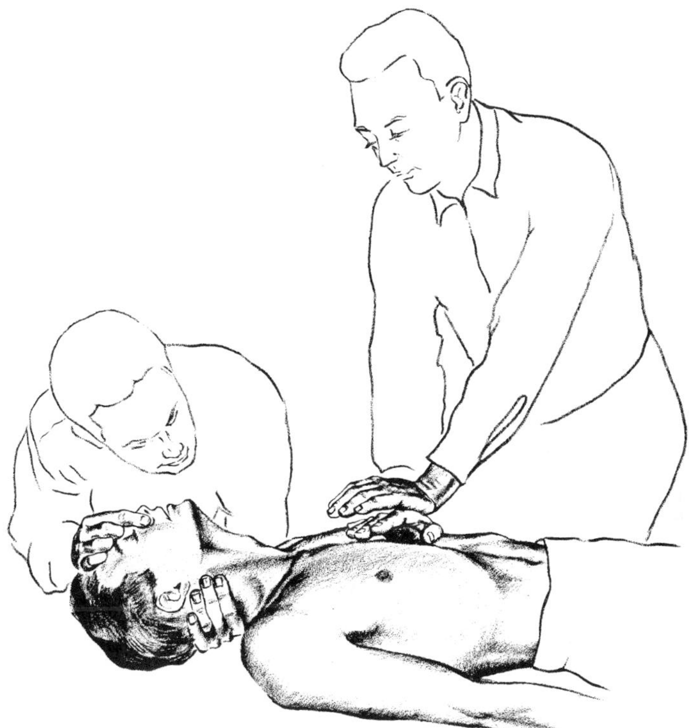

CIRCULATION

After five good lung inflations, if the patient does not start breathing and if the pulse is absent and the pupils are dilated, begin external cardiac compression. This is best performed by two rescuers. One places himself at the side and above the patient's chest. He places the heel of one hand over the lower one-half of the sternum (not including the xiphoid process of the sternum) and places the other hand on top of it. Keeping his elbows straight, he then uses the weight of the upper part of his body to exert 60 to 100 pounds of pressure almost straight downward. This should depress the sternum 1½ to 2 inches. The compression is repeated at a steady rate of 60 times per minute with a smooth, regular action which is 50% compression and 50% relaxation. Care must be exercised to use only the heel of the hand, to keep it in the middle of the chest, and not to let the fingers touch or press on the chest. The other rescuer keeps the head extended at all times and continues artificial respiration.

FIVE RULES OF FIVE

(1) **Start immediately**—always in less than ❺ minutes. The brain can survive without damage for only four to six minutes after breathing stops, only two to four minutes after circulation stops.

(2) Open the airway and inflate the lungs every ❺ seconds.

(3) After ❺ good breaths, if breathing does not resume, the pulse is absent and the pupils are dilated, begin external cardiac compression.

(4) For effective HEART-LUNG RESUSCITATION, inflate the lungs between each ❺ compressions.

(5) **Never** interrupt HEART-LUNG RESUSCITATION for more than ❺ seconds at any time.

Figure 12–3. (*Continued*)

Injuries [from the procedure itself] can be kept to an acceptable minimum if the resuscitator is trained to open the airway adequately, apply expired air ventilation, locate the correct pressure point for closed-chest manual heart compression (lower half of the sternum), and position himself to the side of the victim who should be on a solid surface. Pressure should be applied through the heel of the hand and the sternum pushed in toward the spine about 4 or 5 cm. in adults. The proper positioning of the hands over the correct pressure point reduces the likelihood of injuries. Successful resuscitation can be performed by one person giving both artificial ventilation and circulation, although two qualified persons are preferable. The risk of such complications is acceptably small and the anticipated benefits are great enough to warrant the prompt application of closed-chest cardiopulmonary resuscitation by well-trained individuals in instances of suspected cardiac arrest. Since it is estimated that irreversible changes to the central nervous system occur four to six minutes after cardiac arrest, resuscitation efforts must be begun promptly after the recognition of cardiac arrest.

The above statement was prepared by the American Heart Association. The nurse may learn this procedure through the American Red Cross, through her employer, through a local health agency or some other community resource.

SUMMARY

Anoxia has many causes. The nurse is in a position to assist her patient in many ways. She may perform cardiopulmonary resuscitation, she may help with transfusions, she may play a part in administering oxygen safely and skillfully, she may take nursing measures which help the patient to make his treatment as beneficial and comfortable as possible. Whatever her role may be, it is an important one.

SUGGESTED READINGS

Heart Attack. American Heart Association, 44 East 23rd Street, New York, 10, New York, 1956.

Shafer, Kathleen Newton, et al.: *Medical-Surgical Nursing.* Ed. 3, St. Louis, C. V. Mosby Co., 1964, Chapters 18, 19 and 23.

Sutton, Audrey Latshaw: *Bedside Nursing Techniques.* Philadelphia, W. B. Saunders Co., 1964, Chapters 5, 6, 13, 14.

Wolff, Ilse S.: The Experience. *American Journal of Nursing.* November, 1964, p. C-3.

REFERENCES

American Heart Association. The Closed Chest Method of Cardio-Pulmonary Resuscitation—Revised Statement (Editorial). *Circulation,* May, 1965, p. 641.

Buschle, D. F., and Saklad, M.: Compatible Solution for Administration With Blood. *Anesthesiology,* January, 1953, p. 53.

Cahill, Dorothy: The Nurse's Role in Closed Chest Cardiac Resuscitation. *American Journal of Nursing,* March, 1965, p. 84.

Circular of Information for the Use of Whole Blood (Human) and Packed Red Blood Cells (Human) by Physicians. Prepared by the Committee on Standards of the American Association of Blood Banks, February, 1962.

Coe, Myrtle: Some Roles of Nursing in Cardiac Disease. *Nursing World*, February, 1956, p. 7.

Dorland, W. A. Newman: *American Pocket Medical Dictionary*. Ed. 20, Philadelphia, W. B. Saunders Co., p. A-39.

Fuerst, Elinor V., and Wolff, LuVerne: *Fundamentals of Nursing*. Ed. 3, Philadelphia, J. B. Lippincott Co., 1964.

Guest, Paul G.: Oily Fibers May Increase Oxygen Tent Fire Hazard. *Modern Hospital*, May, 1965, p. 180.

Hall, Lydia, and Alfano, Genrose: Incapacitation or Rehabilitation? *American Journal of Nursing*, November, 1964, p. C-20.

Hazeltine, Louise S.: The Weeks of Healing. *American Journal of Nursing*, November, 1964, p. C-14.

Kinlein, M. Lucille: The Critical Hours. *American Journal of Nursing*, November, 1964, p. C-10.

Leifer, Gloria: *Principles and Techniques in Pediatric Nursing*. Philadelphia, W. B. Saunders Co., 1965, Chapter 8.

Matheney, Ruth V., et al.: *Fundamentals of Patient-Centered Nursing*. St. Louis, C. V. Mosby Co., 1964, Chapter 17.

Nonflammable Medical Gas Systems 1962. NFPA No. 565, National Fire Protection Association, 60 Batterymarch Street, Boston, Massachusetts 02110.

Nuerenberg, David V.: *Guide to Inhalation Therapy Procedures*, ABC Oxygen Rental Service, Inc. 2438 27th Avenue, Minneapolis 6, Minnesota, 1966.

Sutton, Audrey Latshaw: *Bedside Nursing Techniques*. Philadelphia, W. B. Saunders Co., 1964, Chapters 5, 6, 13, 14.

Wood, Edwin C.: Understanding the Patient With Heart Disease. *Nursing Outlook*, February, 1959, p. 90.

13

Care of the Operative Patient

Advances in surgical techniques continue to provide many new avenues of treatment. Aside from making it possible to intervene surgically for formerly inoperable conditions, newer techniques and equipment make old surgical procedures more successful.

It is beyond the scope of this book to do anything but cite a few examples. We are familiar with the blood bank, but preservation of other organs continues to be perfected. Cornea transplants and kidney transplants are possible. Methods of preserving organs over longer periods of time are being developed.

The use of animal and synthetic organs is expanding. In the field of blood vessel surgery, teflon and nylon may be grafted in place of a diseased blood vessel. In the field of orthopedic surgery, specially treated bone of unborn calves is used for bone grafting in spinal fusions and reconstructive facial operations.

Cardiac surgery continues to become more successful with the combined use of artificial heart-lung machines and hypothermia machines. Certain types of congenital and acquired heart defects can be operated on because such equipment provides the surgeon with a "dry site."

New sutures and needles have aided the eye surgeon. The field of electronics is finding a place in the operating room. In all fields, surgical possibilities and successes increase daily.

The operative patient goes through six and sometimes seven phases. They are: the preparatory phase before admission to the hospital, the preoperative period after hospital admission, the operation itself, the awakening from the anesthetic, the postoperative and convalescent period which is often followed by a rehabilitation period. The nurse rarely has an opportunity to become involved in the preparatory phase. On the other hand, she can become more involved with convalescent care than she is at present. As more and more care is given in the home, the nurse in the hospital must become more concerned with convalescent and rehabilitative care.

PREPARATORY CARE

Preparatory care is mainly performed by the physician. He will describe what is to be done, the method of anesthetic administration, what the prognosis is likely to be and the length of time expected for hospitalization and return to normal activity. The physician's office personnel can help the patient with insurance information, what to take to the hospital and details of the day and time of admission.

Aside from information and instructions given by the physician, the patient will receive a host of other informational details from friends, relatives and neighbors. Some of this will be helpful, some will be misinformation, and some may be extremely discouraging. Some people seem to enjoy telling prospective patients a tale about an aunt who died from an anesthesia reaction and never even had her operation. Other kinds of "tips" and words of encouragement, however, are of real assistance. Nevertheless, even helpful advice can be misleading because of the difference between symptoms and reactions even of the same disease.

The patient also has his own fears, his personality reactions and his personal problems. As a result, the patient comes to the hospital with varying degrees of preparation by the physician, a mixture of tales from friends and his own personal characteristics. One of the nurse's first responsibilities is to ferret out the quality and quantity of information possessed by her patient so that she can best assist him. Chapters 7 and 8 also deal with this aspect of care.

THE HOSPITAL PREOPERATIVE PERIOD

Psychological Preparation

The nurse will have to attempt to evaluate the knowledge of her patient so that she can sit down with him and answer his questions, as well as tell him certain things about his postoperative period. If a patient is prepared for having certain symptoms after his surgery, he is less likely to become alarmed by them when they occur.

The patient will be having surgery performed on a particular anatomical system. He may be having orthopedic surgery, gastrointestinal surgery or brain surgery. The reason for the surgery may be to correct a congenital defect, to reduce the effect of an accident, to minimize degenerative changes or to remove a tumor which may be benign or malignant. It may have a restorative or incapacitating outcome. Whether the nurse is a graduate of yesterday or yesteryear, she can help the patient to know some of the things that will happen to him. Because the education of the nurse in the past emphasized procedures, the returning nurse tends to forget how much she can help her patient in ways that are completely unrelated to knowledge of procedures.

Her patient will want to know if he will have pain after surgery and what he can expect to have done for it. He will want to know when he can see his relatives. He will want to know when he can eat and that intravenous fluid is the usual method of replacing loss of fluid during surgery. He will need to know the importance of coughing, turning and early ambulation so that when he is asked to do these things when he is uncomfortable, he will better understand the reasons. He should also know ahead of time that he will at times be asked to care for himself postoperatively to prevent undue loss of strength.

The patient should know in advance whether he will go to a special care unit for a few days or return to his present room after the operation. Relatives should know these things also. The family needs to know where to wait for the doctor so that they can talk to him as soon as possible after surgery. The family should be informed of the approximate length of the operation so that undue worry is prevented. They also should be told whether the patient will stay in a recovery or post-anesthesia room until he is awake from his anesthesia. Patients stay in these areas for shorter periods because they awake sooner with many of the newer anesthetics.

The patient will also want to know how the anesthesia will be administered, by mask, vein or by spinal or local injection. The operating room can give the nurse this information if it is not written on the surgery schedule. At some institutions, the nurse anesthetist or the medical anesthesiologist visits the patient before and after surgery. In this case, the nurse is less responsible for this area of preparation.

The importance of preoperative instruction has been studied in several settings. In a study at Massachusetts General Hospital in Boston, two groups of patients were studied. One group was given special instructions before and after surgery by an anesthetist. The other group did not receive the instructions. The group of patients who received the preoperative instructions required about half as much pain-killing narcotics postoperatively as the other group. This study demonstrated the value of informing patients about postoperative pain, deep breathing, moving and methods of relaxation.

Throughout the preoperative period, the nurse who remains alert to the less obvious signals for help will serve her patients best. A patient may indicate, either directly or indirectly, a desire to see a clergyman. If the nurse senses this need, she will want to inquire whether this is his wish. He may wish to see his own clergyman or the hospital chaplain if there is one. The patient may express anxiety by muscle tremors, hyperactive reflexes, dilated pupils, wet palms, restlessness or rapid pulse. Some patients may not express their fears verbally and so the nurse must not dismiss silence as a lack of anxiety. All behavior is meaningful whether we completely understand it or not. Knowing this can help us to accept our patients even if we do not always have insight into the reasons for certain behavior.

Once the nurse has assessed her patient's individual requirements and given him opportunity to express himself, she is then ready to carry out some of the routine duties common to all patients who are to have surgery. Routines should be periodically examined to make sure that they best serve our patients in the light of present-day methods.

Physical Evaluation

The patient will need a recent physical examination and medical history to make sure that nothing has been overlooked. The physician may have done this in his office, asked an internist to do it, instructed the intern or resident to do it upon admission to the hospital or relied upon a combination of these methods.

The patient will also be required to have a current blood test and urinalysis. Other blood tests may also be requested by the physician. In most hospitals, a chest x-ray is taken either upon admission or just prior to admission. Other evaluative examinations may be required, such as an electrocardiogram, a metabolism test or other x-rays. Some authorities feel that the minimum preoperative laboratory and x-ray work on any preoperative patient over 50 years of age should be a complete blood count, a urinalysis, a chest x-ray, an electrocardiogram, a blood urea nitrogen and a fasting blood sugar.

Either the nurse or the physician will be responsible for inquiring whether the patient has any allergies. In any case the person giving the anesthesia will want to know what they are and how they are manifested. If a patient is allergic to codeine or has asthma, one can readily see that both pieces of information will be vital to his care. The anesthesiologist will also want to know if the patient has had any cortisone during the past six months, as this may affect the patient's reaction to anesthesia.

The nurse will be expected to take the patient's temperature, pulse, respirations and blood pressure. She will weigh the patient and measure his height. She will also make subjective observations and record them. All these evaluation tools will contribute to a physical picture of the patient which will determine his readiness for surgery.

Physical Preparation

Physical preparation of the patient will include preparation of the operative site. This might include a shave, a scrub with a bacteriostatic solution, an internal douche, an enema, eye drops, special baths or any number of other things which will reduce the possibility of infection of the operative area. If the physician does not specifically order what he wants for each patient, the hospital will provide written guides which personnel can follow. Operative skin preps may be done by station personnel or operating room personnel. Assignment of this task varies among hospitals.

With rare exceptions, the patient going to the operating room will not be allowed to have any food or fluid for 8 to 12 hours before the operation. It is imperative that the room or bed be labeled so that water and fluids are not inadvertently given to the patient. Even when the patient knows he is not to eat or drink, he may momentarily forget and accept something.

The physician may request that an indwelling catheter be inserted prior to surgery. If not, the patient should be asked to void before his medication is given.

The patient will usually be given some type of preoperative medication to make him tranquil, to diminish pain, to suppress respiratory secretions and to prevent central nervous system irritation. Older patients usually receive about half the usual dose. It is important that preoperative medications be given far enough in advance of the administration of the anesthetic. When sedation is given an hour ahead of time, it has had an opportunity to relax the patient and has taken effect so that the anesthetist knows the patient's reaction to the drug. If such a medication is given only about 15 minutes ahead of time, the sedation takes full effect after the anesthesia has been administered.

Legal Aspects of Surgical Preparation

John F. Horty, Director of the Health Law Center of the University of Pittsburgh, stated in a talk that the law defines negligence as a failure to use due care. Because standards change with advanced knowledge, due care may be defined differently every decade. If the nurse does not read the label on the medicine bottle before she gives it, she is not using due care. Basically, the law is stating that sound reasonable policies and procedures are carried out to the best of everyone's ability at a certain point in time.

The patient must first of all be properly identified. He should have some identification on his person, such as a bracelet which is usually applied to the wrist but may be applied to the ankle if necessary. Careful identification of patients when they enter the operating room is important to prevent any confusion between patients.

The operative permit must be signed by the patient, parent or guardian. This must be done before the patient has received any sedation so that there can be no possibility of the patient signing it when he is not completely clear mentally. In the case of sterilization, a special permit is usually used instead of the operative permit.

While a hospital can rarely be held liable for the loss of personal property and valuables, it does have a responsibility for careful handling of certain types of property. The patient should not expect the hospital to protect him from loss of expensive jewels, furs and large sums of money. However, when the patient has a small amount of money at his bedside, a watch, wedding ring and perhaps eyeglasses and dentures, the nursing staff should make every effort to protect these articles from loss or breakage.

When a patient goes to surgery, his dentures or bridgework should be placed in a denture box which is placed in his drawer and labeled with his name. Eyeglasses or contact lenses should be placed in a case or box and also placed in the patient's drawer. Watch, rings and billfold should be either locked in the safe or placed in a locked area at the nurses' station while the patient is out of his room and until he is awake.

NURSING CARE DURING THE OPERATION

The operating room nurse performs a rather unique function. She has technical, administrative and teaching responsibilities. They center on maintaining a safe environment, providing up-to-date equipment in good working order, observing good surgical techniques and procedures and maintaining a schedule which utilizes many types of personnel to the greatest benefit to the patient.

Direct contact with the patient who is awake is usually limited. She may or may not go to the patient's room before the operation to talk to him. In most cases, however, the nurse will meet the patient in the operating room, talk to him briefly and check the patient's name and surgical procedure for identification purposes.

Student education in the operating room has changed greatly. Emphasis is no longer on learning skills and procedures. In some programs, the operating room is by-passed completely as a practice area for students. In such programs, the student will observe surgical procedures which are selected for particular objectives related to a particular course. She will learn principles of asepsis. In some programs, the student will follow a patient from his admission, through his operative procedure, through his postanesthetic period and into his postoperative period. The continuity of such learning is beneficial in patient teaching.

The operating room technician is frequently used to assist the surgical nurse. This technician has had a formal or informal course in operating room technique. He or she scrubs for physicians and often circulates for cases of varying degrees of complexity, depending upon the person's ability and length of training. In most operating rooms, the registered nurse is used for administration of the surgery suite and to circulate in rooms where the most judgment and knowledge is required.

THE ANESTHESIA RECOVERY PERIOD

Because the immediate postoperative period is a precarious one for the patient, most hospitals provide a room where the patient can receive constant attention and where emergency equipment is located. Such an area is usually referred to as the recovery room or the post-anesthesia room (P.A.R.).

Initially, operating room personnel must report the nature of the operation performed, the anesthetic agent used, any unusual occurrences during the operation, the presence and position of any tubes and the general condition of the patient. Side rails should be in place, and the patient should be covered with a cotton blanket.

The patient will be positioned so that his breathing will not be obstructed. An "airway" or breathing tube may be used to keep the patient's tongue from blocking his air passage. He should be placed on his side or on his back with his head turned to one side to prevent secretions or emesis from flowing back into the throat. Newer anesthetics make the latter less common than in the past. Gentle throat suctioning may be necessary.

The pulse, respirations and blood pressure will be taken every ten to 15 minutes until they stabilize. They will then be taken every 30 minutes until the patient awakens. It is important to remember that the patient may respond to certain signs and signals even though he is not totally cognizant of his surroundings.

Some patients recall being in a P.A.R. while others do not. For this reason, personnel in these areas must refrain from confidential or "chatty" conversations. Because it is impossible to know the exact level of consciousness of a patient, it is common to find a patient remembering a comment we were unaware that he heard. On the other hand, a patient may repeatedly ask a question indicating he had not understood our answer.

All tubing should be connected to an appropriate suction unless otherwise ordered. It is vital that the nurse watch for kinks in tubing and note the color and amount of all drainage. Urine bags must be noted to make sure of kidney function. Intravenous fluids should be checked for the rate of flow, possible infiltration and possible pressure from the arm board.

The operative site should be checked frequently to make sure there is not excessive bleeding or drainage. Vital signs will serve as a clue to internal hemorrhage.

As patients begin to awaken, they are likely to complain of three things: thirst, backache and being cold. Placing a cotton bath blanket next to the patient's skin will help to provide warmth. To prevent thirst while oral fluids are still being withheld, he may wish to suck a gauze square moistened in cold water. The backache usually comes from being on his back for several hours, and a back rub is greatly appreciated at this time.

During the period of recovery from anesthesia, the nurse must remain with the patient. She must take his vital signs frequently, maintain an open airway, observe his color and observe his general condition. She will also be concerned with any dressings, drainage, intravenous fluid absorption and output. In addition, she will be concerned with his safety and general comfort. Because many possible complications may occur during this period, the nurse will want to report untoward symptoms to the physician immediately.

POSTOPERATIVE CARE

When the patient returns to his room or to the special care unit, he will need continued vigilance and good general nursing care. He will need reassurance and carry-over of the elements discussed during his preoperative care.

Nurses have a tendency either to rely on pain medication too much or to feel they should give it sparingly. Individual considerations are vital. We should not wait until the patient's pain becomes too severe. When a patient experiences pain, he will need reassurance and nursing measures which will relax him such as a change of position and a back rub. These measures are helpful, but a recent operative patient will probably need medication also. It is imperative that the nurse give the medication p.r.n. within a three- or four-hour period. Pain medication can usually be given 30 minutes before the stated interval if nursing measures are not successful. If medication helps the patient for less than three hours, the physician should be notified. He may wish to check the patient for a possible complication or wish to order a different medication.

Patients will need to be turned and coughed every two to four hours. Support of the edge of the operative site will make it less uncomfortable for him when he coughs. These measures help to prevent contractures, decubitus ulcers, hypostatic pneumonia and blood clots. Early ambulation and deep breathing also contribute to the reduced number of postoperative complications.

It is important that the patient have an adequate nutritional intake postoperatively. Intravenous electrolytes and fluids will supplant oral intake during this period whenever necessary. Intake and output is usually measured the first 48 hours after major surgery and/or the administration of general anesthesia.

Signs of the return of urinary and gastrointestinal functions are observed and recorded. Gas pains and distention are frequent postoperative discomforts caused by slow peristalsis. A rectal tube is sometimes inserted to relieve these symptoms if flatus is not being passed spontaneously. Elimination will be noted. The physician will want to know if the patient will need enemas or cathartics. This usually becomes apparent about the third postoperative day. If the patient does not have an indwelling catheter, the frequency and quantity of his voidings should be noted along with a description of the urine.

Dressings must be checked at least once every shift and more often the first day and whenever there is drainage. The nurse will need to know if she may change dressings or merely reinforce them. If a cast is applied, it should remain uncovered until it is dry. If a cast or a circular bandage has been applied, the area beyond it must be checked for swelling, numbness, cold, cyanosis and motion. When such symptoms are present, the part should be elevated, if possible, and the doctor should be notified. The odor of all wound areas should also be noted and reported.

Throughout all phases of the patient's care, accurate recording and description of the patient's condition is essential. The nurse who gears her charting to the individuality and condition of her particular patient will provide a record which is helpful in planning his care.

CONVALESCENCE

I prefer to think of convalescence as the period beginning with the less acute postoperative condition in the hospital and extending to the return of normal activity or the beginning of a rehabilitation program, if there is to be one. The reason for this preference is that it brings the hospital nurse home with the patient mentally. It helps the nurse to realize that she has responsibility for home care even though she does not go home with her patient.

An essential part of the patient's postoperative care is that of preparing him for any rehabilitative aspects of his future during his convalescence. This is obviously related to his age, diagnosis and degree of impairment. Rehabilitative activities may range from the mere readjustment to normal activity after an appendectomy to a totally new physical and vocational alteration of someone undergoing an arm amputation.

The hospital nurse is responsible for helping the patient to prepare for home care and rehabilitation even though she will not be directly involved. The patient will leave the hospital long before these things are completed.

Most patients will require activities which will help them to convalesce as rapidly as possible. They will need to walk and move around so that they minimize loss of strength other than that lost as a result of their surgery. They will need to help themselves as much as their condition permits. Something between inactivity and overactivity is needed for the convalescing postoperative patient.

The patient will need to know if he can bathe or shower when he goes home. He will need to know if he should change his dressings at home. If so, he should be shown how to place a soiled dressing in a paper bag, when his hands should be washed and how to apply clean dressings. He must also know when to return to his physician's office, and he should be instructed about his diet and any medications he takes home.

The nurse will want to know if the patient has family or friends who will be able to help him. In some cases, these persons will need instructions also. It is helpful to ask yourself the following questions while you are giving home-going instructions, "Can this patient carry out the instructions I am giving him? If not, what arrangements can be made to permit him to do so in order that his recovery period be as short as possible?"

REHABILITATION

A chapter has been devoted to this subject, but it is necessary to at least mention it in relation to surgery. Many patients have permanent changes in their lives as a result of an operation.

The patient having a colostomy or ileostomy needs a great deal of instruction both in the hospital and after he has returned home. He will find that he has many questions which did not occur to him while he was hospitalized. Therefore, he needs the name of a public health agency or some other follow-up facility. In larger metropolitan areas, colostomy clubs exist. Such clubs are composed of patients who get together to help one another and to share their experiences. Many times club members visit patients preoperatively. Such a group usually has the support and guidance of one or more physicians. In areas where such groups do not exist, the physician or public health nurse may know of patients who are willing to assist one another.

Aside from patient groups, the physician and nurse may want to refer patients to a public health nursing agency, a vocational counseling organization or a rehabilitation clinic appropriate to the particular need. A social agency might be needed to coordinate referrals or be instrumental in assisting the patient both financially and psychologically.

SUMMARY

The nurse admits her patient. He may have a minor or a major problem. He enters the hospital with a certain amount of accurate information, a few misconceptions and many fears and questions. His background and condition will help to determine the quantity and type of assistance given. She helps him through the various phases of his hospitalization. The anticipatory period with varying degrees of anxiety, the period of total dependence, the period of increasing independence and the return to maximal activity each require different knowledge and skills and contribute to the patient's ultimate recovery. At discharge, the nurse no longer has direct responsibility for her patient, but what happens to him may be directly related to the preparation she did or did not give him while he was still in her charge.

SUGGESTED READINGS

Matheney, Ruth V.: *Fundamentals of Patient-Centered Nursing.* St. Louis, C. V. Mosby Co., 1964, Chapter 8.

Scully, Harold F., and Martin, Stevens J.: Anesthetic Management for Geriatric Patients. *American Journal of Nursing,* February, 1965, p. 110.

Shafer, Kathleen Newton et al.: *Medical-Surgical Nursing.* St. Louis, C. V. Mosby Co., 1964, Chapters 7, 12, 13, 14 and 36.

Sutton, Audrey Latshaw: *Bedside Nursing Techniques.* Philadelphia, W. B. Saunders Co., 1964, Chapters 9 and 10.

REFERENCES

Bonnel, P.: Understanding Surgical Patients. *American Journal of Nursing,* August, 1959, p. 1148.

Collins, Jo Anne K.: Care of the Colostomy Patient. *Nursing World,* March, 1960, p. 24.

Egbert, L. D., et al.: Reduction of Postoperative Pain by Encouragement and Instruction of Patients. *New England Journal of Medicine,* Vol. 270, No. 16, p. 825, April, 1964.

Gardner, Warren: They Will Talk Again. *Nursing Outlook,* June, 1954, p. 314.

Hallinger, Paul, Johnson, Kenneth C., Mansueta, Mario, and Jameson, Carmen: Cancer of Larynx. *American Journal of Nursing,* June, 1957, p. 738.

Horty, John F.: *Legal Implications of Providing Hospital Services.* Speech given in Minneapolis, Upper Midwest Hospital Conference, May 12, 1965.

Keane, Claire Brackman: *Essentials of Nursing.* Philadelphia, W. B. Saunders Co., 1964, Chapters 5 and 8.

Leithauser, D.: Early Ambulation. *American Journal of Nursing,* April, 1950, p. 203.

Matheney, Ruth V.: *Fundamentals of Patient-Centered Nursing.* St. Louis, C. V. Mosby Co., 1964, Chapter 8.

Owens, Evelyn: From One O.R. Nurse to Another. *American Journal of Nursing,* February, 1963, p. 106.

Parrott, John: Nursing Care of the Endarterectomy Patient. Lecture given at St. Barnabas Hospital, Minneapolis, October 9, 1964.

Scully, Harold F., and Martin, Stevens J.: Anesthetic Management for Geriatric Patients. *American Journal of Nursing,* February, 1965, p. 110.

Shafer, Kathleen Newton, et al.: *Medical-Surgical Nursing,* St. Louis, C. V. Mosby Co., 1964, Chapters 7, 12, 13, 14 and 36.

Sholtis, L.: Nursing the Elderly Surgical Patient. *American Journal of Nursing,* December, 1951, p. 1256.

Skinner, John F.: The Cardiac Patient as a Surgical Risk. *Hospital Medicine,* May, 1965, p. 7.

Squibb Company, *Boplant.* October, 1964.

Young, Lucie S.: O.R. Experience for Students. *Nursing Outlook,* December, 1964, p. 47.

SPECIALIZED TEXTBOOKS

Bordicks, K. J.: *Nursing Care of Patients Having Chest Surgery*. New York, Macmillan Co., 1963.

Davis, David M., and Warren, Kenneth C.: *Urological Nursing*. Ed. 6, Philadelphia, W. B. Saunders Co., 1959.

Hooper, Reginald: *Neurosurgical Nursing*. Springfield, Ill., Charles C Thomas, 1964.

Peddie G., and Brush, F.: *Cardio-Vascular Surgery—A Manual for Nurses*. New York, G. P. Putnam's Sons, 1961.

Wiebe, Anne E.: *Orthopedics in Nursing*. Philadelphia, W. B. Saunders Co., 1961.

14

Care of the Patient Needing Rehabilitation

"Medical rehabilitation is the clinical process by means of which the disabled person is restored to a state of optimal effectiveness and given an opportunity to enjoy a meaningful life."* There are many definitions of rehabilitation, but all of them either state or imply that there are three major facets of rehabilitation: prevention of further impairment, restoration of as much function as possible and the preservation of existing abilities in order that they may be used maximally. The emphasis of rehabilitation is on ability, not disability.

Neither the concept of rehabilitation nor the practice of rehabilitation is totally new, but the emphasis, the body of knowledge and the need for broader application become greater every day. Physical medicine and rehabilitation has been a rather isolated branch of medical and nursing education for too long. Because rehabilitation concepts and techniques can be incorporated into the care of a majority of patients, it is at last finding a place in the basic education of both medical and nursing students. As our life span lengthens, our population will contain a greater percentage of older citizens. As more acute illnesses are either prevented or successfully treated, the amount of chronic disease will continue to rise. It is, therefore, up to every nurse who will be working with patients to have some concept of the goals of rehabilitation, the roles of the many persons who may be involved and a general acquaintance with the nursing role in particular.

POSSIBLE MEMBERS OF A REHABILITATION TEAM

The principal reason for incorporating rehabilitation into general medical and nursing education is that there are degrees of patient need.

*Hirschberg, Gerald G., Lewis, Leon, and Thomas, Dorothy: *Rehabilitation*. Philadelphia, J. B. Lippincott Co., 1964, p. 6.

It is not necessary to send every patient in need of rehabilitation to a specialized center, nor does every hospital need such facilities. When the need exists, the patient should naturally be sent to an area where all possible facilities and personnel are available to him, but many patients can be helped in less specialized surroundings if personnel are adequately educated. It is also true that the amount of time required for rehabilitation of a patient can be greatly reduced if personnel caring for him during his acute illness are properly instructed.

In order to give the refresher an idea of the number of facets of rehabilitation, it might be helpful to know who conceivably might participate in the care of a person needing it. No one patient will need all services, but a rehabilitation center makes these services available because all their patients will need more than one service. This is a truly multidisciplined patient service requiring the team approach.

The primary and most important member of the team is the patient. From the beginning of his accident or illness, he needs to become involved in helping the other team members to understand his goals and disappointments and in planning and learning some of the steps in achieving the greatest possible restoration of abilities.

Possible members of a rehabilitation team, besides a doctor and a nurse, are: a social worker, a physical therapist, an occupational therapist, a speech therapist, a psychologist, a minister, a vocational counselor, an engineer, an orthotist (maker of braces, splints and self-help devices), a prosthetist (maker of artificial parts for the body) and a teacher. A variety of medical specialists may be used: the physiatrist, the psychiatrist, the internist, the orthopedic surgeon, the neurologist, the obstetrician, etc. The physiatrist usually functions as the team leader, so to speak.

When a patient first enters into a rehabilitation program, an evaluation of his condition and potential needs is made. A current research study is concerned with the problem of locating predictors concerning the outcome of a rehabilitation program for patients with cardiovascular disease. The evaluation of the patient not only includes obvious things, such as an adequate history (social, physical and psychological) and physical examination to determine the exact amount of incapacitation, but also includes vocational studies if the patient is not likely to be able to pursue his present occupation, psychometric studies for aptitude and intelligence if indicated, and psychological tests if a need for psychological treatment or support seems especially indicated. Some authorities say that as many as 50 per cent of their patients never obtain maximum use of their abilities for psychological reasons, so that help in this area may be vital.

Paramedical services are selected after the initial evaluation of the individual patient has been completed. Realistic goals must be set for each patient. Employment counseling is obviously going to be of little benefit to a 75-year-old hemiplegic, but it may be a primary need for a

35-year-old hemiplegic. The amount of brain damage in terms of mental functions must also be taken into consideration in the selection of rehabilitation goals. For elderly persons, the ability to care for themselves physically may be the very thing which will permit them to live in dignity. In other words, goals are matched to the patient's predicted future. They must be re-evaluated at intervals so that the goal can be changed according to the patient's progress, his psychological readiness, any alteration in the course of his disease or impairment and any other new factors which may arise.

The nurse is in a rather strategic position in rehabilitation work. She often becomes the coordinator of the many services which converge on the patient. She is the one person who sees him 24 hours a day and is the only one who can provide the crucial element of continuity. Her observations may not only be a determinant for certain aspects of treatment, but her nursing care is frequently an adjunct to other care. For example, she will give her patient an opportunity to practice some of the things he has learned from a speech therapist. She will want to position her patient so that physical therapy aims are fostered. The role of the nurse as a rehabilitation coordinator is not just an administrative role: it is a direct patient care role requiring a great deal of information.

DISEASES WHICH MAY REQUIRE REHABILITATION

Strictly speaking, every patient can be said to have need for rehabilitation. Be that as it may, the conditions which are listed here are the ones which require some kind of rehabilitation program, even if it is informally planned, requiring only a few disciplines, or of a relatively short duration.

Poliomyelitis once accounted for a large number of adults and children requiring rehabilitation. One of the most exciting examples of modern medical achievement is the development of the Salk and Sabin vaccines which reduced the incidence of poliomyelitis over 97 per cent in only a few years. The major case load of patients requiring rehabilitation as a result of this disease are follow-up polio victims who contracted the disease before the vaccines were developed.

Patients with cardiovascular disease, particularly those having had a stroke or a heart condition require a program of rehabilitation. Patients who have suffered strokes will need training in ambulation, self-care, possible speech training and vocational evaluation to see whether their occupation is compatible with their condition. In the case of patients with heart disease, a slow, steady increase of physical activity is planned and observed after a period of rest is prescribed by their physician. Cardiac work-up programs are becoming as common as teaching the stroke victim how to get in and out of a wheel chair.

A metabolic disorder such as arthritis, hematologic diseases such as purpura, hemophilia and polycythemia vera, poison victims and such conditions as osteoporosis and osteomalacia can all benefit from physical therapy. Patients with muscular, neurological and neuromuscular diseases require continued care. Diseases such as multiple sclerosis involve remissions and exacerbations so that rehabilitation goals must alter with the condition of the patient.

Patients with spinal cord disease or injury, such as the paraplegic and quadriplegic, require intensive rehabilitation programs because their lives are altered drastically. Surgical patients who have had a mastectomy, thoracic surgery or a laryngectomy will require special help. The patient who has had a laryngectomy will need speech assistance and the patient who has had a mastectomy or thoracic surgery will require special breathing and shoulder joint exercises. Patients who have had fractures or burns will need to know the best methods of regaining the strength and function of a limb which has been immobilized over a period of time. Special programs are also necessary for amputees. In this area the Army Prosthetics Laboratory and the Navy Prosthetics Laboratory have done remarkable work using doctors and engineers in the development of artificial limbs which are more functional, more comfortable and more pleasing esthetically.

Further listing of conditions requiring rehabilitation programs would be fruitless. However, knowing the range of conditions which can benefit from rehabilitation measures makes it clear why it is so important that this field become integrated into all nursing care.

REHABILITATION NURSING

In an effort to liberate rehabilitation nursing from the isolation of specialization, a recent course for freshman nursing students was called "Basic Nursing Care." Elements of rehabilitation nursing are basic to the care of all patients. One of these aspects has already been dealt with in Chapter 11, "Care of the Patient's Skin." Another facet was discussed in Chapter 8, "Teaching Today's Patient." Certain aspects of basic nursing care, however, are required in more depth for the patient who will require a rehabilitation program.

Bed Rest and Deterioration

"Look at a patient lying long in bed. What a pathetic picture he makes! The blood clotting in his veins, the lime draining from his bones, the scybala stacking up in his colon, the flesh rotting from his seat, the urine leaking from his distended bladder, and the spirit evaporating from his soul."* The author of this graphic picture is describing the

*Asher, R. A. J.: Dangers of Going to Bed. *British Medical Journal*, December 13, 1947, p. 967.

evils of an "overdose" of bed rest, deterioration caused by bed rest, not disease. The nurse has an important role to play in preventing many of these side-effects.

Psychological reaction to bed rest may be that of depression or dependency. During an acute illness, dependency is normal and needed, but to have it persist into the chronic stage of an illness causes unhappiness on the part of the patient, frustration for his family and blocking of rehabilitation goals. Mental and psychological stimulation can help the patient as his disease passes beyond the acute phase.

Loss of muscle strength and mobility must be prevented. Because one part of the body must be immobilized does not mean that other parts need the same treatment. It takes longer for an injured part to heal than it does for a healthy part to deteriorate. Therefore, secondary deterioration unrelated to the disease needs to be prevented. The patient will need to exercise uninjured parts to prevent disuse atrophy.

Proper positioning of the body is vital. The patient must be kept in good body alignment while he is in bed. Pillows should be used discriminately. If a patient is sitting in bed with his head pushed forward by pillows, they should be removed and/or repositioned. Pillows under the knees can cause flexion contractures which are completely unrelated to the patient's condition. In one study, it was found that it took 52 days to regain full range of motion of a limb which had been immobilized for seven days, and 300 days for a limb which had been immobilized for only 21 days.

Proper positioning requires the use of certain accessory equipment. This might include a felt or firm innerspring mattress, a footboard and half rails used by the patient for controlling movements. When a footboard is used, there should be space between it and the end of the mattress so that the patient's heels are not resting on the mattress. If a footboard is not used, top bed linen should be loose to prevent foot drop. Bed boards may also be placed under the mattress to obtain additional firmness to help support the spine and to make moving on a bed easier for the patient. Hand rolls, pillows and trochanter rolls may also help prevent external rotation of the hip, internal rotation of the arm or clawlike hand positions.

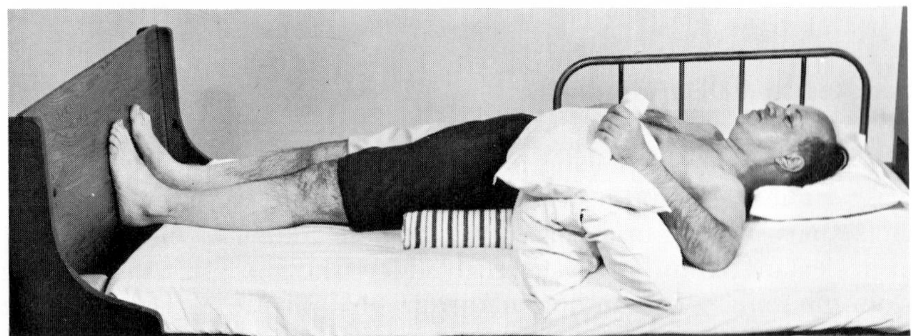

Figure 14–1. *Footboard for patient's bed. (Courtesy American Rehabilitation Foundation, 1800 Chicago Ave., Minneapolis, Minnesota 55404.)*

Lack of activity can also cause thrombophlebitis and hypostatic pneumonia. During bed rest greater amounts of nitrogen and calcium are excreted. The loss of nitrogen causes decubitus ulcers which have already been discussed. Calcium is lost from the bone matrix which goes eventually to the kidneys where calcium salts form kidney stones. The loss of calcium can also make patients prone to pathological bone fractures. Positioning, good body alignment and frequent turning are all required to prevent adverse conditions caused by bedrest.

General Guides for Moving Patients

GOOD BODY MECHANICS. Certain basic rules of good body mechanics can prevent injury to personnel. Working with patients who have diminished strength and mobility requires the use of guides which can be adapted to the individual patient and circumstance. Efficient use of the body in stooping, lifting, carrying, pushing, pulling and reaching can prevent fatigue as well as injury and strain. Key points are:

1. Stand close to the object which is to be moved.
2. Stand with feet apart with one foot slightly ahead of the other in order to provide a broad base of support and balance.
3. Keep back as straight as possible and bend hips and knees when stooping to lift or replace an object.
4. Keep the load as close to the body as possible.
5. Avoid any twisting of the body or spine.
6. If an object can be pulled, it is generally preferable to pushing it.

PATIENT COMFORT. There are certain points to be utilized in order to give the patient maximum comfort when he is being moved. Key points are:

1. Grasp an extremity at the joint if the patient has muscle pain.
2. Grasp an extremity above or below the joint if the patient has joint pain.
3. Do not allow hands to rest on a pressure area or incision.
4. Whenever a patient cannot help himself to turn and move, use a folded sheet placed from the shoulders to below the knees to change his position.
5. Whenever more than one person assists the patient to move, simultaneous motion is required for patient comfort. Counting "one, two, move" is a helpful method of accomplishing this.
6. When a patient is being moved up in bed, make sure that the arms are crossed over the chest.
7. If a leg is paralyzed, make sure that it is properly supported during any movement. In some instances, it may be crossed at the ankle on top of the good leg.
8. Be careful not to bump the patient's feet or head when lifting him up or down in the bed.

9. Instruct the patient to lift his head when he is being raised or lowered in bed in order to increase the ease and comfort of the movement.
10. In the case of hemiplegia, the patient can be positioned on his back, his stomach and his good side.

Passive Range of Motion

Range of motion is the extent of motion within a given joint. In order to prevent unnecessary loss of range, certain exercises may be indicated. If the patient is able, he should be encouraged to do certain exercises himself. If this is impossible, the nurse or physical therapist must exercise the patient, so to speak. In this case, it is called passive range of motion (P.R.O.M.).

The nurse will usually require a physician's order to do passive range of motion for her patients. When she receives the order, she will be concerned with the joints of the shoulder, the elbow, the wrist, the fingers, the hip, the knee, the ankle and the toes. For a detailed description of exercise of each joint, the reader is referred to *Rehabilitative Nursing Techniques*, booklet No. 3, published by the American Rehabilitation Foundation in Minneapolis.

There are several general concepts of passive range of motion which are needed by the nurse before she learns the mechanics of the procedure. The nurse must remember to use good body mechanics to prevent fatigue. For most exercises, the patient is in the supine position, preferably using no pillows. It is important to have the patient close to the edge of the bed on the side on which the nurse is working. The patient's clothing should be kept from restricting any motions.

Extremities are usually supported and held at the joint, except for patients with arthritis. All movements should be made slowly and smoothly and should not exceed the patient's existing range of motion. In other words, these are not stretching exercises. Movements must be kept within a pain-free range and are usually done three times a day.

Bowel and Bladder Training for Hemiplegics

Whenever possible, bladder training is preferred to the use of a catheter. It reduces the possibility of infection and helps the patient's morale. After removal of the catheter, the patient is initially placed on a commode or bedpan every two hours during the day and every four hours during the night. Bedding or clothing is protected whenever there is any leakage of urine. Fluids are often reduced during initial training and omitted after supper. The length of time between voidings is increased until a satisfactory regular interval has been established.

Bowel training also is accomplished by establishing a regular hour, usually right after breakfast. The patient may be taught to insert a glycerin suppository or a similar aid about 30 minutes before evacuation. Patients must be checked for fecal impaction whenever results are inadequate. The success of a bowel and bladder training program is very important to the patient's sense of dignity.

Psychological Consideration

Although the social worker, psychologist or psychiatrist, occupational therapist and vocational counselor are responsible for psychosocial aspects of patient care, the nurse also has a part to play. She must encourage patients to relinquish unhealthy adjustments to disabilities. The patient may well be anxious and depressed. Some may have accompanying brain damage. Some patients will deny the implications of their disease for the future or react by withdrawing or becoming unmotivated and disinterested in their rehabilitation program.

The delicate balance of dependence and independence is especially critical for the handicapped person. Too much help can affect unfavorably his sense of worth just as too little help can increase his feeling of dependence. Many patients express the hope that friends and family will not help them unless they ask to be helped. This is important to know and to work out with the family. It points out the reason for teaching as many tools for independent living as possible.

Some patients reach higher degrees of rehabilitation success when they are in their home setting. For this reason, it is important that nursing personnel observe the effect of visits by relatives. This may give clues about the potential success of early home care as opposed to a longer period of institutional care.

Rehabilitation units should provide as homelike an atmosphere as possible. Patients should be dressed, well-groomed and not allowed to remain in bed so that they do not "feel sick." Sitting rooms and dining rooms are important parts of such units. Patients need the stimulation of activity, social interchange and recreation. This can prevent frequent dozing, which may come from boredom and is likely to interfere with adequate night-time rest.

It is also important for the nurse to know that certain conditions, such as hemiplegia, can cause mood swings which are physical in nature rather than psychological. The nurse will be challenged by her role in helping patients to assume as much normalcy as possible. She will need to listen carefully to her patient, as he may indicate a need or desire to talk to a clergyman or psychiatrist or express some other wish. Her responsiveness to his needs can greatly influence his ultimate acceptance and adjustment.

Teaching Activities of Daily Living (A.D.L.)

Exercise, massage, heat, gait training, braces, feeding devices and

GREATER NEW YORK INTERAGENCY REFERRAL FORM
Hospitals, Physician – Public Health Nursing and Other Health Agencies

A. 1. From *General Hospital*

Address *555 Main Street*

Tel. No. *MA 5-2424* Ext. *7851*

Name *M. Smith, R. N.*

Service-Dept. *Private-Surgery*

Sun.-Nights call ______ Dept. ______ Ext. ______

2. To *Visiting Nurse Assoc.*

Address ______

Date of Referral *12/20/62*

3. Hosp. No. ______

Patient *John Doe* Sex *M* OPD No. ______

Birth Date *1908* SMWD Sep. SSD No. ______

Husb. or Father ______ Wife or Mother *Mary*

Address *200 State Street*

Floor *1st* Apt. *1A* Tel. *GE 1-2345*

Hosp. Adm. date *12/3/62* Disch. date *12/20/62*

Next appt. date *12/27/62* In Clinic (name) *Private – M. D.'s office*

D. of W. No. & Category ______

Report needed (date) ______

B. Medical diagnosis and prognosis: (Other significant medical factors)

Cancer of the Bladder. Surgery performed on 12/5/62. Cystostomy and ilso-bladder done.

Diabetes Mellitus—controlled.

Physician's Orders and Instructions: (Including bedrest, exercise, bathroom privileges, diet, etc.)

Cleanse distal suture line with H_2O_2 (peroxide) and apply dry sterile dressing daily for one week.

Vitamin B_{12} 1 cc (1000 micrograms) by intramuscular injection once weekly.

Diabetic diet.

Patient to be provided with (check)

Diet list ______ **Rx** ______ **Medication** ______ **Equipment and Supplies (specify)** ______

John Jones, M.D.

Signature of Physician

C. Report by Hospital Nurse, Physical Therapist, Dietitian, Occupational Therapist (Observations, results of teaching). Please add signature and title.

Mr. Doe was admitted to hospital knowing his diagnosis and aware of the surgery to be performed. He has adjusted quite well to the postoperative situation. He can care for his ileostomy bag and equipment but cannot cope with his dressings. The private physician will see the patient at home and in his office.

Mr. Doe's wife and two grown children are willing to cooperate in caring for him.

Figure 14–2. *Sample referral form. (From Wensley, Edith:* Nursing Service Without Walls. *National League for Nursing, 10 Columbus Circle, New York 19, N. Y. 1963.)*

D. Report of Medical Social Worker

Not known

Plans:

Date________________ **Signature**________________

E. Report by Public Health Nurse and/or other worker in community agency

The abdominal incision appears to be healing well. There is no longer any drainage from it and the nurse will now visit 3x weekly. Mr. Doe and his family have responded well to suggestions for interim care. He seems to be gaining strength and now spends more time ambulating about house and is assuming more self-care responsibility.

Nutrition and dietary advice given were well received and the family are now interested in further help from nutritionist.

The family relationships are close and the atmosphere seems conducive to a good surgical recovery and adjustment to Mr. Doe's limitations.

Plans: *Nurse will continue to visit three times weekly until incision is healed. Injection is given as directed once weekly.*

S. Brown, PHN

Agency *Visiting Nurse Assoc. of Brooklyn* **Signature /s/** *Sally Brown*

Address *894 Flatbush Avenue, Brooklyn* **Date** *January 18, 1963* **Tel. No.** *IN 2-2710*

Figure 14–2. *(Continued)*

other forms of therapy and assistance all become meaningful when the patient becomes able to comb his hair, feed himself, transfer himself in and out of a wheel chair, bathe himself, earn a living and carry on the many activities of daily living which we take for granted and do automatically. The nurse on the rehabilitation station or in the hospital and the public health nurse are in a unique position to see how much activity is performed by the patient independently and to know how much and what kind of assistance he requires.

The nurse will teach and help patients to practice these activities. Rehabilitation nursing does not consist of "doing" things "for" patients. The nurse must consciously restrain herself from assisting the patient in anything but to help himself except when physical limitations interfere or learning is still taking place. If a patient is well motivated, he often can do things which authorities find almost unbelievable based on physical findings alone.

Follow-up of Patients

Follow-up of patients who are sent home from a rehabilitation program is vital. Many studies indicate that patients regress in their level of achievement. Much regression could be prevented by follow-up guidance in dealing with problems encountered early in their arrival home. Patients may be asked to do things which are impossible because of the physical setup of their homes. They may receive the wrong kind of help or lack help from their family because of poor understanding of goals or unreal aspirations concerning rehabilitation. The practice of spending weekends at home with family involvement while the patient is still hospitalized tends to reduce the number of these problems. Vocational problems may arise. Any number of unforeseen complications may occur. Follow-up for re-evaluation at regular intervals is necessary if a rehabilitation program is to be considered complete.

In order to make follow-up possible, there must be some form of communication between the institution and the public health agency. The person who follows up the patient after discharge must have a clear picture of the patient's abilities, motivations and needs at the time of discharge. She must know the goals of the rehabilitation program for the particular patient or she will have nothing with which to compare her evaluation of the patient's progress. She will need to know many details in order to play an effective part in the patient's continued achievements. Communication between hospital and home can be done in writing, by telephone, by conference, by having the public health nurse visit the patient in the hospital or by having the hospital nurse visit the patient in his home. The method of communication is far less important than the content of communication.

SUMMARY

Although rehabilitative techniques and treatments are not new, they are being better integrated into all types of care and more widely used because of the increase in chronic disease and the greater number of older citizens. Once a patient is evaluated for speech, hearing, vision, mental activity, physical potential and other pertinent aspects concerning his future, members of his health team are selected on the basis of his needs. For most patients, rehabilitation programs are long. It is vital for the nurse to know her roles: that of teaching, coordination, support and prevention. The goal for all patients is "not to add years to life but to add life to one's years."

SUGGESTED READINGS

Fuerst, Elinor V., and Wolff, LuVerne: *Fundamentals of Nursing*. Ed. 3, Philadelphia, J. B. Lippincott Co., 1964, Unit 4.

Nayer, Dorothy D.: Skin Grafts: The Patient. *American Journal of Nursing*, November, 1964, p. 98.

Sutton, Audrey, L.: *Bedside Nursing Techniques*. Philadelphia, W. B. Saunders Co., 1964, Chapters 12 and 17.

See list of readings for patients at end of Chapter 8.

REFERENCES

Asher, R. A. J.: Dangers of Going to Bed. *British Medical Journal*, December 13, 1947, p. 967.

Fuerst, Elinor V., and Wolff, LuVerne: *Fundamentals of Nursing*. Ed. 3, Philadelphia, J. B. Lippincott Co., 1964, Unit 4.

Gregg, Dorothy: Anxiety—A Factor in Nursing Care. *American Journal of Nursing*, November, 1952, p. 1363.

Hirschberg, Gerald G., Lewis, Leon, and Thomas, Dorothy: *Rehabilitation*, Philadelphia, J. B. Lippincott Co., 1964.

Kessler, Henry H., and Kiessling, Edward A.: The Pneumatic Arm Prosthesis. *American Journal of Nursing*, June, 1965, p. 114.

Kottke, Frederic J., and Blanchard, Russell S.: Bedrest Begets Bedrest. *Nursing Forum*, Vol. 3, No. 3, p. 56, 1964.

Krusen, Frank H.: *Concepts in Rehabilitation of the Handicapped*. Philadelphia, W. B. Saunders Co., 1964.

McCown, Pauline P., and Wurm, Elizabeth: Orienting the Disoriented. *American Journal of Nursing*, April, 1965, p. 118.

McCulough, H., and Farnham, Mary: *Space and Design Requirements for Wheelchair Kitchens*. Agricultural Experiment Station Bulletin No. 661, Urbana, University of Illinois, 1960.

Niesenbaum, Leonard, Levenson, Carl, and Kimbel, Philip: Multidisciplinary Team in Special Unit Helps Rehabilitate Emphysema Patients. *Modern Hospital*, January, 1965, p. 91.

Nursing Outlook, A Community Hospital Rehabilitation Unit (Editorial). February, 1965, p. 40.

Park, Wilford E., and Moe, Mildred I.: Rehabilitation Care in Nursing Homes. *Public Health Reports*, July, 1960, p. 605.

Peterson, Jean C., and Olsen, Ann P.: *Language Problems After a Stroke*. Minneapolis, American Rehabilitation Foundation, 1965.

Preston, Tonie: Meeting the Needs of Nursing Home Residents. *Nursing Outlook*, December, 1964, p. 44.

Rehabilitative Nursing Techniques, American Rehabilitation Foundation, Minneapolis,
1. Bed Positioning Transfer Procedures for the Hemiplegic. 1962.
2. Selected Equipment Useful in the Hospital, Home or Nursing Home. 1962.
3. A Procedure for Passive Range of Motion and Self-Assistive Exercises. 1964.
4. Self-care and Homemaking for the Hemiplegic. 1964.

Rusk, Howard A.: *Rehabilitation Medicine*. Ed. 2, St. Louis, C. V. Mosby Co., 1964.

Schoening, Herbert, Hannan, Vivian, Plass, Jean and Fahland, Beverly: Basic Nursing Care. Telecourse Study Guide 1964-65, Channel 2, St. Paul, Minnesota.

Shafer, Kathleen N., et al.: *Medical-Surgical Nursing*, Ed. 3, Section 4, St. Louis, C. V. Mosby Co., 1964.

Sutton, Audrey L.: *Bedside Nursing Techniques*. Philadelphia, W. B. Saunders Co., 1964, pp. 802–808, Chapters 12 and 17.

Warshaw, Leon J., and Lembright, Katharine A.: The Cardiac in Industry. *American Journal of Nursing*, November, 1964, p. C-26.

15

Prevention of Hospital Infections

Unsafe bacterial contaminations in hospitals have been the subject of many articles in popular magazines and newspapers, but there is seldom reference to the continuous, active programs conducted by modern hospitals to combat the never-ending battle against nosocomial contamination. A nosocomial infection is defined as a hospital-acquired infection which may be caused by any number of microorganisms. The staphylococcus is the most widely known among laymen.

There are many reasons why hospitals have infection problems. Some are known and some are unknown. Protective and preventive procedures are based on what is known about nosocomial infections, the problems of eradication and the facilities available to an institution.

THE HOSPITAL AS A TREATMENT CENTER

The very nature of hospitals brings together a combination of factors that increases the possibility of infection. Patients who have an infection, are subject to infection or are debilitated are all under one roof. For example, a patient with severe pneumonia is likely to be admitted to a hospital just as is the patient with leukemia or severe anemia. This combination of patients obviously must be dealt with in the safest possible manner.

Many of us are incubating bacteria within our bodies. This is no problem to us nor is it likely to cause disease when we (or others) are in good health. Should we become ill or debilitated, such bacteria may become pathogenic and precipitate an infection. In such a case, we did not "catch the infection" out of the blue. Thus, bacteria may cause disease in one person and not in another.

One authority tells us, "When microorganism meets man, an infection is not inevitable. Whether or not an infection occurs depends upon a permutation and combination of factors in the invading microorganisms, the environment and the host."* In other words, the possibility of the occurrence of infection in a particular person is dependent upon his general physical condition, his environment and the organism itself. This statement suggests to us the need for careful handling of dressings, good isolation techniques, proper methods of handling excreta and soiled articles and adequacy of sterilization for the prevention of spread of infection. Good patient care then includes proper medical aseptic techniques on the part of all personnel caring for patients either directly or indirectly. Frequent hand washing cannot be overemphasized.

MUTATION

With the ever-increasing use of antibiotics and chemotherapeutic agents, bacteria are undergoing a continuous mutation. That is, the form and chemical composition differ from that of the original organism. Bacteriologists now see many mutants. A great number of these new strains are resistant to chemotherapeutic and antibiotic agents.

Because of this, the search for new products to combat bacterial disease is very prevalent today. There is a definite trend among physicians to be cautious in the use of antibiotics. In order to have an effective antibiotic available when a patient really needs one, physicians do not wish to prescribe one for every sore throat and cold. Before starting treatment (except in the case of severe infection), many physicians recommend that the organism be identified by culture and that a drug sensitivity test be run on the organism to determine which drug will be most effective in the treatment of a particular patient. There is often great pressure on physicians, however, to use antibiotics. The public knows they are available and is, therefore, critical whenever an antibiotic is not prescribed for an infection.

The most common organisms found in hospitals are gram-positive staphylococcus, fungus, virus and gram-negative organisms such as *Escherichia coli, Aerobacter aerogenes,* Pseudomonas, and Proteus. Although the staphylococcus organism is common, the other organisms are appearing more frequently than they did in the past. Thus, there is not only mutation of microorganisms, but there is also change in the types of organisms found.

In summary, the development of new strains of bacteria increases the need for new and more potent antibiotics and chemotherapeutic agents to stop further mutations.

CONCERNS OF INTERRELATED SERVICES

Architect and Builder

As more and more information about nosocomial infections becomes available, future hospitals can be planned and built to minimize

*Balsley, Marie: Study of Today's Changing Hospital Environment Shows New Directions for Infection Control. *Hospitals,* May 16, 1965, p. 19.

the possibility of spread of infection. Suitable work areas which separate the storage, delivery and pick-up of clean and used equipment can be built into an institution. Traffic patterns can be studied to prevent contaminated and clean equipment from traveling through the same corridors. Adequate numbers of hand washing facilities must be available. Every patient area and work area requires at least one hand washing facility. Foot pedal or knee-operated faucets are often used.

A few years ago, I was visited by a nurse from Calcutta. She was interested in an isolation procedure for a particular area in her 3000-bed hospital. This area had 50 patients and one wash basin at the end of the hall. Sometimes three or four of the patients had a contagious disease, and there were usually only two nurses on duty. Such a situation clearly demonstrates the need of adequate physical facilities for carrying out a safe and effective procedure.

A new approach in the prevention of infection is to build "maze" entry into vital areas such as the operating room, the delivery room and the nursery. This makes it possible to enter these areas only by going through a section with showers and dressing rooms where clothes must be changed.

Modern architectural plans usually provide for separate isolation rooms or units. Special work rooms are provided also.

Engineers continue to work on air control. Humidity and temperature can influence the life of organisms. Separate ventilation systems are often provided for the areas in which patients with infectious diseases are housed. This air usually goes directly out of the building rather than being recirculated into the total system. Special air exchange systems may be used for critical areas, such as nurseries, operating rooms and delivery rooms. Bacterial studies of air samples determine the success of these systems.

It is interesting to see how an engineering innovation can alter a nursing procedure. In the past, part of the terminal isolation procedure included airing the room for 24 hours after the discharge of a patient. If a hospital has an air exchange system, this is no longer necessary because the air in the room is exchanged every eight to ten minutes.

Multiple nurseries are often built on the obstetrics unit as a means of reducing the possibility of infection. Each nursery is smaller than usual, accommodating about 12 infants. In this way, nursery use can be rotated in order to allow cleaning at specified intervals. Even smaller nurseries for only two to four infants are sometimes built adjacent to the mothers' rooms.

The Laundry

Handling of soiled linen in the nursing areas is of vital concern to the overall picture of infection control. It is becoming increasingly important that linen be held away from the nurse's uniform and that it be bagged on the floors as a protective measure before it travels through the corridors. Cultures have revealed that the bacteria count in a room increases whenever linen is changed. For this reason, nurses should not shake linen out over a bed. Soiled linen should be removed from the bed by folding it up, and clean linen should be unfolded onto the bed to minimize the amount of air being "stirred up" by daily activities.

Some institutions close linen chutes at intervals to hose them down with a germicidal solution. Hospitals are being built without linen chutes. Laundry personnel who handle dirty linen do not handle clean linen and vice versa. If they do, they are asked to shower and change clothes after handling soiled articles.

The recent development of a soluble laundry bag can help with the disposition of contaminated linen. The management of wet contaminated linen continues to be something of a problem. Large amounts of wet linen seeping through regular laundry bags is a source of contamination. Wet linen in the soluble bag can also be a hazard. Selective use of such a new item is required to maximize its value.

Care of linen in the laundry is important. Use of water of high temperature along with bacteriostatic ingredients and adequate washing and rinsing cycles are all important to the production of linen which is clean esthetically and bacteriologically. This is another area in which handling of clean and dirty items can be separated by architectural planning.

The Housekeeping Department

Whether general housekeeping is the main concern of the housekeeping department or whether it is shared by the nursing department, rigid standards and techniques need to be utilized. Each institution will select one or two good germicidal solutions to be used. They will be picked for their effectiveness and their reaction to the material being cleaned.

Floor mopping must be scheduled and the schedule must not be related to visible dirt. A machine which scrubs and dry vacuums the floor is available. Besides daily mopping, operating room floors are mopped between cases. Isolation areas are usually mopped at least once a shift. Germicidal floor mats at the entrance to operating rooms, delivery rooms, intensive care units and nurseries may be used in conjunction with regular mopping to minimize bacterial counts.

Sinks, toilet areas, storage shelves and refrigerators in all areas of the hospital are also routinely cleaned. Sinks are cleaned several times a shift in some areas. Shelves may be cleaned daily in the nursery and weekly in a utility room. Procedures are geared to each area.

Discharge units, whether isolated or not, require complete cleaning. Germicidal solutions are used to wipe off the telephone, the signal cord, the radio pillow speaker and the paper towel holder as well as the more obvious things, such as the bed, the mattress or the furniture. Fogging machines which can produce a germicidal vapor that penetrates all areas of a room are on the market for terminal cleaning of isolation areas.

The Dietary Department

The dietary department must be concerned with the separation of clean and dirty food areas. Dietary personnel need to check and maintain an adequate dish washing method, which provides for the removal both of food particles and bacteria. Paper dishes and disposable eating utensils can be used for patients in isolation to prevent the return of contaminated dishes to the kitchen. In spite of these "disposables," the department must maintain high standards, as there may be cases of infectious disease which are unrecognized and therefore unisolated.

The Nursing Department

Nursing personnel are responsible for careful observation of patients so that signs and symptoms of possible infection can be recognized and reported to the physician as soon as possible. They need to be especially cognizant of possible wound infections which may be manifested by fever, pustular drainage, wound odor or improper healing.

The nursing department is responsible for teaching its procedures to all new personnel. If a patient is placed in isolation, the nurse is responsible for rigid technique to keep the infection from spreading. She will need to teach colleagues who are less familiar with the procedures. Isolation procedures vary greatly. They are geared to the physical facilities of the institution, the policies concerning the disease involved and the approved and adopted procedures of medical and nursing staffs. A major objective in all procedures is to provide a barrier to the spread of an organism whether its source be in the trash, linen, air, excreta, equipment, food or personnel. It is also vital to prevent the entrance of any organism to another area such as the nursery or a burn unit which might be considered to require a reverse isolation technique or a so-called protective isolation procedure.

Nursing personnel can be vital in the prevention of the spread of infection, not only by carrying out good isolation technique, but by carrying out good general aseptic technique in the care of all patients. They can make sure that, when a dressing is changed, the soiled dressing is placed in a waterproof bag, the wound is carefully inspected, hands are washed and care is used to apply the clean dressing. The dressing cart is being replaced in some places by individual dressing trays. If a cart is used, it needs to be carefully protected from contamination or soiling.

The use of an individual thermometer technique for each patient decreases the chance of cross infection. Care in disposing of used tissue is important. In the 1940's, general aseptic technique was relaxed because of the development of antibiotics. As time goes on, general aseptic technique almost gains a more important place because of antibiotics! The fact that prevalent microorganisms are more virulent and have an increased resistance to antibiotics makes these measures even more important.

While the nurse should not be put in the position of policing aseptic techniques and isolation care, she is in a strategic position to help non-nursing personnel. X-ray and laboratory personnel are often faced with the job of carrying out techniques which they seldom use. Usually these persons do not resent assistance. This is also true of physicians who find themselves in the awkward position in which they are expected to know the isolation technique of several different hospitals. They are more likely to be perplexed than careless. Thinking that a faucet handle should be kept clean, a physician may turn it on with a paper towel and off with his hands, only to find that that particular hospital considers its faucets dirty, so he should have turned them on with his hands and off with a clean paper towel. No one way is correct, but there must be a consistent method used by personnel in a particular area in order to make a procedure serve its purpose.

The Laboratory

The modern hospital laboratory has the task of obtaining routine random culture samples of areas and equipment which might be sources of pathogenic organisms. The nursing department is responsible for requesting a culture whenever a cleaning technique is suspected of being faulty. Culture data are reported to the nursing department and records are filed. Recommendations for the elimination of the focus of infection are proposed and tried. Areas cultured might include the operating room floor, the water supply, the nursery sink, a clean thermometer, a clean sheet or any number of other places or things. This kind of vigilance helps us to know the effectiveness of techniques and to locate potential hazards.

OVERALL HOSPITAL INFECTION CONTROL

Because continued mutation of microorganisms demands constant vigilance in order to prevent hospital infections, most institutions have created an Infection Control Committee. Such a committee is usually composed of representatives from the medical staff, the nursing staff, the administrative staff and the laboratory. The pathologist, if there is one on the hospital staff, usually chairs the committee. The committee is concerned with study, discussion, identification, recognition and prevention of the problem. This will include some system of identifying and reporting cases of hospital infections. Sometimes both the nursing service and the laboratory will be asked to keep daily records. The committee is also responsible for studying the adequacy of the infection control program and techniques. At the University of Kansas Medical Center, a committee such as this was also given the right to rule on disputes between various categories of personnel about the need for adhering to established techniques. The number of disputes decreased when the committee was given this power.

One other method of controlling infection is to have an active health service and education program for employees. Aside from annual physical examinations and chest x-rays, health services might offer immunization for smallpox, diphtheria and tetanus in addition to polio and influenza. Employees at hospitals need to be instructed to remain away from patients when they have colds, especially in such areas as the operating room, delivery room, postanesthesia room, nursery, intensive care unit, burn area and certain pediatric sections. It is also important that employees do not work in any of these areas if they have any kind of skin infection or draining wound. Mantoux testing and chest x-ray follow-up are recommended for employees exposed to tuberculosis patients whose disease was undiagnosed and who, as a result, were not properly segregated.

Research into the prevention and cause of hospital infections is vital. An eight-year study at Johns Hopkins Hospital identified several factors associated with postoperative infections. These included wound contamination by unsterile viscera during surgery, a higher incidence of infections during January and February and a higher incidence of infections in patients who had chest surgery, burns or congenital heart failure and in those who were already debilitated or had an infection elsewhere.

Another study demonstrated that an individual sheds more bacteria into the air from his skin after a shower than before a shower! Undoubtedly the future will teach us that we presently have many misconceptions. In the meantime, every clue that is revealed will aid us in knowing which general aseptic techniques and which special adaptations will be best for protecting our patients.

SUMMARY

Although all the causes of nosocomial infection are not known, all evidence points to the fact that no one department can be held responsible for their prevention. It is up to the administration of the hospital to make sure that every department takes its responsibility seriously and that the hospital as a whole is organized to study and to protect its patients to the best of everyone's ability.

SUGGESTED READINGS

Luschen, Mildred: Technique and Temperament Made the Difference. *American Journal of Nursing*, October, 1964, p. 103.

Matheney, Ruth V., et al.: *Fundamentals of Patient-Centered Nursing*. St. Louis, C. V. Mosby Co., 1964, Chapter 11.

Sutton, Audrey Latshaw: *Bedside Nursing Techniques*, Philadelphia, W. B. Saunders Co., 1964, Chapter 7.

REFERENCES

Balsley, Marie: Study of Today's Changing Hospital Environment Shows New Directions for Infection Control. *Hospitals*, May 16, 1965, p. 19.

Beal, Charles B.: Plastic Bubble Isolates Patient Anywhere in Hospital. *Modern Hospital*, January, 1965, p. 83.

Burke, John F.: Boston Concept Uses Air and Plastic for Burn Isolation. *Modern Hospital*, January, 1965, p. 80.

Cole, William R., and Bernard, Harvey R.: Quantitative Air Sampling, A Contrast with the Settling-Plate Method for the Study of Bacterial Air Contamination in Operating Rooms. *Surgery*, May, 1962, pp. 658-662.

Edgeworth, Dorotha: Nursing and Asepsis in the Modern Hospital. *Nursing Outlook*, June, 1965, p. 54.

Ellerbe, Thomas F., and Henslin, Rod: O.R. Asepsis Is Goal of Texas Burn Center Plan. *Modern Hospital*, January, 1965, p. 81.

Fuerst, Elinor V., and Wolff, LuVerne: *Fundamentals of Nursing*. Ed. 3, Philadelphia, J. B. Lippincott Co., 1964.

Ginsberg, Frances: Management of Burned Patients Is Challenge to Aseptic Care. *Modern Hospital*, January, 1965, p. 116.

Henning, Mildred: Infection Problem Dissolves in the Laundry. *Nursing Home Administrator*, March/April, 1965.

Letourneau, Charles: Nosocomial Infection. *Hospital Management*,
Part I—February, 1957, p. 41.
Part II—March, 1957, p. 52.
Part III—April, 1957, p. 56.

Lewis, Charles E.: Evolution of an Infection Control Program. *Hospitals*, April 16, 1965, p. 64.

Lichter, Jeanne M.: Infection Control in Maternity Units. *Nursing Outlook*, August, 1964, p. 32.

Speers, R., Jr., et al.: Increased Dispersal of Skin Bacteria Into the Air After Shower-Baths. *Lancet*, February 27, 1965, p. 478-480.

Vesley, Donald, and Brask, Marion: Environmental Implications in the Control of Hospital Acquired Infections. *Nursing Outlook*, December, 1961, p. 742.

Yanis, Bertha Meade: A Laboratory Evaluation of Fogging. *Hospital Management*, August, 1965, p. 102.

16

Guides for Administering Medications

Several hundred new medications enter the market each year. Millions of dollars are spent annually for research in new drugs, improvement of old drugs and better understanding of their biochemical actions. Pharmaceutical companies conduct a great deal of this research.

Certain standards and controls are placed on the manufacture and sale of drugs by the 1906 Federal Food, Drug and Cosmetic Act which has been amended several times in order to provide regulations which are in keeping with the problems of the times. The act designated the Pharmacopeia of the United States of America, referred to as the U.S.P., and the National Formulary as the sources of official drug standards. Enforcement of this act is a responsibility of the Food and Drug Administration.

What about all these new drugs? It is obvious that a full-time practicing physician or nurse cannot learn all about all the new drugs which reach the market. It is, therefore, necessary to have some method by which a practicing physician or nurse can have current drug knowledge. A publication, such as *The Dispensatory of the United States of America*, the *American Hospital Formulary Service*, the *Modern Drug Encyclopedia* or the *Physicians' Desk Reference to Pharmaceutical Specialties and Biologicals* (commonly referred to as the P.D.R.), must be available to those working with patients and medications. Some drugs are accompanied by a description of the drug and written instructions. The hospital pharmacist is an excellent resource for further information. It is vital that up-to-date information be available to persons needing it.

WHAT TO STUDY

If you are returning to your profession, you will find that most refresher courses will include classes which deal with the most important new drugs currently in use. If you do not have a refresher course available before returning to nursing, you will need to develop a guide. It will do little good to study a pharmacology book without some frame of reference. You might well find yourself studying drugs which are rarely used by the group of physicians providing medical care for your area.

The best place to begin is with your patients. Each time you take care of a patient, jot down the medications which are being given, look them up in whatever source is available and study the drug dosage, its effect and its expected action in relation to the particular patient. In this way, tedious and often unsuccessful rote memorization is avoided.

Unless you are working with a very specialized group of patients, concentrate your energies upon groups of drugs which are used frequently. Drugs will have a chemical name, a generic name and a brand name. The generic name of a drug becomes its official name and is listed as such in official publications. A drug may be known by its generic name or its trade name. An example is meprobamate, the generic name for Equanil and Miltown, which are both trade names. If you work in a hospital where Equanil is used, it is conceivable that you would never know it as meprobamate or Miltown.

Study the emergency drugs available in your area. This is an excellent way of learning what drugs the institution provides for emergency care of patients.

Pay special attention to the newer drugs which are used most commonly. Because of frequent usage, learning of antibiotics, anticoagulants, psychotherapeutic agents, synthetic narcotics, synthetic nonnarcotics, and hormones will be rapid. Antineoplastic or carcinostatic drugs are also beginning to be used more frequently.

You will soon discover also that it is easy to study drugs in relation to a disease. A brief glance at most modern textbooks will make it clear that drug therapy is included as part of the discussion of medical and nursing treatment of most diseases.

In deciding what drugs to study, select what is related to a particular patient, a particular disease and current usage in a particular institution. This will keep the learning of drugs from becoming an overwhelming and seemingly impossible task.

The Hospital Formulary

The Hospital Formulary System is being developed by many institutions. Such a system is developed through a Pharmacy and Therapeutics Committee, which is composed of physicians representing various sections and specialties of the medical staff. The pharmacist is a member *ex officio*. The initial purpose of such a committee is to select and evaluate drugs which are to be kept in the pharmacy of the hospital. Drugs are selected on the basis of drug quality, therapeutic effect and patient safety. They are listed by their generic names. Physicians are then requested to order drugs by the generic name. Provisions for permitting physicians to order nonformulary drugs vary from hospital to hospital.

Once the formulary is established, the Pharmacy and Therapeutic Committee reviews its drugs at intervals and selects and evaluates new drugs. Such a committee usually makes stipulations about telephone and verbal orders. They also establish which drugs should have automatic stop orders. In hospitals where such a committee does not exist, the medical staff has usually established a policy concerning these matters. A hospital policy may state that a telephone or verbal order may only be given to the charge nurse and that it must be signed within 24 hours after it has been given. An automatic stop order policy may state that all antibiotics, anticoagulants and narcotics must be discontinued automatically at the end of 48 hours unless the physician re-orders them.

There are several benefits from the use of a formulary system. Physicians know that the drugs they are using have been reviewed and studied, and they know that they have readily obtainable drug information. The system also controls the pharmacy drug stock. Economy is gained by mass purchasing and avoidance of duplicate stocks of the same drugs. Nurses become better acquainted with the drugs which are used because the same drug is not being ordered under several names, which would compound her problem.

What to Learn About a Drug

Its Action. The nurse will want to know what the response to a drug should or might be. The biochemical and physiologic action of drugs upon cells is not always completely understood. Drugs may have a local effect on skin or mucous membrane, which might be astringent, antiseptic, irritating, soothing or neutralizing. Systemic actions will either stimulate or depress cell activity or cell function.

The drug will be given in order to obtain a therapeutic effect. There may be side-effects which were not intended. Side-effects may merely be annoying to the patient or they may actually be harmful to him. A peculiar response to a drug, occurring only in one particular patient, is called an idiosyncratic effect. A patient may be hypersensitive to a drug due to sensitization from former doses. Because of the potential danger of such a reaction, it is important to ask patients at the time of admission if they have any known drug allergies or have ever had serious reaction to drugs. Some patients may have a drug tolerance. This is an acquired reaction from former use in which the patient requires a larger dose in order to obtain a therapeutic effect from the drug. Some drugs interact with each other, creating a response which is not typical of the drug when it is given in conjunction with some other drug. The nurse must, therefore, be watchful for untoward drug reactions.

THE DOSE. When the nurse studies a particular drug, she must be aware of the recommended range of dosage. Dosage is based on the weight and general condition of the patient. Sex is sometimes considered a factor and the temperament of the patient is often taken into account. Excitable persons sometimes require a smaller dose. Route of administration affects the dosage as does the time a drug is given in relation to meals. A drug is absorbed more quickly if it is given before a meal, and in the case of some drugs, it is therefore more effective when taken on any empty stomach. In the case of an irritating drug, it might better be given after a meal.

Most drugs wear off in three or four hours. This depends upon the route of administration and the form of the drug. It is important that the nurse space medications around the clock so that the patient maintains a fairly stable amount of drug in his system. This is one reason why an antibiotic, for instance, would be ordered q. 8h. rather than t.i.d. In order to provide a more constant drug level in the body, the Spansule, Gradumet or Timespan has been developed. These are gelatin capsules for oral administration and contain drug particles covered with materials requiring varying lengths of time to dissolve. Thus, continued amounts of drug are liberated at intervals over a period of time.

In order to reduce the possibility of contamination of injected medication, multiple-dose, rubber-stopper vials are being used less commonly. Single dose ampules are replacing them. The sealed glass ampule is made in various doses so that the nurse can usually find an ampule which contains the exact dose she desires. She merely draws the desired dose into the syringe. This has another advantage in terms of accuracy, as the nurse has to calculate a drug dosage less often. Most ampules are scored at the neck, making the ampule file an almost forgotten tool. The top of the ampule can simply be snapped off without loss of medication.

METHOD OF ADMINISTRATION. The nurse will also need to know the method of administration of a drug. Many drugs can be administered by mouth, vein, injection or topical application. It is imperative that the nurse know what route the physician requested and that she make sure that she has the medication in the form properly prepared for that particular route.

Confusion in this area is exemplified by the mistake of a mother who took her toddler home from the hospital recently. The child was recovering from an ear infection and the mother was told to give the child Achromycin drops every eight hours. They were oral drops and the mother put them in the child's ear. Personnel also need to be aware of these possibilities when they give medications. Is an oral tablet being used for a hypodermic injection? Does the label read, "for intravenous use?"

A Drug Study Sheet

When studying medications, the nurse might find it helpful to use one of the tools used by students—the Drug Study Sheet. It can be made without any special form if the principal information is sought. The following headings might be written across the top of a plain sheet of paper and used whenever new drugs are encountered:

Suggested Drug Study Sheet

PATIENT NAME	DIAGNOSIS	DRUG AND USUAL DOSE	ROUTE OF ADMINISTRATION	PURPOSE; EXPECTED REACTIONS	SIDE-EFFECTS

Review of Weights and Measures

Metrology, the science of weights and measures, continues to plague the nurse. The apothecary system is still used along with the metric system, and sometimes household measures are thrown in to add to the confusion. Fortunately, household measurements are not used very often. The metric system is becoming the method of choice and eventually will replace the apothecary system. In the meantime, the nurse will need to review equivalents of the two systems so that she can convert from one system to another whenever necessary. Since both systems provide dry and liquid measures, it will expedite learning to recall that there is numerical similarity between some of the measurements. It will also help the nurse if she carries a small conversion table in her pocket when there is none available in her work area. Many drug companies supply such tables to nurses free of charge.

Review of Arithmetic Conversions

It is sometimes necessary for the nurse to work out simple arithmetic problems. A simple review of conversion of per cents, decimals, fractions and ratios may be helpful.

FRACTION TO RATIO AND RATIO TO FRACTION. Changing back and forth from fraction to ratio is very simple. The fraction line is merely changed to a colon or vice versa, as the case may be. In other words, the fraction $1/2$ becomes the ratio 1:2 and the ratio 1:4 becomes the fraction $1/4$.

PER CENT TO DECIMAL AND DECIMAL TO PER CENT AND FRACTION OR RATIO. When changing per cent to a decimal and back to per cent again, remember that per cent means the number of parts of 100.

Table of Approximate Equivalents

LIQUID MEASURE

HOUSEHOLD		METRIC		APOTHECARIES'
		1000 ml. (cc.)	=	1 quart
		500 ml. (cc.)	=	1 pint
1 glass	=	250 ml. (cc.)	=	8 ounces
2 tbsp.	=	30 ml. (cc.)	=	1 ounce (8 drams)
1 tbsp.	=	15 ml. (cc.)	=	4 drams
1 tsp.	=	4 ml. (cc.)	=	1 dram (60 minims)
15 gtt.	=	1 ml. (cc.)	=	15 minims
1 gtt.	=	0.06 ml. (cc.)	=	1 minim

DRY MEASURE

	METRIC		APOTHECARIES'
	30 gm.	=	1 ounce
	4 gm.	=	60 grains (1 dram)
(1000 mg.)	1 gm.	=	15 grains
	60 mg.	=	1 grain
	10 mg.	=	1/6 grain
(1000 mcg.)	1 mg.	=	1/60 grain
	0.5 mg.	=	1/120 grain
	0.4 mg.	=	1/150 grain
	0.3 mg.	=	1/200 grain
	0.2 mg.	=	1/300 grain

(The above table has only selected equivalents. It does, however, contain all that is necessary in most instances.)

Decimal places are as follows:

.1 = 1/10 or 1:10
.01 = 1/100 or 1:100
.001 = 1/1000 or 1:1000

When converting per cent to a decimal the decimal point is moved two places to the left. If there is no decimal in the per cent, it is assumed to be at the end of the per cent.

49% becomes .49
49.5% becomes .495

When converting a decimal to per cent, the decimal is moved two points to the right:

.0003 becomes .03%
.30 becomes 30%

FRACTION TO PER CENT AND PER CENT TO FRACTION OR DECIMAL. When changing per cent to a fraction the per cent becomes the denominator (100) and the number becomes the numerator: 5% is 5/100 (1/20).

When converting a fraction to per cent, divide the numerator by the denominator, move the decimal two places to the right and add the % sign.

$$\frac{1}{2} = 1 \text{ divided by } 2 = .50 = 50\%$$

If you had wanted to obtain a decimal, you would have done the same thing and stopped when you had the decimal.

PER CENT TO RATIO AND RATIO TO PER CENT OR DECIMAL. Since per cent means parts of 100, 50% becomes 50:100. In all cases ratios and fractions should be reduced to the simplest term so that 50:100 becomes 1:2.

When converting the ratio to per cent, divide the first number of the ratio by the second: 1:20 becomes .05 or 5%.

SUMMARY. In order to change 1:5 to a fraction the colon is changed to a virgule (/), and 1:5 becomes 1/5. In order to change it to a decimal, five is divided into 1 to become .20. In order to change .20 to per cent, the decimal is moved two places and becomes 20%.

Reversing this, 20% becomes a decimal by moving the decimal point to the left to become .20. It becomes a fraction by using 20/100 (reduced to 1/5) and becomes a ratio by changing the virgule to a colon or 1:5. The nurse will find practice problems at the end of the chapter.

Common Types of Arithmetic Problems

The nurse is faced with far fewer calculations and arithmetic problems than in the past. Prescriptions are supposed to be filled by the pharmacist in the prescribed dosage whenever possible. They are prepared so that the patient could give himself the medication as he would at home. This ideal is reached many instances. Of the few problems which the nurse is likely to encounter, all but one involves setting up a proportion.

DRUG ON HAND IN SOLUTION. Formula: Dose ordered: amount solution needed :: dose on hand: amount solution for the dosage on hand. Problem sample: The vial of Demerol is labeled 50 mg./cc. The ordered dose is 75 mg. How many cc. must be given?

$$75 : X :: 50 : 1$$
$$50X = 75$$
$$X = 1\tfrac{1}{2} \text{ cc.}$$

A dosage of 1½ cc. must be given.

PREPARING A SOLUTION FROM A FULL STRENGTH SOLUTION. Formula: Amount of drug: finished solution :: %:100.

Problem sample: How much full strength Vesphene is needed to make 1 liter of 2% Vesphene?

$$X : 1000 :: 2 : 100$$
$$2000 = 100X$$
$$20 = X$$

An amount of 20 cc. is required to make a quart of 2% Vesphene.

Problem sample: How much full strength Burow's solution is required to make 2000 cc. of 1:30 Burow's solution for skin packs?

$$X : 2000 :: 3 : 100$$
$$6000 = 100X$$
$$60 = X$$

Doses From Tablets. Rule: Divide the desired dose by the dose on hand to determine the part of a tablet or the number of tablets required.*

Problem sample: Morphine sulphate gr. 1/12 is ordered. The stock tablet is gr. 1/8. How much of the tablet should be given?

$$\frac{1/12}{1/8} = 1/12 \times 8/1$$ (Remember to invert the divisor when dividing fractions!)

$$= 8/12 \text{ or } 2/3 \text{ of the tablet.}$$

Once the amount of the tablet is known, the amount of diluent may be decided upon. The patient should receive between ½ cc. and 1½ cc. of solution for hypodermic injections. Depending upon the fraction one will decide whether to calculate the diluent in cc. or minims. In the case of 2/3, it is easier to calculate 2/3 of 30 minims than it is to calculate 2/3 of 2 cc. Therefore, dilute the drug in 30 minims; 2/3 of 30 minims is 20 minims. The patient will receive 20 minims after 10 minims have been expelled from the syringe. CAUTION: Calculated doses should always be checked by another person to see that the arithmetic is correct and that the proper amount of solution has been expelled. We are all capable of making an error in arithmetic.

Regulating Rate of Intravenous Solutions. Intravenous fluids can be dangerous to a patient if they are given at too rapid a rate. They can be of little help to a patient if they are administered too slowly. Physicians will usually note how many hours they wish a particular fluid to run. An order might read: Give patient 2000 cc. electrolyte fluid in the next eight hours. The nurse will need to know how many cc. per hour and how many drops per minute. Eight hours divided by 2000 cc. means that about 250 cc. fluid should be given each hour. According to our table there are 15 drops/cc. (15 × 250 = 3750 gtt./hr.). Dividing 3750 gtt. by 60 minutes means that the fluid should run at 62 gtt./min. CAUTION: The nurse should always check the stated number of drops per cc. on the label of the intravenous tubing box. Drops vary in size. Pediatric sets may be gauged so that there are 50 drops to 1 cc. Many tubings give 10 drops per cc. In the latter case, the above problem would be solved by having 2500 gtt./hr. or 41 gtt./min.

Reminders About Drawing Up Insulin. There is one vital reminder about obtaining the proper dose of insulin. The unit strength on the bottle must match the unit scale on the insulin syringe. When the

*From Krug, Elsie E.: *Pharmacology in Nursing*. Ed. 9, St. Louis, C. V. Mosby Co., 1963.

bottle reads 40 units, it contains 40 units per cc. If it reads 80 units, it means that it contains 80 units per cc. The scales on the syringe will also be marked. The side which reads 40 U. means that it is calibrated for 40 units to 1 cc. The scale on the other side of the syringe may be marked for 20 or 80 units. Insulin syringes come with different combinations of scales which are plainly marked.

If 20 units of insulin are drawn from a 40 unit bottle, the 40 unit scale of the syringe should be used, making the amount of solution to be injected 1/2 cc. If 20 units of insulin is removed from an 80 unit bottle, the 80 unit scale of the syringe should be used and the amount of solution to be injected is then 1/4 cc. THE QUANTITY OF SOLUTION VARIED BUT THE DOSAGE DID NOT.

Review of Abbreviations

Table 2 lists abbreviations which are commonly used and accepted. There are other abbreviations which can be classified as regional or

Table 2. **Abbreviations**

ABBREVIATION	MEANING	ABBREVIATION	MEANING
aa	of each	per os	by mouth
a.c.	before meals	p.r.n.	as needed
ad lib.	as desired	pulv.	powder
amt.	amount	q.d.	every day
aq.	water	q.h.	every hour
b.i.d.	twice a day	q. 2 h.	every two hours
b.i.n.	twice a night	q. 3 h.	every three hours
c.	with	q.i.d.	four times a day
cc.	cubic centimeter	R_x	take
caps.	capsule	s.	without
comp.	compound	ss.	one half
dil.	dilute	S.S.	soap suds
D.W.	distilled water	sig.	write on label
elix.	elixir	sol.	solution
ext.	extract	s.o.s.	if necessary
fl./fld.	fluid	stat.	immediately
Gm.	gram	syr.	syrup
gr.	grain	tbsp.	tablespoon
gtt.	drop	tab.	tablet
(H)	by hypodermic	t.i.d.	three times a day
h.s.	hour of sleep	t.i.n.	three times a night
Kg.	kilogram	tr./tinct.	tincture
L.	liter	tsp.	teaspoon
liq.	liquid	ung.	ointment
m.	minim		
mcg.	microgram		
mg.	milligram		
ml.	milliliter		
noct.	at night		
non rep.	do not repeat		
o.d.	right eye		
o.s.	left eye		
oz.	ounce		
p.c.	after meals		

institutional. Liberal use of abbreviations often degenerates into a kind of shorthand system, which may be completely incomprehensible to the reader. In such a case, a medical record would have dubious meaning in a court of law. An example of this kind of shorthand is, "O.O.B.s.i.e." This is a sentence which was found in the nurses' notes of a patient's chart. Translated, it means, "Patient was out of bed without ill effects." Such liberties make accepted lists of abbreviations necessary.

The practicing nurse will know many abbreviations which are accepted by her employer such as B.M.R., T.P.R. or EKG. Many others are unacceptable. Generally speaking, an abbreviation should have a common meaning for everyone using it and should never degenerate into a carelessly written communication.

WHO ADMINISTERS MEDICATIONS?

Medications may be administered by the physician, the registered nurse, the licensed practical nurse, a medication technician or the patient himself. The decision as to who administers the drug depends on many factors, such as the nature of the drug, the type of institution and the policies set by that organization.

The Patient

When the patient is allowed to administer his own medications, it is assumed that the patient is reliable mentally and intellectually. He must understand when to take his medication, at what intervals and how much to take.

Some psychiatric patients, patients with poor vision and those who are physically weak or who have moments of confusion should not be allowed to take their own medications. Subcutaneous and intramuscular drugs are usually given by the nurse. Exceptions to this might be the diabetic or asthmatic who must give himself "shots" at home. In this case, however, the nurse should assist the patient to measure and administer his injections so that he can learn as much as possible while he is hospitalized.

When patients are allowed to take their own medications, the nurse must guard against dismissing them from her mind. She must know what drugs her patients are taking and that they are actually being taken regularly and on time, and she must remember to observe for untoward effects as she would if she were administering them. She must not forget her role as teacher in this area, and she must be alert to patients who would be better protected by having her administer the medications.

The Physician

The physician will usually give all intravenous medications in a larger institution. Policies often must be made on the basis of necessity and available personnel. This is not as inconsistent as it sounds. If a nurse is taught proper technique and potential hazards and has a good knowledge of the drug being administered, there is no reason why she cannot give many intravenous drugs.

Whenever a drug is known to cause an untoward reaction, a physician should be on hand in case there is need to order a drug which would immediately counteract the reaction. In this case, one is more concerned about the availability of a physician in case a new order is required than with the actual injection itself.

In large teaching institutions, nursing students may never learn to administer intravenous injections because the medical students need to "get the experience." In small hospitals the nurse may give almost all the intravenous injections. In a hospital where there is a resident medical staff, whether it be interns, residents or paid physicians, the physician will usually be called to give any medication which is injected directly into the vein.

The Nurse

The Practical Nurse. The practical nurse gives many medications. At some hospitals the practical nurse gives medications with restrictions. In other words, she might only give oral medications, or she might give oral medications and selected intramuscular injections. At other institutions she may administer all medications, usually with the exception of intravenous drugs.

The Registered Nurse. The registered nurse may be the only person permitted to give medications, or she may give the ones which the practical nurse is not permitted to give. Whether or not the R.N. administers medications, she is responsible for knowing what medication her patients are receiving and why they are receiving it, and she must be cognizant of expected as well as unexpected reactions.

The Medication Technician

Another approach has been to functionalize medications. Practical nurses or special aides are sometimes trained in metrology, arithmetic and some pharmacology so that their one and only duty is to give medications. Their job title may be medication technician. Some hospitals have found this system to be successful. It relieves bedside personnel of this duty, but it does not relieve them of the total responsibility.

Changes to Be Considered

Medication administration requires a great deal of the personnel's time. It is treatment which takes the nurse away from the bedside for several hours a day. Indirect patient care is usually defined as that time spent by personnel doing things for patients but not in their presence. This task consumes more time away from the patient than some people recognize. Ordering drugs every few days, counting narcotics, maintaining the floor stock (aspirin, castor oil, etc.), checking the medication card against the Kardex, reading the label three times, preparing the medication and charting the medication all consume a great deal more time than the actual administration of the medication to the patient, which can be considered direct patient care.

Besides this, drugs are coming in preparations which can be administered without dosage calculation in most instances. The unit dose system is being tried and used in many places. In this system the pharmacy interprets the order from the chart, prepares the medication and sends it to the nursing station labeled for the patient at each hour the patient is to receive it. Other systems involve subpharmacies on each floor so that the nurse never needs to order drugs.

The unit dose system challenges an old familiar rule "If you pour it and prepare it, you give it." Divided responsibility usually should be challenged. However, if the division of responsibility is clear, then the problem is mitigated. If the pharmacist always prepares medications and the nurse always dispenses them to the patient, then it is clear that an error of a wrong drug falls to the pharmacist and an error of a wrong patient falls to the nurse.

It is true that for many, giving medications has become easier and safer because of new developments in drug systems and drug preparations. Medications are also more numerous. The nurse will not need to review arithmetic if she works where the pharmacist prepares drugs, but her knowledge about the effect of drugs must be no less accurate regardless of who dispenses them.

Reminders on Giving Medications

This book has made a point of excluding procedures. While the following is not a step-by-step procedure, it does contain most of the ingredients of a medication procedure. It is included because the average nursing procedure does not include these reminders which refreshers have found helpful.

General Safety

1. Discontinue conversation with others while checking medication cards and preparing medications.

2. Never give a medication from an unlabeled bottle or one that is illegibly labeled.

NOTE: The nurse never labels or relabels medications.

3. No medication is given without a physician's order.

4. Know the expected effect and possible toxic reactions of the drugs you are administering.

5. Know the usual dosage of the drugs you are preparing and check with the nurse in charge or the physician if you think the maximum dosage has been exceeded.

CAUTION: Remember that children, small or thin adults, and older persons require smaller doses.

6. When calculating a dosage, always ask another person to check your arithmetic for any possible error.

7. Do not give medicines prepared by another nurse.

8. Make sure that you are giving the right medication to the right patient by checking the patient's identity. Check the bed tag, room tag or preferably the identification bracelet, if he is wearing one. If identification must be obtained verbally, ask the patient what his name is. If you ask, "Is your name Mr. Jones?" a potential error may result if he was preoccupied or did not hear you or you may have misinterpreted a "yes" for a "no."

9. Remain with the patient until he has taken the medication unless hospital policy gives you other guidelines.

10. Never leave a tray of medicines unattended. Keep the tray with you.

11. Break and throw away all disposable needles and syringes when you have finished with them. Hospital waste baskets and trash cans are favorite places for persons who need narcotics to look for syringes.

Care in Preparation of Medications

1. Check the patient's drug allergies against any ordered medications.

2. Read the medicine card and Kardex carefully making sure that the entries are identical in all respects.

NOTE: If there is a discrepancy or an entry is illegible, check the original physician's order in the patient's chart.

3. Read the label of the medication container three times:

When removing it from the shelf
Before pouring the medicine
Before returning it to the shelf.

4. Oral liquid medications:

a. Before pouring an emulsion or a suspension, shake the bottle well.

b. Measure the exact amount by holding the container at eye level.

c. Pour with label upward to avoid soiling it.

d. Wipe mouth of bottle dry before replacing the cover.

e. Avoid pouring medicine back into a bottle.

f. Dilute bad tasting liquid medications with about ½ ounce of diluent unless they have a local effect, such as cough medicine.

5. Tablets and capsules:

a. Pour tablets into the bottle cap or a spoon rather than using your fingers to remove them from the bottle.

b. Do not divide pills or tablets.

NOTE: This should be done by a pharmacist.

6. Injections:

a. Always read instructions for dilution to make sure that the proper diluent is used.

b. If the amount of diluent is not written on the instructions, label the amount of drug per cc. so that there is no question about the strength of the dosage in the bottle.

c. Be sure to return drugs requiring refrigeration to the refrigerator immediately after use to prevent loss of drug strength.

7. Replace caps on bottles immediately after obtaining the medicine.

8. Never mix drugs unless specifically ordered to do so.

CARE IN ADMINISTRATION OF MEDICINES

1. Give medications on time (within 30 minutes of the specified interval is usually considered on time).

2. Give milk with any oral antibiotic which tends to create gastric irritation.

3. Assist weak and helpless patients as indicated.

4. Rotate sites of intramuscular injections for patient comfort.

5. If an intramuscular dose is more than 2 cc., split the dose and give two injections to alleviate discomfort at the site.

CHARTING MEDICATIONS

1. Record all narcotics and barbiturates in the Narcotic Book.

2. Chart all p.r.n. medicines immediately after giving them.

3. Chart medicines *after* they have been given.

IN CASE OF MEDICATION ERROR. In case a medication error is made, it should be immediately reported to the charge nurse who will notify the physician. The wrong dose, the wrong medication, the wrong patient, the wrong route of administration or the wrong time are the major causes of error. The nurse should familiarize herself with the procedure expected by her employer when an error is made. Usually an Error Report is required, which serves a twofold purpose. It gives the nurse an opportunity to analyze the reason for her error, and it provides the institution with proper records and a method of studying potentially weak spots in procedures. In order for Error Reports to have a useful purpose, personnel should be conscientious about reporting all errors in writing as well as verbally.

SUMMARY

When you go back to nursing, you will need to review drugs in a manner which will not make the project too overwhelming. First of all, morphine sulfate, codeine sulfate, Seconal and aspirin are still being used and so every drug you encounter will not be new. If drugs are studied a few at a time and in relation to a specific patient with a specific condition, learning new drugs will be made easier. Thus, if you live in North Carolina, you will not find yourself studying drugs which are used in Colorado under a different name. If a hospital does not have a formulary, learning generic names may not always be helpful.

Reviewing common abbreviations and learning those which are used at your institution will be helpful. Mathematics should be reviewed according to the kinds of problems which are encountered at the institution where you are employed. If you keep these specific things in mind, giving all the new drugs will be much easier than you imagined.

PRACTICE PROBLEMS IN ARITHMETIC
(Answers at end of problems)

A. Addition:

(1) 15 +49 (2) 486 +585 (3) 1/4 + 1/2 = (4) 1/2 + 1/2 =

B. Subtraction:

(1) 238 −199 (2) 63 −59 (3) 1/2 − 1/4 = (4) 2/3 − 1/6 =

C. Multiplication:

(1) 243 ×967 (2) 1000 ×100 (3) 2/3 × 3/4 = (4) 1/4 × 3/4 =

D. Division: (Carry answer out to the second decimal.)

(1) 1.24) 1.892 (2) 0.064) 8

(3) 1/4 ÷ 1/3 = (4) 4/5 ÷ 1/10 =

E. Which is the smallest number in each group?

1.	1/150	1/200	1/120
2.	1/8	1/3	1/4
3.	3/16	2/32	1/64
4.	1/6000	1/3000	1/4000
5.	1/15	1/35	1/25
6.	0.05	1.5	0.005
7.	0.16	1.6	0.016

F. Convert the following into their equivalent values:

	Fraction	Ratio	Decimal	Per cent
(1)	3/8	______	______	______
(2)	______	1:5000	______	______
(3)	______	______	0.1	______
(4)	______	______	______	.1%

G. Complete the following equivalents:

(1) 1 cc. = ____minims
(2) 30 cc. = ____ounces
(3) 1 Gm. = ____mg.
(4) 1 ml. = ____ cc.
(5) 4 cc. = ____drams
(6) 1 Gm. = ____grains

H. Work out the following problems:

1. 75 mg. of Demerol is ordered. The vial of Demerol is labeled 50 mg./cc. You will give ____cc.
2. How much full strength Burow's solution is required to make 200 cc. of 1:25 Burow's solution for derm packs? ________
3. How much full strength Vesphene is needed to make 1 liter of 2% Vesphene? ________
4. How many tablets of 0.5 Gm. sodium salicylate will you need to give gr. XXX of the drug?________
5. The order of morphine sulphate gr. 1/20 is written. The stock tablet available is gr. 1/6.
   Amount of tablet needed ________
   Amount of diluent used ________
   Amount given to patient ________
6. 1000 cc. of intravenous fluid is ordered to run in over a period of eight hours. How many cc. must run in each hour? ______ How many gtt./min. must be regulated to achieve this order?______
7. The medication card reads "codeine gr. 1/2 p.r.n." The bottle reads "codeine 15 mg."
   How many tablets will you give? ________

Answers

A. 1. 64
2. 1071
3. 3/4
4. 1

B. 1. 39
2. 4
3. 1/4
4. 1/2

C. 1. 234,981
2. 100,000
3. 1/2
4. 3/16

D. 1. 1.52
2. 125
3. 3/4
4. 8

E. 1. 1/200
2. 1/8
3. 1/64
4. 1/6000
5. 1/35
6. 0.005
7. 0.016

F.

1.	3:8	.375	37½%
2.	1/5000	.0002	.02%
3.	1/10	1:10	10%
4.	1/1000	1:1000	.001

G.		H.		
1. 15		1. $1\frac{1}{2}$ cc.	5. 3/10
2. 1		2. 8 cc.	2 cc.
3. 1000		3. 20 cc.	6/10 cc.
4. 1		4. 4 tab.	6. 125 cc.
5. 1			31 gtt/min
6. 15			7. 2 tablets

SUGGESTED READINGS

Jarratt, Virginia: The Keeper of the Keys. *American Journal of Nursing*, July, 1965, p. 68.
Krug, Elsie E.: *Pharmacology in Nursing*. Ed. 9, St. Louis, C. V. Mosby Co., 1963, Chapter 5.

REFERENCES

American Journal of Nursing News Item, Iowa Tries New System of Drug Handling. July, 1964, p. 50.

Anderson, Ellen M.: *Workbook of Solutions and Dosage of Drugs*. Ed. 2, St. Louis, C. V. Mosby Co., 1960.

Beckman, Harry: *Pharmacology—The Nature, Action and Use of Drugs*. Ed. 2, Philadelphia, W. B. Saunders Co., Chapters 1, 2, 3, 5 and 13.

Durbin, Richard L., and Brewer, Myrdas: 24 Hour Pharmacy is Best Prescription. *Modern Hospital*, June, 1965, p. 126.

Fuerst, Elinor V., and Wolff, LuVerne: *Fundamentals in Nursing*. Ed. 3, Philadelphia, J. B. Lippincott Co., 1964.

Goostray, Stella: *Problems in Solution and Dosage*. Ed. 2, New York, Macmillan Co., 1952.

Keane, Claire B., and Fletcher, Sybil M.: *Drugs and Solutions*. Philadelphia, W. B. Saunders Co., 1965.

Krug, Elsie E.: *Pharmacology in Nursing*. Ed. 9, St. Louis, C. V. Mosby Co., 1963.

McClain, M. E.: *Simplified Arithmetic for Nurses*. Ed. 2, Philadelphia, W. B. Saunders Co., 1960.

Pellegrino, E. D.: A Physician Appraises the Formulary System. *Hospitals*, January 1, 1965, p. 77.

St. Barnabas Hospital, *Nursing Procedure Book*, 1963.

Simon, Gilbert J.: Hospital Formularies: History, Philosophy, Implementation. *Hospital Topics*, April, 1965, p. 75.

Skelly, Esther G.: *Medications for the Nurse*. Albany, Delmar Publishers, Inc., 1960.

17

Fluid and Electrolyte Balance

The refresher as well as the practicing nurse often finds fluid and electrolyte balance a baffling subject because basic physiology and chemistry have long been forgotten. In order to be able to make more pertinent patient observations and to be more cognizant of safety measures required to carry out related treatments and nursing care, it will be helpful to review a few basic facts associated with the subject.

Generally speaking, fluid and electrolyte balance refers to the volume, composition and position of water and electrolytes found in a state of health. It is the result of a miraculous synchronization of body activities based upon mechanisms which continually adjust the loss and restoration of body elements.

ELECTROLYTES

An electrolyte is a molecule which dissociates itself into two or more particles (ions) in solution. This process of dissociation into separate components in water is called ionization. In other words, NaCl becomes Na^+ and Cl^- when placed in water. When urea and dextrose are placed in water, they do not break down and are therefore nonelectrolytes. When ionization occurs, the number of positively charged ions (cations) equals the number of negatively charged ions (anions). Cations are bases and anions are acids.

Electrolytes may be measured by obtaining blood samples. The unit of measurement for plasma electrolytes is the milliequivalent, which is abbreviated mEq. Because sodium, chloride and potassium are the most commonly studied plasma electrolytes, it is helpful to know their normal values. Approximate norms are sodium 137 to 147 mEq, chloride 100 to 110 mEq, potassium 4 to 5.5 mEq.

FLUIDS

Sixty per cent of the body weight of an adult is water. Body fluids are located inside cells, surrounding cells and in the blood stream. The fluids of these three compartments are separated by the cell membrane and the capillary wall. These two membranes are semipermeable, which means that water can flow freely back and forth through the membrane while electrolytes pass only under certain conditions. When water passes through a membrane it always passes in the direction of the fluid which has the highest concentration of electrolytes. Another way of expressing it is by the principle, "Water goes where salt is." It is important to remember this concept.

Isotonic solution is a solution which has the same salt concentration as plasma. Therefore, when isotonic solution is introduced into the blood stream, relatively little exchange occurs between the plasma and the red blood cells. When a hypotonic (a solution with less salt than plasma) solution is introduced, fluid enters the cells causing them to burst. If a hypertonic (a solution with less salt than plasma) solution is used, fluid will leave the cells causing them to shrink. From this, it is clear why near-isotonic solutions are used in intravenous therapy.

Cellular or Intracellular (Inside the Cells) Fluid

Two thirds of the body fluid is inside the cells. The cell membrane separates cellular fluid from other body fluids. The chief ion of cellular fluid is potassium.

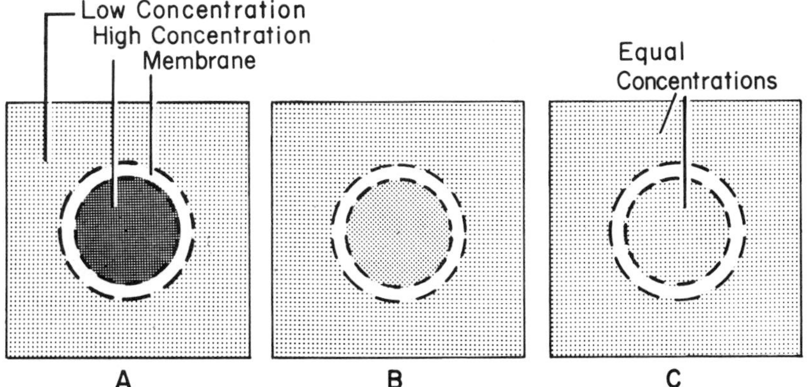

Figure 17–1. *Osmosis. A, The solution within the membrane has a higher concentration of salts than the solution on the outside. B, In the process of osmosis, water flows into the solution of high concentration until the concentrations are equalized (C). (From Routh, Joseph I.:* Fundamentals of Inorganic, Organic and Biological Chemistry. *Ed. 5, Philadelphia, W. B. Saunders Company, 1965.)*

Extracellular Fluid (Outside the Cells)

One third of our body fluid is found outside the cells where the major ions are sodium and chloride, which approximate sea water. It is sometimes called man's "inside sea." There are two compartments of extracellular fluid, plasma and interstitial fluid, which have a similar electrolyte composition except that protein is found in plasma in a higher proportion.

INTERSTITIAL FLUID. Accounting for about 15 per cent of the body weight, this fluid surrounds and bathes the cells of the body. It is separated from plasma by the capillary wall and from the cell by the cell membranes.

VASCULAR FLUID (PLASMA). This accounts for about 5 per cent of the body weight. Because it is possible to measure the composition of plasma, it is this fluid which is studied in clinical practice in the laboratory. From these findings, inferences about other fluids and electrolytes are made.

ACID-BASE BALANCE

Whether a fluid is acid or alkaline depends on the concentration of hydrogen ions. Acid-base balance is maintained at the ratio of one part acid to 20 parts base. Acids have a higher concentration of hydrogen ions than bases. Acid-base balance is chiefly determined by the ratio of carbonic acid (regulated by gas exchange in the lungs) to bicarbonate (regulated by metabolic and renal ion exchange). This can be measured by the pH. A pH is considered neutral at 7, acid below this figure and alkaline above this figure. The pH of blood is normally between 7.35 and 7.45, slightly alkaline. Certain substances in the blood, called buffers, resist change in the pH when acids and bases are introduced. Acid-base balance can also be measured by the carbon dioxide combining power of blood which is normally about 25 mEq.

Respiratory Acidosis and Alkalosis

Carbon dioxide originates from carbonic acid of blood. Thus, when a patient hyperventilates, he is blowing off greater amounts of acid (carbon dioxide) and creating respiratory alkalosis of the extracellular fluid. When a patient has inhibited respirations, there will be a tendency to acidosis, as the patient is not blowing off enough carbon dioxide to maintain the delicate balance. The latter occurs when a patient has emphysema or pneumonia. This has particular importance to the nurse, as her observations of respiratory function take on greater significance when this phenomenon is understood.

Metabolic Acidosis and Alkalosis

When the body loses or retains alkali by nonrespiratory routes, metabolic acidosis or alkalosis occurs. Alkalosis occurs when acids such as HCl have been lost because of vomiting. Acidosis occurs when bases are lost as a result of diarrhea or when there is an accumulation of acids in the body as in the case of diabetes or kidney disease.

BODY REGULATORS OF FLUID BALANCE

We do not eat and drink exactly what our bodies require for the maintenance of health. As a result, the body must separate what is needed from what is not needed. Certain organs are largely responsible for this task. The lungs have already been mentioned in the role of regulating acid-base balance of extracellular fluid. The kidneys and certain glands are even more vital.

The Kidneys

The kidneys are the most important organs concerned with maintaining fluid and electrolyte balance. Microscopic nephrons, approximately one million in each kidney, perform two remarkable tasks. They receive water and electrolytes from the blood stream and then select how much water and which electrolytes must return to the blood stream, sending out its discards in the form of urine. If the kidney fails to function normally, a disturbance in fluid and electrolyte balance results. Potassium accumulates in the blood stream which depresses the heart and may ultimately cause heart block and cardiac arrest.

The Glands

The Adrenal Glands. The adrenal glands interact with the kidney. They secrete the hormone aldosterone, which affects retention of sodium and excretion of potassium. When these glands are underactive, the sodium level falls and water retention is impaired. When they are overactive, they cause retention of sodium and water and remove too much potassium.

The Pituitary Gland. The posterior lobe of the pituitary gland produces the antidiuretic hormone (ADH), which conserves water by enhancing reabsorption of water in the tubule of the kidney.

The Parathyroid Glands. The parathyroid glands regulate the calcium level in extracellular fluid. When these glands are removed or destroyed, tetany will occur. When they are overactive, the serum calcium level will rise and excess calcium will be deposited in the kidney causing the formation of stones.

Differences in Fluid and Electrolyte Requirements of Infants

Weight is not an adequate determinant for fluid and electrolyte requirements. Figures for infants and small children are not proportionately smaller than those used for adults. For example, it is obvious that if a 150-pound adult requires 2000 cc. of fluid a day, a 15-pound infant will need more than 200 cc. of fluid per day. Fluid and electrolyte requirements are more commonly based upon surface area of the body. A newborn infant has about three times more skin surface in proportion to his weight than an adult. Therefore, physicians find it more satisfactory to use tables which determine fluid requirements on the basis of skin surface area. Such tables can also be used for adult requirements.

The infant's kidney differs from that of the older child or adult. The kidney is not fully developed at birth, and for this reason it is less able to excrete excess fluid and electrolytes. Phosphates are especially difficult for the immature kidney to handle. In prescribing fluid therapy for premature and newborn infants, one must take these factors into consideration.

The metabolic rate of infants is higher and is shown in their proportionately greater output. Infants, therefore, need proportionately more fluid to carry off proportionately greater waste products.

Fluid distribution also differs. While about 60 per cent of an adult's weight is fluid, about 77 per cent of an infant's weight is fluid. Forty-five per cent is cellular fluid in both the adult and the infant. The rest is extracellular fluid which means that the infant has almost twice as much extracellular fluid as an adult. About half of an infant's extracellular fluid is exchanged each day compared with about one fifth of that of an adult. Therefore, an infant has twice as much extracellular fluid to lose and can lose it more than twice as fast.

Because of these factors, fluid and electrolyte imbalances in infants and young children must be treated quickly. A dehydrated person is somewhat like a fish out of water in that cells are not being properly bathed by extracellular fluid to maintain life. When the amount of extracellular fluid decreases, plasma depletion will result in shock and eventual death if the process is not reversed. While this can occur in any patient, it can occur more quickly in the pediatric patient. This is the reason why severe dehydration is considered an emergency on pediatrics.

General Comments on Treatment of Fluid and Electrolyte Problems

Fluid and electrolyte problems are associated with most diseases. Certain conditions, however, require special attention to these needs.

Severe diarrhea, vomiting, burns, diabetic acidosis, the period of fast after major surgery, salicylate poisoning, heat exhaustion and shock are examples of such conditions.

The general aim of fluid therapy is threefold: first, to correct previous losses; second, to correct continued losses; and third, to maintain daily requirements. The physician bases his decisions on some of the following things.

The history of the patient will identify the symptoms and reveal their duration. The physical examination will reveal the general condition of the patient. The weight, age, blood pressure and other vital signs will be considered in determining the amount of fluid to be given. Laboratory study of the blood sodium, chloride, potassium, hemoglobin and CO_2 combining power and a urinalysis will also assist him.

There are many types of solutions. Each company manufactures somewhat similar fluids under different trade names just as drug manufacturers do. It is the responsibility of the nurse to learn the purpose of the fluids which are used at her particular institution.

A few general statements can be made about the purposes of certain types of fluids.

Carbohydrate solutions provide calories and prevent protein breakdown. They may be given with or without electrolytes. Protein solutions are used to replace protein losses. Plasma or a plasma substitute can be used to replace plasma while whole blood is used when there is also a loss of red blood cells. Hydrating solutions usually consist of dextrose in half strength or quarter strength saline without potassium and are used until urine output is assured. Replacement solutions provide fluid, carbohydrate, saline and either no potassium or low potassium. Molar lactate replacement solutions are used in the treatment of acidosis. So-called maintenance solutions usually contain carbohydrate and low electrolyte levels.

Once the physician has started treatment, it is up to the nurse to carefully record and report the patient's condition as well as to see that therapy is carried out safely and correctly. The physician will recalculate fluid needs on a continuing basis until the body can again take over the job of maintaining its own fluid and electrolyte balance.

NURSING CARE OF PATIENTS RECEIVING FLUID THERAPY

Oral Fluids

Oral intake is obviously the route of choice whenever possible. An ingenious nurse may be able to prevent a patient from needing parenteral fluids. If she cannot do this, she may at least be able to shorten the length of time that a patient will require parenteral fluids. Feeding pediatric patients and encouraging adult patients to take fluids often takes time, ingenuity, patience and subtle methods of persuasion.

There are certain contraindications for giving oral fluids aside from the obvious ones of recent surgery or lack of consciousness. A patient who has a burn or a traumatic injury may be very thirsty and desire fluids. Because such patients are losing protein, electrolytes and water through the wound, it is imperative that the patient's thirst be satisfied only if nausea and vomiting do not accompany oral intake. If vomiting occurs, oral fluids should be withheld to prevent an already existing fluid and elctrolyte problem from becoming worse.

Patients who have gastrointestinal suction may also be thirsty. Oral fluids should not be given as the water will simply wash out valuable electrolytes. Hard lemon candies or sucking a wet cloth may help alleviate thirst until parenteral fluid therapy has relieved the symptom. Explanations for lack of fluids must be presented without frightening the patient.

In the case of potassium deficit, as occurs in salicylate poisoning or mild diarrhea, fruit juices and milk which are high in potassium should be given if the patient tolerates oral fluids. If the patient is suffering from sodium depletion, such as a patient receiving intensive hot pack therapy, salty broths can be given unless, of course, his sodium is restricted for some reason. In general, the nurse should find a fluid which the patient likes and offer it in a quantity and at a frequency which is tolerable whenever oral fluids are not contraindicated.

Proctoclysis

The rectum is sometimes selected for giving fluids over a short period of time. This method is contraindicated if there is diarrhea or colon or rectal surgery.

The rate of flow for a proctoclysis needs to be adjusted to the rate of absorption. Assuming the tube is in the rectum, expelled water indicates that the rate of flow is too rapid. The patient should be checked frequently for comfort and position of tube. Temperature of solution should be maintained a few degrees above body temperature. This can be accomplished by placing in the proctoclysis can a 4 ounce prescription bottle filled with water 108° F.

Subcutaneous Fluids

Subcutaneous infusion is also used for short-term therapy. Restraints should be used only if the patient, such as a child or confused adult, is likely to dislodge the needles and hurt himself. The rate of flow should be slow at first in order to have an opportunity to observe how rapidly absorption is taking place. The physician may order a preparation to increase the rate of absorption. The nurse must remain alert to signs of pallor and mottling of the skin which might indicate impending shock. If these signs are noted, the fluid should be clamped off and the physician notified immediately.

Intravenous Fluids

Intravenous fluid administration may be accomplished in several ways. The most usual way is to insert a needle or polyethylene tubing into a vein. The cutdown and scalp vein infusion are often used in pediatrics. Common sites of injection are the antecubital area, the dorsum of the hand and the saphenous vein of the leg. Physicians prefer not to use the latter site in older patients with thrombophlebitis.

The nurse must be aware of the possible dangers of intravenous fluid therapy. First of all, in order to prevent the introduction of infection, good aseptic technique is required when a needle or tubing is inserted. The nurse must know how much fluid is to be given within a specified length of time. She must then calculate the number of cc. to be given each hour.

The nurse caring for the patient receiving intravenous fluids must make the following observations:

1. Make sure that the prescribed fluid is prepared for administration. Procedures for identification of fluid and patient should be identical with those for administering medications. Some hospitals use a regular medication card for parenteral fluid administration.

2. Make sure that the patient is voiding before potassium is given. Accumulation of potassium can cause renal shutdown and heart block so that this observation is vital.

3. Once the fluid has been started, check the patient every 20 minutes for the following:

   a. General comfort

   b. The site of injection and surrounding area for possible infiltration, pressure sores or redness which may indicate a beginning phlebitis

   c. The amount of fluid remaining in the bottle and the drip chamber for the rate of flow

   d. Signs of overhydration, such as edema, restlessness, apprehension, dyspnea, headache or back pain.

4. If symptoms of overhydration occur, clamp the tubing so that the fluid is running at only a few drops per minute in order to keep the tubing open and call the physician immediately.

5. If the fluid is not running properly, check the tubing for a possible kink and the air filter for a possible plug, and try raising the height of the bottle.

Signs and Symptoms to Be Noted

Dehydration. When a patient is admitted to the hospital or when his fluid intake is not adequate, the nurse must know the symptoms of dehydration: thirst, dry mucous membranes, flushed and dry skin with poor turgor, sinking eyes (especially noted in children), diminished urine output and fatigue. Apprehension, nausea, changes in heart activity and headache indicate an accompanying loss of electrolytes.

Overhydration. Symptoms of overhydration must be looked for during fluid therapy. They include restlessness, edema of the face (especially the eyelids), the feet and hands, dyspnea, headache, back pain and apprehension.

Blood Transfusion Reaction. Reactions to fluid and electrolyte solutions are not usual. The nurse on occasion, however, will see a transfusion reaction which is manifested by chills, dizziness, dyspnea and itching of the skin. If these symptoms are seen, the transfusion should be stopped. The physician should be notified immediately and the laboratory usually wishes to be called also.

Shock. The underlying mechanism in shock, whether it is caused by burns, hemorrhage or crush injuries, is a shift of extracellular fluid from plasma to the interstitial compartment. Symptoms include pallor, tachycardia, low blood pressure, apprehension, cold extremities and unconsciousness in severe cases.

Intake and Output

Balance of intake and output is important. The amount of fluid taken by mouth and the amount of urine excreted approximately equal each other in a state of health. Other losses include about 200 cc./day in the feces and about 800 cc./day through the lungs and skin. These losses about equal the amount of fluid taken as a part of our food and that created by oxidation of food.

Water loss through the lungs and skin varies with the temperature and humidity of the environment. Insensible perspiration is that which is lost through evaporation. Sensible perspiration is that which is seen and creates moisture on the skin. When a person has visible perspiration or has a fever, his water requirements are substantially increased.

Water and electrolyte loss through vomiting or diarrhea also create disturbances which must be replaced if they occur to any degree. When a patient is put on intake and output, it is vital that the nurse understand that this is not a perfunctory chore imposed upon the nursing staff. When the nurse is asked to keep an intake and output record, she is being asked to report on kidney function and loss of electrolytes through symptoms such as perspiration, vomiting or diarrhea. She is also expected to note drainage from wounds, to report suction drainage accurately and to be equally scrupulous in her record of intake, whether it is by mouth, vein or tube.

Accurate records are a vital part of good nursing. This aspect of fluid balance cannot be overemphasized. It is the nurse who observes, reports, measures and records intake and output. Every fluid ordered by a physician is influenced in part by her recordings. It is the responsibility of the registered nurse to explain the importance of this record as it relates to patients, personnel and visitors. Accuracy is imperative, although one cannot help but speculate about its priority rating when one sees the night nurse struggling with inaccurate and incomplete intake and output slips kept by her colleagues.

Intake and output records are usually kept on surgical patients, on those with burns, kidney disease and some heart ailments, and on anyone receiving parenteral therapy. The doctor will order intake and

Name
Room

INTAKE & OUTPUT WORK SHEET

Date____________________

FLUID MEASUREMENTS

Carafe	500cc	Glasses		Ice cream	75cc
Coffee cup	150cc	Ice chips	50cc	Jello	40cc
Coffee pot	250cc	Juice - meal	75cc	Sherbert	75cc
Creamer - large	75cc	Nourishment	120cc	Soup bowl	120cc
Creamer - small	20cc	Water	200cc		

11-7				7-3				3-11			
INTAKE				INTAKE				INTAKE			
Time	Type	cc Given	cc Taken	Time	Type	cc Given	cc Taken	Time	Type	cc Given	cc Taken
				Break							
								Dinner			
				Lunch							
TOTAL				TOTAL				TOTAL			

OUTPUT			OUTPUT			OUTPUT		
Time	cc Urine	Other Type-cc	Time	cc Urine	Other Type-cc	Time	cc Urine	Other Type-cc
Total			Total			Total		

Figure 17–2. *Sample intake and output record used in St. Barnabas Hospital, Minneapolis, Minnesota.*

24 HOUR I. V. RECORDING

NAME ______________________

AGE ______________ DIV. ______________

RECORD NO. ______________ DATE ______________

	SOLUTION	AMOUNT				TOTAL ABSORBED		RATE	
TIME	TYPE	BEFORE FLUID ADDED	ADDED	TOTAL IN BURETTE	ABSORBED SINCE LAST RECORDING	PLASMA OR BLOOD	FLUID	GTTS. PER MINUTE	INI-TIALS

I. V. TO RUN ______ GTTS/MIN. ______ CC/HR.

REMARKS:

TOTALS

NORMAL SALINE	CC
BLOOD	CC
PLASMA	CC
	CC
	CC

Figure 17–3. *Sample parenteral fluid record. (From* Care of Children in Hospitals, *American Academy of Pediatrics, 1801 Hinman Ave., Evanston, Illinois, 1960.)*

output when he wishes it, but the nurse should keep track of it on her own when she sees signs and symptoms which would make it valuable to the patient.

Daily intake and output records are usually more accurate if each shift totals its own fluids. Another reason for having eight-hour totals is to have immediate information available for the physician who is recalculating fluid requirements every eight hours. Many hospitals also have a special parenteral fluid sheet which is an actual part of the chart.

Recording and observing output must be equally accurate. When an output record is required, urine should be measured. The color, odor and general appearance need to be noted. Pain or discomfort when the patient voids must also be known and reported. Number and description of stools need to be included on the record. Excessive perspiration needs to be known. Vomiting must be described in terms of color, odor, estimated amount and consistency.

Suction drainage must also be described in terms of color and amount. One aspect of suction output is often overlooked by the nurse. Whenever a suction is irrigated, irrigating fluid must be recorded as intake in order to present an accurate picture.

Surgical patients may receive fluids during surgery which are not recorded. The nurse in the recovery room or operating room must remember to include this on the chart.

SUMMARY

The nurse caring for patients receiving fluid therapy has a special challenge in the area of written and oral communications. Careful observations are vital. General knowledge of the most outstanding causes of imbalance will help the nurse to communicate pertinent information promptly to the physician.

SUGGESTED READINGS

Burgess, Richard E.: Fluids and Electrolytes. *American Journal of Nursing*, October, 1965, p.90.

Snively, William D.: *Sea Within*. Philadelphia, J. B. Lippincott Co., 1960.

REFERENCES

Brickman, Doris A.: Some Pointers on I.V. Therapy. *R.N.* August, 1961, p. 38.

Christensen, Halvor N.: *Body Fluids and the Acid–Base Balance*. Philadelphia, W. B. Saunders Co., 1964.

Clatworthy, H. William, Jr., and Stewart, Mary M.: Intravenous Therapy for Infants and Children. *American Journal of Nursing*, May, 1957, p. 630.

Colle, Eleanor, and Paulsen, Elsa Proehl: Response of the Newborn Infant to Major Surgery. *Pediatrics*, Vol. 23, June, 1959.

Cooke, Robert E., Fluid Therapy in Surgery of the Newborn. *Pediatrics,* Vol. 23, June, 1959.

Elman, Robert: Fluid Balance from the Nurse's Point of View. *American Journal of Nursing,* April, 1949.

Farr, Hollon: Fluid and Electrolyte Balance—with Special Reference to the Gastrointestinal Tract. *American Journal of Nursing,* July, 1954, p. 826.

Fielo, Sandra B.: Teaching Fluid and Electrolyte Balance. *Nursing Outlook,* March, 1965, p. 43.

Fluids and Electrolytes, Abbott Laboratories, North Chicago, Illinois, 1960.

Jacob, Stanley W., and Francone, Clarice Ashworth: *Structure and Function of Man.* Philadelphia, W. B. Saunders Co., 1965, Chapter 16.

MacBryde, Cyril Mitchell: *Signs and Symptoms.* Philadelphia, J. B. Lippincott Co., 1964, Chapter 30.

Maddock, Walter G.: Some Fundamentals in Water and Electrolyte Balance. *Ohio State Medical Journal,* May, 1949, p. 462.

Moyer, Carl A.: *Fluid Balance,* A Clinical Manual. Chicago, Year Book Medical Publishers, Inc., 1952.

Parenteral Administration. Abbott Laboratories, North Chicago, Illinois, 1959.

Routh, Joseph I.: *Fundamentals of Inorganic, Organic and Biological Chemistry.* Philadelphia, W. B. Saunders Co., 1965.

Shafer, Kathleen N., and others: *Medical-Surgical Nursing.* Ed. 3, Section 6, St. Louis, C. V. Mosby Co., 1964.

Simple Intravenous Fluid Therapy in Young Children. *What's New,* 1956, No. 196, p. 5.

Snively, William D.: *Sea Within.* Philadelphia, J. B. Lippincott Co., 1960.

Wolf, Edith S.: The Nurse and Fluid Therapy. *American Journal of Nursing,* July, 1954, p. 831.

Worthen, H. G., and Raile, R. G.: Fluid and Electrolyte Balance: II. Parenteral Fluid Therapy in Infants and Children. *Minnesota Medicine,* August, 1954, p. 558.

18

Common Types of New Equipment and Supplies

It is very frustrating and often undermining for the refresher—or anyone else, for that matter—to be unable to handle a piece of equipment. If it occurs in the presence of a patient, it is doubly upsetting, as the patient may exhibit a sense of uneasiness. In most cases, such an experience is totally unnecessary, especially if there has been an adequate orientation or in-service program. Needless to say, being confronted with a new piece of equipment alone for the first time at the patient's bedside is a less than ideal situation in which to learn about it.

Many times the item creating an embarrassing situation is as simple as a new kind of clamp on intravenous tubing. This is one reason why a hospital is loathe to change products unless the product in use is unsatisfactory. Besides, prices for hospital supplies of comparable quality are quite similar. When one gets used to many types of new supplies, however, one gains enough experience to learn new product adaptations very quickly.

There is an endless number of products available for use in hospitals. Some are labor-saving devices, some aid in the prevention of cross infection, some aid in the treatment and comfort of the patient, and some merely make certain tasks a great deal easier. I will mention only some of these items in order to acquaint the refresher with the variety of things available.

DISPOSABLES

Disposables refer to supplies which are used once and then discarded. These supplies intended for single use have several advantages. Sterility is better guaranteed. Time spent in preparation of trays and the carrying out of procedures is reduced or eliminated. In most cases they are more convenient for the nurse to use. Some items are cheaper, but some create additional cost. There are many factors which each institution must consider before deciding to add new disposable items to its inventory. It is not in the province of this book to discuss these considerations. It is interesting, however, to know that central service departments handle about five times the number of items with about one half the number of personnel than they did ten years ago. This has been largely due to disposables.

Increased use of disposables creates two very serious problems. First of all, there is greater need for storage space. Sometimes products must be refused because of lack of space. More frequent delivery of smaller amounts of supplies sometimes alleviates the problem. The purchasing department of the hospital has the responsibility of maintaining an adequate inventory for the hospital so that personnel do not run out of supplies. Both the nursing stations and the central service department or the hospital storeroom must have adequate shelving to accommodate supplies for varying lengths of time.

Secondly, disposing of disposables becomes a problem. In fact, a disposable disposer is manufactured. More personnel may be needed to handle trash. It can cause problems among personnel who we may forget are involved. At one hospital the night trash man became enraged at the day trash man because he started leaving a cart load of trash to be burned every night. The day trash man was not loafing on the job and was very defensive. What neither they nor their supervisor knew was that the nursing department had recently started using disposable 2 cc. syringes, disposable enema equipment and disposable underpads all at once. This had created two additional loads of trash per day. The day trash man had been able to handle one extra load, but not two.

There is another important aspect of disposing of disposables. Narcotic addicts and children may find hospital trash available outside of buildings awaiting removal. This has become such a problem that the American Public Health Association suggests that needles and syringes be crushed, destroyed by heat, or buried in separate containers in sanitary fill. Nurses are asked to break needles off at the syringe or to break the needle and to separate the barrel from the plunger when they are being discarded.

Paper Products

Paper drinking cups may be available in patient bathrooms. This reduces the possibility of mix-up, as patients in multiple-bed rooms have no need to take a drinking glass to the bathroom with them. They are also available for guests who, in years gone by, have been seen drinking from the patient's glass. In most cases the patient still uses a drinking glass, but it can more assuredly be considered his own when paper cups are available nearby.

The medicine glass has been replaced by a paper cup of the same size and shape with measurements printed on the side. It is wise for the nurse to note the printing on these cups as once in awhile a shipment arrives with blurred markings. Plastic medicine cups are also used and in some instances are cheaper and more accurate than paper ones. Either one saves the nurse the task of washing medicine glasses. It is obviously a cleaner method when one recalls the conditions under which the nurse used to wash these glasses. Small paper soufflé cups or similar items are available for taking pills to the patient.

Paper slippers, similar to scuffs, are manufactured for patients. It is surprising how many patients routinely arrive at a private hospital without robe or slippers. While paper slippers are not ideal, they do serve a function when nothing else is available.

Paper masks may be used in surgery, in nurseries, in isolation and for protective isolation. Paper masks come in a variety of sizes and shapes and differ in filtration ability. Few hospitals use many washable cloth masks anymore. Cloth masks are usually made available for the few persons who have a personal liking for them. The better grades of paper masks provide better protection because they contain several filtration layers and new filtration materials. Careless handling and prolonged wearing of the same mask is still not recommended. Esthetically, it is more pleasant to put on a mask which has never been worn by anyone else, regardless of the soundness of the laundry procedures.

Paper dishes and paper utensils are being used for isolation patients. This, too, saves many steps and provides a better barrier for the prevention of cross infection.

Paper specimen containers are commonly used. The urine specimen jar has become a urine specimen container (paper or plastic). The sputum cup is a half-pint carton. The large specimen pails are gallon cartons. Washing such items in the service rooms or laboratory or C.S.R. is no longer necessary, and another possible health hazard for personnel and patients is eliminated.

Paper underpads (small, medium and large) are used instead of cloth underpads for giving enemas or when drainage or incontinence exists. Again, this saves the amount of laundry, lessens the amount of soiled linen transported through the chutes and halls and probably means that the patient is drier, because a soft paper underpad can be changed more easily and more rapidly than foundation linen on the bed. Disposable diapers are also manufactured. Disposable sheets and gowns are being studied.

Some hospitals use sterile paper drapes in the operating room and delivery room. Because of the variety of individual differences in procedures among hospitals, physicians and nurses, this is a difficult area for manufacturers to standardize. As a result, the use of paper drapes is less common than might be expected. Paper drapes also have varying degrees of absorption qualities. The combined use of paper with plastic is sometimes thought to be the answer to providing an effective bacterial barrier. Many hospitals are presently using a plastic drape under the regular cloth drape to lessen the danger of contamination from a drape which becomes soaked with drainage. As these products become more varied, they will undoubtedly be used more commonly.

The paper drinking straw has replaced the hazardous glass drinking tube. The T-binder now comes in paper. The bath mat is paper. When you enter a hospital, be alert to these products so that you become aware of the "paper revolution," so to speak.

Autoclave tape is an extra check on autoclave adequacy. Packs are secured with tape instead of string. The tape changes color if the sterilization process has been successful.

Autoclave envelopes of various sizes and shapes are available for wrapping items. Some are even self-sealing. They replace the specially made wrappers which were made in the linen room. Bedside bags for disposing of the patient's tissue wipes eliminate the need for folding and pinning newspaper bags on the bed. Paper bags to dispose of perineal pads are available in patient bathrooms, as well as in public rest rooms.

Plastics

SYRINGES AND NEEDLES. Disposable plastic syringes have become available by mass production. As a result, most hospitals find that it is cheaper to use them in place of glass syringes. Needles are made of various metals. The advantage of using the disposable needle is that the needle is always sharp and never plugged with a foreign protein which the "needle girl" did not discover and remove. Sterility and cleanliness are virtually assured.

NARCOTIC PILL COUNTER. Do you remember counting pills in a bottle while they rolled around? Various kinds of counters are available. One is a plastic rotating disk which holds each pill in a numbered slot. Counting narcotic pills requires only a quick glance at the disk. This particular gadget was invented by a nurse.

TUBING. Intravenous tubes, enema tubes, gastric tubes, drainage tubes, suction tubes, oxygen tubes and many others are made of plastic. Again, cleanliness is assured. Adequate cleaning of tubing had limitations even with the best techniques. These items have completely replaced rubber tubing with few exceptions. Plastic gastric tubes are sometimes harder to swallow and sometimes more irritating to the mucosa. Because of this, the physician may prefer a rubber tube. With greater perfection of plastic, this will undoubtedly become less of an exception. Rubber is commonly used for urethral catheters, also. At the present time, plastic is less often used for gastrointestinal tubes and urethral catheters.

OXYGEN SUPPLIES. Oxygen masks are rarely rubber today. Many types of oxygen masks (with and without rebreathing bags), oxygen catheters and oxygen cannulas are all made of plastic. Oxygen tubing is traditionally distinguished by its green color.

Bags. The variety of sizes, shapes and uses of plastic bags almost reach infinity. Wastebaskets are lined with them so that refuse may be removed, sealed, disposed of without handling and transported through corridors without exposure to the air before final incineration. Surgical dressings are collected in them so that moisture cannot soak through a bag and transmit infection. They may be used to cover patients' plants when patients go home in the cold weather. They are used to collect patients' belongings. They are used for everything that someone wants to use them for. Plastic bags, or possibly waxed paper bags, are used to collect refuse from isolated rooms. They are used to carry and to cover hot packs. Soft plastic enema bags, douche bags and drainage collection bags are almost routinely used instead of cans or jars. Even blood and plasma may come in plastic bags rather than bottles.

Dissolvable laundry bags are being tried in some hospitals. They are placed directly into a washer, and the bags disintegrate during the washing process. The success of this depends on the way in which the washer can manage possible residue.

Disposable Sitz Bath. A plastic basin is made which can rest on the toilet bowl (with the toilet seat raised). The patient sits on the basin which is filled with warm water. A bag containing warm water drains into this basin slowly to create an exchange of warm water. They are ideal for home use and for isolation patients who need frequent sitz baths.

Adaptors. Gone are the days of cut fingers which have tried to remove tight tubing from a glass adaptor. Plastic adaptors replace glass whenever possible for reasons of accident prevention.

Cloth and Other Combined Materials

Dressings. Absorbable paper and gauze may cover the patient's wound. Absorbable sponge rubber is also used for dressings. Dressings such as 4 × 4's (fluffs), abdominal pads and several others are packaged together by the manufacturer for change of dressings on wounds from which there is profuse drainage.

Dressings are held in place by paper or plastic tape. Tape sensitivity is far less common because most tapes have some degree of porousness.

The carefully cut butterfly which had to be flamed now comes in individually wrapped papers like Band-aids. They come in several sizes.

Nonadhering dressings are prepared in various sizes, shapes and mixtures of materials. The side of the dressing which is placed on the wound will soak up drainage and at the same time will not adhere to the wound. Some dressings are treated with an antibiotic so that a dressing also becomes a treatment. Even prepackaged dressings moistened with Burow's solution are manufactured.

Some types of surgical wounds can be closed with special tape rather than sutures. When this is possible, the advantages are that stitch removal is unnecessary, the possibility of stitch abscess is eliminated, and pain is reduced when a small wound needs to be closed in a physician's office or an outpatient department. Petrolatum strips, formerly hand prepared and autoclaved in a stainless-steel boat, now comes in individually foil-wrapped packages. These petroleum dressings are sterile and come in many sizes.

PREPACKAGED SETS. There is an endless number of prepackaged trays, all of which used to be prepared in the dressing room or the central service room (C.S.R.). Most hospitals use at least some of these trays. Few hospitals consider total use of these items economical to the patient or feasible in terms of storage space. Available are catheterization sets, Foley catheterization sets, enema sets, spinal trays, operative prep trays, bladder irrigation trays, dressing change sets, spinal anesthesia trays, as well as many others. A prepackaged set of equipment for a particular procedure is very helpful to the nurse if everything she needs is actually included in the package.

In summary, the boom in disposable items has contributed to work efficiency and assures sterility of many supplies used by hospitals. As a refresher, you will find that in most cases, disposables will make your job a great deal easier.

THE PATIENT'S ROOM

When a patient is admitted to the hospital, he needs a short course in the use of the "gadgets" surrounding him. Everything is simple to use, but an elderly patient, an overly anxious patient or one who is slightly confused needs help to keep the buttons from becoming overwhelming. When you first see these things, you will need a thorough explanation. It is vital to remember that the patient will need the same, especially since it has become second nature to you. A patient's room may have more or less equipment than is described here, depending on the age of the hospital.

The Radio

A pillow speaker is available for each bed. This provides radio for one patient without disturbing anyone else, as it has a built-in volume control. Generally, the radio receives three or four local AM stations available to the area plus a station which has piped in Musak. This station is controlled by the hospital. Hospitals with a religious affiliation often broadcast their worship services on this station. The radio is usually furnished free of charge.

Television

Most new hospitals have built-in, wall-mounted television sets.

They are often not owned or operated by the hospital. If they are not, a local commercial company owns and operates them. In most cases, there is a daily charge for the service. Provision for the cost of this makes a very nice gift for a hospitalized friend.

The Bed

As already mentioned in Chapter 3, a great convenience to the nurse and a service to the patient is the bed which can be raised and lowered in height. Some of these beds are electric, and some are cranked up and down by hand. Hospitals with this kind of bed usually have a policy stating that the bed must be in the low position at all times except when the nurse is attending the patient. Patients with fractures, surgery or any kind of incapacity can usually get in and out of bed more safely and more comfortably from a low bed. When these beds are used, the old step stool is no longer a necessary hazard.

If the bed is electric, the patient's head and/or knee can be raised and lowered by pressing a button. Usually the button is made available to the patient so that he can change his position as he wishes without calling the nurse. The control buttons are operated by personnel when the patient cannot do it for himself. If a patient misuses the control buttons, they can be made inoperable. Some models are retractable, which means that the patient does not find the bedside cabinet behind him when he raises the head of the bed. The bed adjusts for this.

Side rails are usually part of the bed. They no longer are brought in and out of rooms and attached and removed from beds according to the patient needs. Some hospitals purchase half rails and some purchase full rails. If a hospital has upper half rails, lower rails can be added if they are considered necessary. The advantage of half rails is that a majority of patients, regardless of age, like to use them. They hold onto them to balance themselves getting in and out of bed. Many persons think they are advantageous for the elderly confused patient who tries to get out of bed. They feel these patients are less likely to hurt themselves if they fall from a low bed rather than over the additional height of a rail. There are many studies analyzing the merits of half rails versus full rails. Numbers of falls and injuries from falls have been compared, and it was found that each type of rail has certain advantages. When the half rail is used routinely, some hospitals have given up the arbitrary policy which requires everyone over a certain age to have side rails. While this is hard for some to accept, it seems, in general, wise to let the nurse decide to use side rails according to the condition of her patients. A 20-year-old with a head injury is in far greater need of side rails than a spunky, clear-headed 80-year-old with a broken wrist. This particular subject illustrates how a traditional policy may not always best serve a patient. It is an example of the kind of decision which is being left to the nurse's good judgment based on her knowledge and observations.

Electronic Bedside Cabinets

Newer hospitals are installing audiovisual centers at the bedside. These units contain space for bedside utensils and towels and washcloth. In addition, physiological monitoring, telephone, radio, television and an intercom system to the nursing station are all part of the unit.

THE NURSING STATION

Automation has come to the nursing station in several very common forms. Other comments about some of these innovations have been made in Chapters 3 and 4.

The Pneumatic Tube

Most new hospitals build in a pneumatic tube system. Charts, orders, requests, small unbreakable items and messages can be sent to and received from departments all over the hospital.

The Intercommunication System

The intercommunication system (intercom) serves as a voice communication from the patient's room to the nursing station. When the patient pulls the signal cord at his bed, a light outside his door turns on and his room number lights up on a panel at the desk. The secretary at the desk speaks to the patient, receives his request and relays it to personnel. If the person who says, "May I help you?" is not a nurse, it is important that the patient understand this. If the patient does not, he may visualize a nurse visiting at the desk and taking her time to get his bedpan.

Nurses often fail to take advantage of the intercom for themselves. They can save many steps. As an example, instead of going to the desk to ask someone to order a piece of equipment, the nurse can call the request to the desk, thus utilizing both the intercom and the station secretary to the patient's advantage.

Intercoms have many different features according to the manufacturer. Any intercom, however, is a mixed blessing. If nursing personnel ignore the light over a patient's door and let the secretary handle all the calls, it can delay patient care, rather than expedite it. It is an aid to patient care when it is not substituted for personal attention when the nurse is nearby.

In addition to voice communication, visual communication can be obtained through closed-circuit television.

The Addressograph

The addressograph saves much clerical time. A plate, much like a charge-plate, is made for each patient at the time of his admission. The information imprinted on the plate depends on the needs of the individual hospital. The patient's name, hospital number, physician's name and room number are usually considered necessary information.

Use of the addressograph requires caution, as it can be a source of error. If the person using the apparatus stamps a request with the wrong plate, a white blood count may be ordered for Mrs. Smith instead of Mrs. Jones. Since this can be a source of error, personnel should be encouraged to be especially careful in its use.

Monitoring Devices

Monitoring devices which can keep track of a patient's vital signs are beginning to be used for the patient with coronary disease, the acutely ill patient, the major surgical patient and any patient requiring frequent checks of temperature, pulse, respiration, blood pressure and electrocardiogram. Few nurses have ever used such equipment. Thorough instruction would be needed by anyone using monitors.

Computers

The computer can transcribe physicians' orders, make charges and remind the nurse to give her medications. It can be used for patient billing, inventory control, menu planning and storage of patient records among other things. A few hospitals are doing research with computers and data processing equipment under research grants. Others are already beginning to use them for certain functions with expectation of expanding their use.

EQUIPMENT USED FOR TREATMENT

The kinds of equipment used for treatment are vast in number, and the information in this section does not pretend to be complete. This is a field where the older nurse and the new graduate have something in common. They both feel insecure. A nurse must rely upon her employing institution to provide assistance for operating equipment. Material provided by the manufacturer is often inadequate without additional explanation, description and/or demonstration. A company often tends to use technical engineering terms in its instructions. One or two words, such as coupler, may stand as a barrier to the nurse's understanding. No matter how old the nurse is, she will experience the use of a new piece of equipment, small or large, every few months. Therefore, no matter how thorough an orientation may be, each one of us will be learning something new at frequent intervals. As the experience of new equipment becomes common, it seems less awesome. One soon finds that new things are often new arrangements of old things, so that one can quickly adapt old knowledge to learning the new. Here are but a few examples.

Aquamatic K Pad

The Aqua K pad can virtually replace the hot water bottle if dry heat is needed on a continuous basis. It can also reduce many problems associated with the application of hot packs. The apparatus has two main parts. One is a plastic pad with veinlike compartments inside. The other is a small container holding water. It is electric and the two parts are connected by small hoses. A gauge can be set so that water continuously circulates through the pad at a certain temperature, usually about 105° F. It can be used as a simple heating pad to apply dry heat, or it can be wrapped around moist wool to keep a hot pack hot. It is one of several products which simplify the application of hot packs.

Alternating Pressure Mattress

The alternating pressure mattress is the length and width of the mattress on the bed. It too is plastic and has veinlike compartments running lengthwise. Attached is a pump which expands and deflates every other vein alternately and is used to prevent bedsores. It is only about one inch thick and is placed on top of the regular mattress. It is covered by a sheet which acts as the bottom sheet of the bed.

Thermal Blanket

This equipment also consists of two-veined mats or so-called blankets similar in size to the alternating pressure mattress. One is placed on top of the mattress. The other is placed over the patient who lies between the two blankets wrapped in a sheet, so that his skin does not directly touch the blankets. These blankets are attached by hoses to a fairly large piece of equipment having temperature control dials. Alcohol circulates through the blankets. It can be used to raise or lower body temperature. It is more usual, however, to use it to lower the temperature of a patient with an abnormally high temperature.

Circle Bed

The circle bed serves the same purpose as the old Foster frame. It has a frame on which the patient lies when he is on his back and a frame on which he rests when he is prone. It is used for patients who are difficult to turn, as in the case of a cervical fracture or a burn. It permits change of linen with minimal pain or discomfort to the patient. If the patient is to be turned front to back, the posterior frame is locked into place with the patient between the two frames. He is then turned a half circle so that he is lying on the posterior frame. The anterior frame is then removed until the patient is again turned.

Bennett Respirator

The Bennett respirator is one of several types of respirators which perform the functions of helping the patient to breathe or of giving aerosol treatment to a patient with asthma, emphysema or bronchiectasis. This machine operates under positive pressure with oxygen. It can provide air and pressure to the patient to help him to breathe without his participation. If it is used for aerosol treatment, the patient may learn to operate it himself. This should be of comfort to the nurse who thinks she cannot learn to use such machinery. If the machine model is highly complicated, an anesthetist, an inhalation therapist or a nurse recently trained in its use may need to be consulted.

Croupette

The Croupette is a high-humidity tent used in the pediatric department. The humidity is forced into circulation either by a motor or by oxygen. A properly operating humidity tent brings rapid relief to the infant or child in respiratory distress due to swollen mucosa.

MISCELLANEOUS SUPPLIES AND EQUIPMENT

Among hundreds of other items are the electronic thermometer, piped-in wall suction and plastic utensils which eliminate the noise of metal utensils. The plastic bedpan also eliminates the problem of the cold bedpan. Automatic doors, such as those in many supermarkets, reduce the awkwardness of getting large pieces of equipment through doors and prevent the age-old problem of bumping litters into doors. Disposable examining gloves and disposable surgical gloves are manufactured. Special dumbwaiters are made to handle large equipment. Hydraulic lifts and stretchers reduce the amount of back-breaking lifting needed to care for patients. Motorized wheel chairs, oxygen recording devices and microscopes that can be used to see unstained tissue are other items. Further enumeration of equipment would be pointless. The nurse will learn to operate the equipment used in her hospital and/or area. It would be fruitless to learn how to operate equipment you might never use. The nurse needs to be somewhat familiar with the existence of the main kinds of available equipment, but she need not nor cannot know how to operate anything she has never seen or used.

SUMMARY

Vast numbers of new items, small and large, are invented and manufactured every month. Some of these never become successful and some develop into items used every day by many of us. What was used yesterday may become obsolete today. Knowledge of equipment belongs in the realm of in-service education. Orientation may familiarize you with what is used in your work setting, but in-service education, formal or informal, will help you to become familiar with new equipment as it is put into use.

REFERENCES

George, Joyce Holmes: Electronic Monitoring of Vital Signs. *American Journal of Nursing*, February, 1965, p. 68.

New Conveyor System Moves All Supplies. *Modern Hospital*, February, 1965, p. 93.

Sutton, Audrey L.: *Bedside Nursing Techniques.* Philadelphia, W. B. Saunders Co., 1964, Chapter 2.

Tetreault, Rosemary F., and Nieto, Eugene J.: Should We Use Disposables? *Hospital Management*, June, 1965, p. 91.

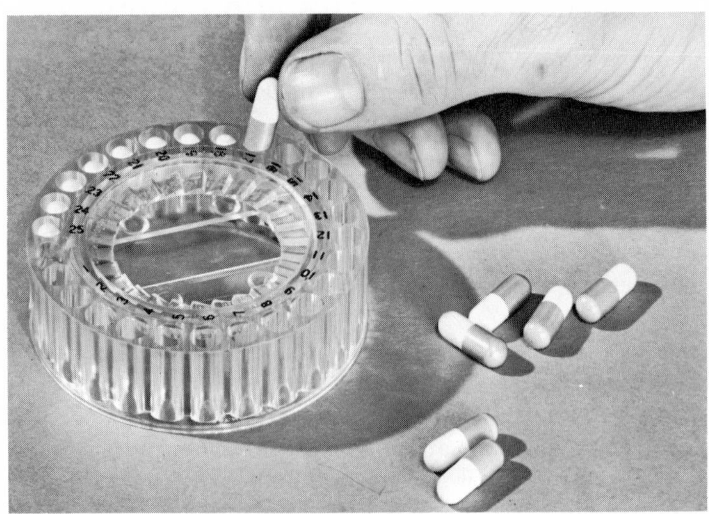

Figure 18–1. *Narcotic counting device. (Courtesy American Hospital Supply Corporation, 2020 Ridge Ave., Evanston, Illinois.)*

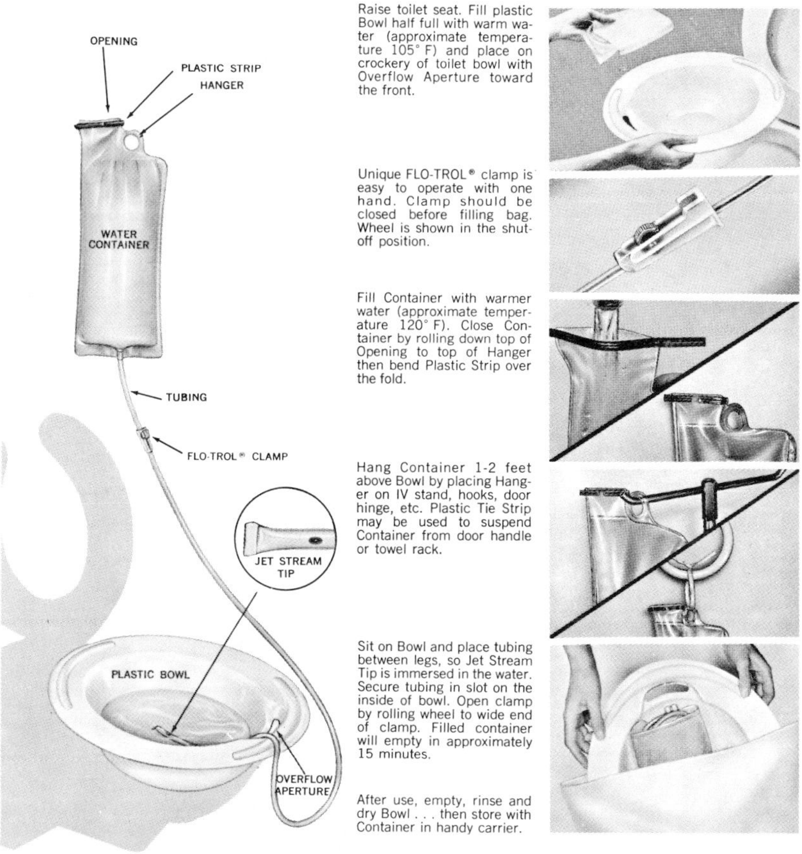

OPENING

PLASTIC STRIP

HANGER

WATER CONTAINER

TUBING

FLO-TROL® CLAMP

JET STREAM TIP

PLASTIC BOWL

OVERFLOW APERTURE

Raise toilet seat. Fill plastic Bowl half full with warm water (approximate temperature 105° F) and place on crockery of toilet bowl with Overflow Aperture toward the front.

Unique FLO-TROL® clamp is easy to operate with one hand. Clamp should be closed before filling bag. Wheel is shown in the shut-off position.

Fill Container with warmer water (approximate temperature 120° F). Close Container by rolling down top of Opening to top of Hanger then bend Plastic Strip over the fold.

Hang Container 1-2 feet above Bowl by placing Hanger on IV stand, hooks, door hinge, etc. Plastic Tie Strip may be used to suspend Container from door handle or towel rack.

Sit on Bowl and place tubing between legs, so Jet Stream Tip is immersed in the water. Secure tubing in slot on the inside of bowl. Open clamp by rolling wheel to wide end of clamp. Filled container will empty in approximately 15 minutes.

After use, empty, rinse and dry Bowl . . . then store with Container in handy carrier.

Figure 18–2. *Disposable sitz bath. (Courtesy Travenol Laboratories, Inc., Morton Grove, Illinois.)*

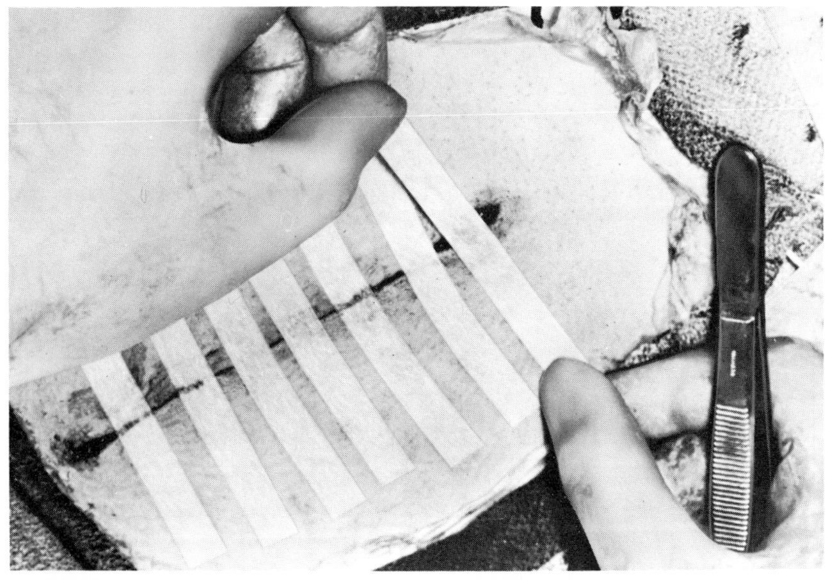

Figure 18–3. *Steri-Strip is a nonsutural skin closure. (Courtesy Minnesota Mining and Manufacturing, St. Paul, Minnesota.)*

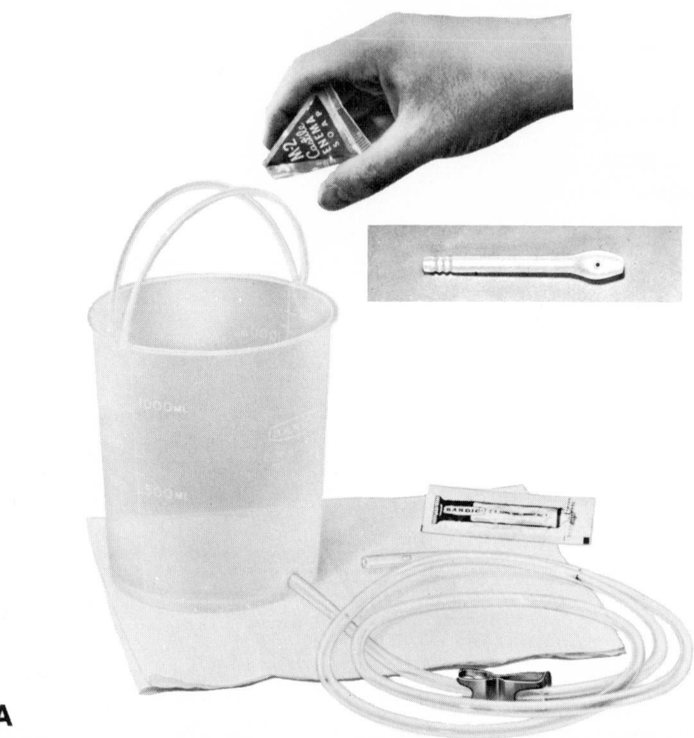

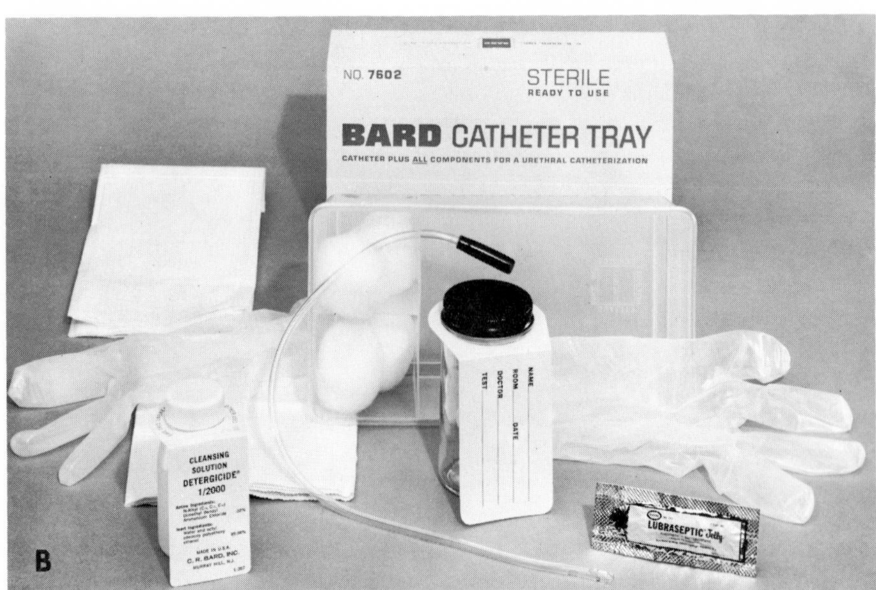

Figure 18–4A. *Disposable enema set. (Courtesy C. R. Bard, Inc.)*
Figure 18–4B. *Prepackaged catheterization tray. (Courtesy C. R. Bard, Inc.)*

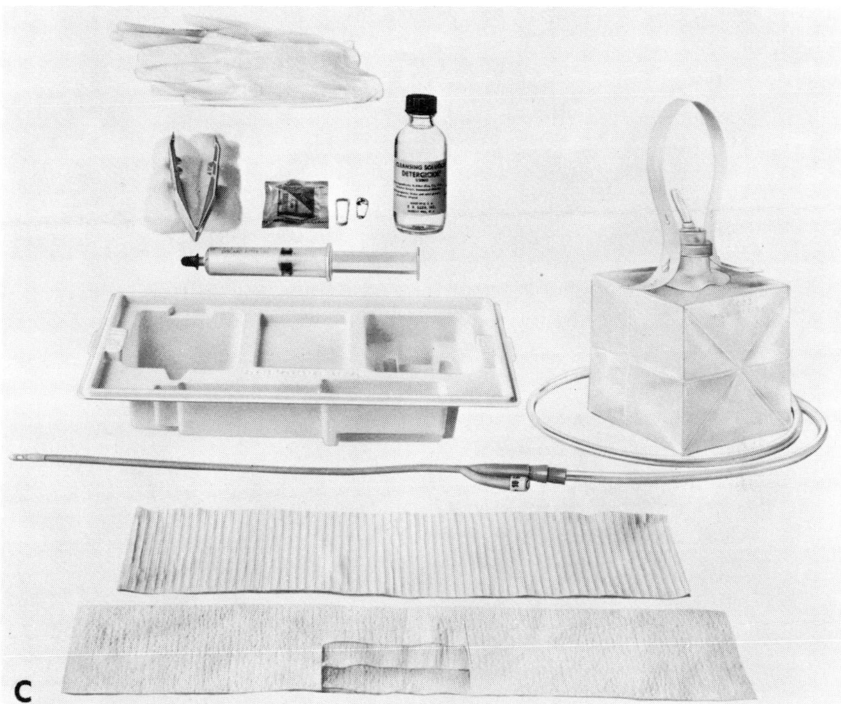

Figure 18–4C. *Foley catheterization tray. (Courtesy C. R. Bard, Inc.)*

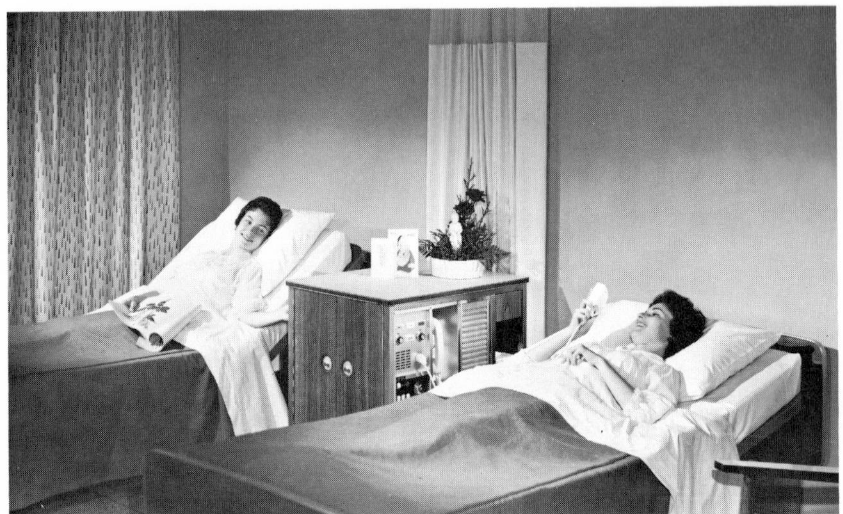

Figure 18–5. *Semiprivate room scene showing double electronic bedside unit.*

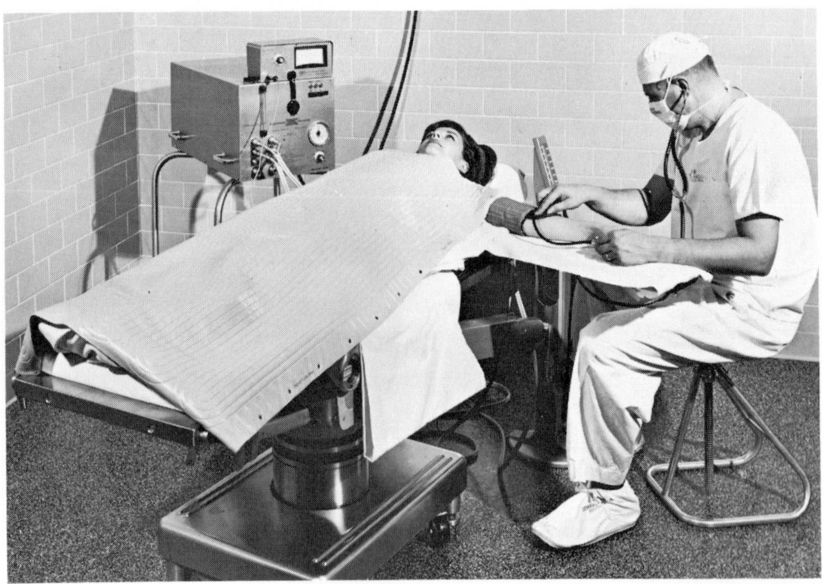

Figure 18–6. *The Aquamatic K thermia machine and blanket may be used to raise as well as lower body temperature. (Gorman-Rupp Industries, Inc., Bellville, Ohio.)*

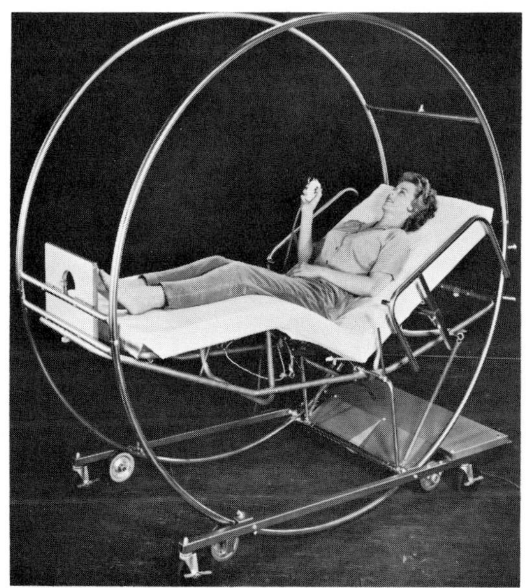

Figure 18–7. *CircOlectric bed. (Stryker Corporation, Kalamazoo, Michigan.)*

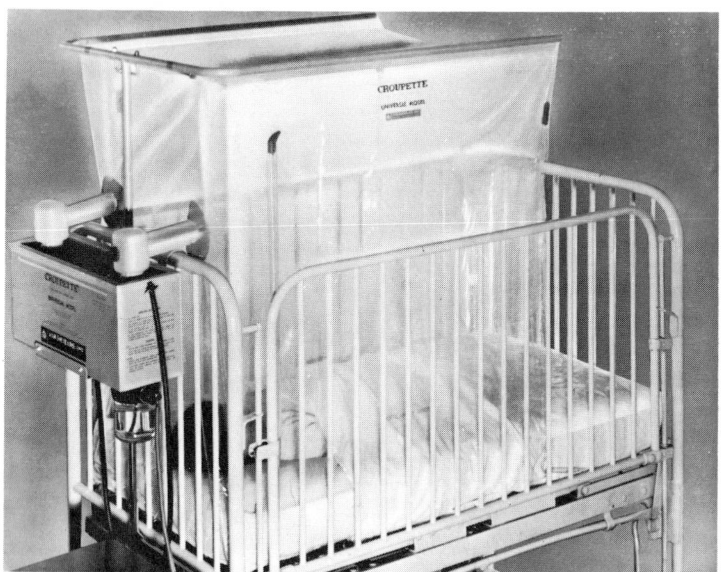

Figure 18–8. *High humidity Croupette is used for infants with respiratory difficulties. (Courtesy Air Shields, Inc., Hatboro, Pennsylvania.)*

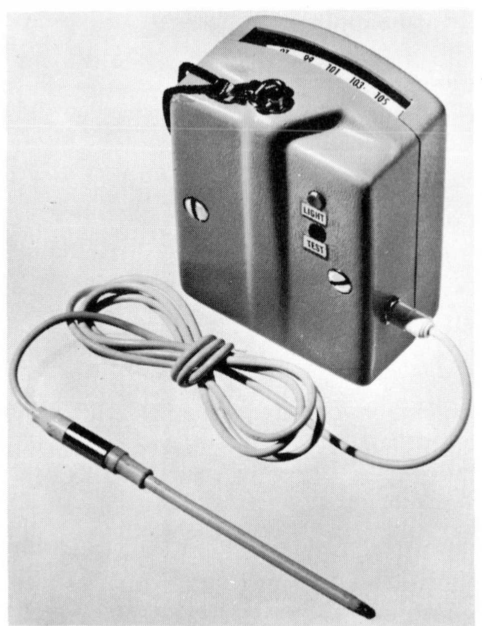

Figure 18–9. *Electronic thermometer. (Courtesy John Bunn Corporation, 1298 Main Street, Buffalo 9, New York.)*

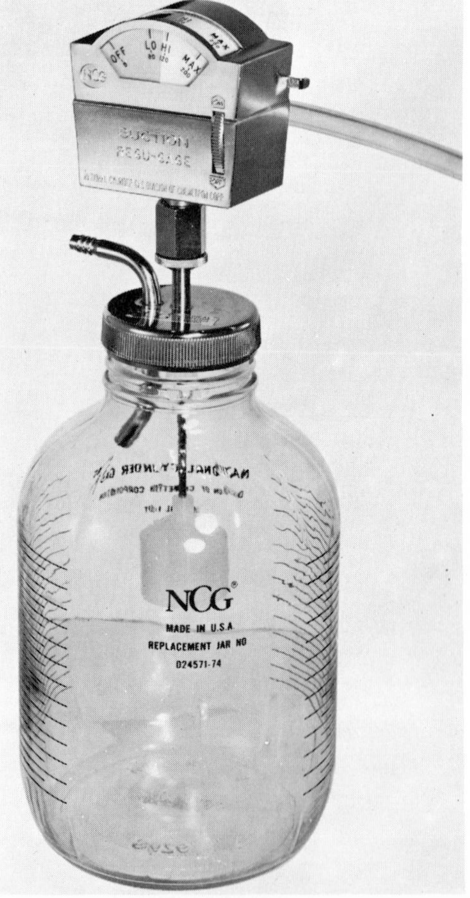

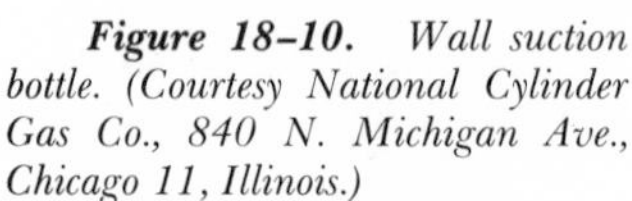

Figure 18–10. *Wall suction bottle. (Courtesy National Cylinder Gas Co., 840 N. Michigan Ave., Chicago 11, Illinois.)*

19

Major Changes in Care of the Mother and Infant

The scope of obstetric nursing has broadened to include maternal and child health care. In the broadest sense, the subject has been described by some as beginning before conception and continuing through the menopause and old age.

The refresher will have to be content with the knowledge that the subject of maternity nursing has become more inclusive and then accept the more conventional manner of this chapter. There will be no attempt to review obstetrics. For the nurse who wishes to return to this field of nursing, a review of a good up-to-date textbook is a must. Recommendations are listed at the end of the chapter.

FAMILY PLANNING AND BIRTH CONTROL

The population explosion of the world is occurring to the greatest extent in countries least able to handle the problem. It is estimated that the population of Latin America will increase 187 per cent by the year 2000, while that of North America will increase 58 per cent. Such disproportionate growth rates accompanied by declining death rates has brought the subject of birth control under the scrutiny of political leaders, economists, educators and religious leaders of the world. As a result, public policy has changed, and it is now considered appropriate to make information about birth control available to the public on a voluntary basis. Previously, this information was only available on a private basis.

In 1958, New York made information about contraception available to the public on a voluntary basis, exempting Catholic nurses and doctors. The United States makes information about contraception and the devices available to countries asking for this aid. Although there is not always whole-hearted backing of all these policies, individual choices about these decisions are usually possible now. Many states still do not allow what has become public policy.

Neither coercion nor argument is suitable to this subject. Professional persons are not expected to inject their personal beliefs. Information about the rhythm method as well as other methods is available at birth control clinics. It is up to the individual to choose the method which is appropriate to his personal and religious views.

INFERTILITY PROBLEMS

Approximately 10 per cent of all married couples have a problem of infertility. About 40 per cent of these are due to problems in the male and about 60 per cent are due to problems in the female. Many diagnostic studies are now available to help locate the cause of the problem which in many cases can be corrected.

A specimen of seminal fluid can be examined. The woman can be examined for basal metabolic problems, ovulation and patency of the ovarian tubes. The length of sperm life in the vaginal tract can be determined.

A culdoscopy examination may be done to evaluate ovarian function and tubal patency. This particular examination is also used to diagnose ectopic pregnancy, pelvic inflammatory disease, endometriosis and ovarian cysts and tumors. Some exploratory laparotomies can be avoided by this examination which is done in the operating room under surgical asepsis without the use of anesthesia. A vaginal examination is done first. Next, 20 cc. of methylene blue is injected into the cervix. The dye spreads to the fundus, the uterine isthmus and the fallopian tubes. These organs are then visualized with the instrument known as a culdoscope.

Many couples are being helped to bear children. The inability to bear children is often accompanied by guilt and anxiety. Should the nurse care for any of these patients, she will find that they are in great need of psychological support and encouragement.

FAMILY-CENTERED MATERNITY NURSING

A great deal has been written about what is known as family-centered maternity care. The basic concept goes against many routines and restrictions which have been traditionally practiced in obstetric departments. The aim is to permit the family unit—mother, father and new infant—to be together rather than separated at a time when they can give one another emotional support. In institutions where family-centered care is provided, the birth of a baby brings a family closer together.

When a hospital concentrates its attention on the family rather than just on the patient, the father is included at all phases. The father remains with the mother throughout her labor. In some cases he is allowed in the delivery room, also. This decision is made jointly by the parents and the physician, who take many factors into account. The physician has the final say on this particular aspect of the care. The father is also free to be in the room when the infant is fed, and he may hold the baby when he so desires. The infant may be brought to the room as the mother wishes.

Another feature of family-centered nursing is that the same nursing staff cares for both the mother and the infant, so that instructions and care are not segmented in such a way that the mother and the infant become separated. No increase in infections has been reported from this type of staffing.

St. Mary's Hospital, in Evansville, Indiana, has reported the reactions of physicians, nurses and patients to this plan which was carefully studied and planned at that institution. Traditional concepts were not easy to change, but the plan continues and the families who have experienced this system would have it no other way. While many hospitals have been reluctant to make as many changes as were made at St. Mary's, the concept of family-centered nursing has had an influence on most up-to-date obstetric departments to some degree. This will be clearer after reading the next few pages.

PRENATAL CARE

Improved prenatal care facilities continue to increase and to be better utilized by the public. Continued reduction of maternal and infant death rates is attributed to better prenatal care. Some abortions may be prevented by early medical evaluation.

Prenatal medical care can be obtained from a physician, a clinic, a hospital or other health facility. Besides medical care, there is a great deal of care and information which is vital to the patient's welfare. Because of this, an important part of the work done by the public health nurse is related to antepartum care of patients who come to her attention.

The birth rate declined during the depression of 1929 and then went to an all-time peak in 1947. Even though the birth rate in the United States is declining at the present time, it may be impossible to provide the public with enough physicians to care for future patients. The place of the trained nurse-midwife will undoubtedly grow. She is permitted to give direct care under the authority delegated to her by a physician, usually an obstetrician. The nurse-midwife may handle normal conditions and is trained to recognize abnormal conditions which she refers to a physician.

The First Prenatal Examination

It is usually suggested that the mother make her first visit to the physician about three weeks after the time she misses her first menstrual period. She will have a physical examination, and a medical history will be taken. Some physicians take external pelvimetry measurements. A serology, a red blood count, hemoglobin and Rh factor will be determined. Blood typing is usually done, also. A urinalysis is done at this and at each succeeding visit. The mother's weight and blood pressure are also checked at each visit.

An important part of any history of the mother is to know what drugs she is taking. The famous thalidomide tragedy in the early 1960's showed how important it is to know the action of drugs on the fetus of a pregnant woman. The thalidomide incident illustrates one other important but less prominent aspect of drugs taken during pregnancy, that is, that 80 per cent of the women taking thalidomide had normal babies. Other genetic and environmental factors, while unknown, are also involved. According to most authorities, the greatest danger is during the first trimester. Authorities also caution against panic at this time.

Follow-up Examinations

The mother is usually asked to return for a checkup every month for the first seven months, every two weeks during the eighth month and weekly during the ninth month. Patients are asked to report immediately symptoms such as vaginal bleeding or leakage, blurred vision, headache, marked swelling of the legs and hands, abdominal pain or persistent vomiting. Frequent follow-up permits the initiation of any necessary preventive measures at a time when they will be most helpful.

During the last trimester, an internal pelvic examination is done. If there is need for an x-ray, it is usually considered a safe procedure because x-ray techniques have improved so that the amount of exposure to radiation is considered negligible. Multiple diagnostic examinations by x-ray are not recommended, however. X-ray pictures may be taken after the first trimester and are done for reasons such as diagnosis of a multiple birth or a fetal death, determination of the size of the infant's head or determination of possible fetal abnormalities.

If the mother has Rh negative blood, the father's blood is also examined. If his blood is Rh negative, nothing more need be done. If it is Rh positive, however, the mother's blood will be examined at intervals to see if a sensitivity is being built up, causing erythroblastosis in the infant.

If fetal death seems likely, intrauterine transfusions to prevent fetal anemia are now being done. Intrauterine transfusions are given by injecting blood or packed red blood cells into the peritoneal cavity of the fetus. It is then absorbed into the blood stream. This procedure is relatively new.

A diagnostic aid, the amniocentesis, is available. This procedure is performed much like a paracentesis. Approximately 20 cc. of amniotic fluid is aspirated and examined. The results of this examination help the physician to determine the need for possible intrauterine transfusion or the feasibility of early induction of labor if the period of gestation has been long enough.

Parent Classes

Prenatal classes are conducted by a variety of agencies and institutions. The Red Cross, private hospitals, clinics, public health agencies and some voluntary agencies may conduct prenatal classes for parents. It is often assumed that the only persons needing such classes are parents who are having their first baby, those who are uneducated or those in the low economic group. This is not true. Educated persons need to learn the content of parent classes just as much as uneducated parents. Interestingly enough, many doctors and nurses attend these classes, especially for their first child.

Information about the anatomy and physiology of pregnancy is given to provide a better understanding of what will be happening to the mother during the next few months. The importance of an adequate diet and the necessity of trying to keep the weight gain to about 20 pounds is stressed. Maternal clothing is described. Suggestions for the infant's layette are given. Exercises to help the mother to relax, to control her breathing and to train muscles for the expulsion of the baby are usually demonstrated to make labor and delivery more comfortable. A description of what to expect during labor and delivery prepares parents for an experience which otherwise might be frightening. Hospital facilities may be toured. The father is an important part of these classes. He learns what is expected of him. In most cases he is allowed to be with his wife throughout labor and, in some cases, during delivery.

Prenatal Care of the Unwed Mother

Contrary to public opinion, the unwed mother is usually unsophisticated and lacks knowledge of sex. In 1959, 52 of every 1000 births were born to unwed mothers, and the highest percentage of these mothers were under 15 years of age.

A group of unwed teen-age mothers in a low economic and culturally deprived area was studied. Special conferences were held for them.

Discussions were geared to about an eighth-grade level and subjects were preselected but left flexible enough so that the desires of class members could be incorporated easily. Apathy and defiance were often an expression of futility. They were afraid to show their fears lest they betray ignorance. Their greatest psychological needs were to be understood, to gain acceptance and to be aided in developing their self-esteem. Many of these girls returned to school and kept their babies.

Unwed mothers are in need of prenatal care and will need the advice and help of a medical social worker. Some may wish to go to a home, such as those provided by the Florence Crittenton Mission, Roman Catholic agencies or the Salvation Army. Others may live at home or work in private homes away from their own locale. Whatever the decision, it is vital that they receive physical and psychological help during their pregnancy as well as help in making appropriate decisions about their future and that of the baby.

LABOR AND DELIVERY

Labor

In 1940, 56 per cent of all births occurred in a hospital, and in 1959, 96 per cent occurred in a hospital. Hospital environments usually allow more privacy; hospitals are cleaner and provide equipment which is readily available for emergency care of the mother and the infant. The availability of hospitalization insurance is also an important factor contributing to this change.

Parents who attended prenatal classes have learned the signs and symptoms of labor so that the physician is usually notified in ample time. Naturally, there are patients who have short labors, but even then both the patient and the physician are usually prepared, if an adequate history has been taken. When the mother arrives at the hospital, the father is asked to provide any admission information which has not already been obtained. The physician usually sends prenatal records to the hospital several months in advance. As a result, the hospital has ample time to obtain admitting data a month or two ahead of time.

Upon arrival at the hospital, the mother is taken immediately to the labor room, examined and prepared for delivery. An electrocardiogram of the fetal heart can be done, or the fetal heart can be monitored if it is deemed necessary. The father can join the mother and is frequently allowed to remain with her during her labor. The mother is rarely left alone during labor for more than a few moments.

The refresher will be likely to notice one other thing which will be different to her. The patient may have less pain and therefore receive less sedation during her labor. Many women have learned exercises during their prenatal period. Some women have read Dr. Grantly Dick Read's book, *Childbirth Without Fear*, which stresses the interaction of fear, pain and tension. His general contention is that if fear and tension can be removed, pain is prevented. While his concepts are not wholly adopted, his influence is felt in the modern-day practice of obstetrics in many cases. The patient who has learned to control her breathing, exercised to strengthen certain muscles and has her husband at her side usually needs less sedation and anesthesia during her labor.

Another kind of antepartal preparation for childbirth is called the Lamaze method, also known as psychoprophylactic painless childbirth. It is based on learning a conditioned response to pain. The expectant mother is taught a technique of accelerated, shallow respirations. She learns that this is to be her response from the beginning to the end of a contraction.

A decompression apparatus has been developed to relieve the discomfort of contractions. A negative pressure dome fits over the mother's abdomen and is operated by her. As a contraction begins, the mother presses a button which causes air to leave the dome. This in turn raises the abdominal wall and relieves the discomfort of the contraction. This apparatus reduces resistance to labor contractions and therefore reduces the length of labor. Many patients who have used it have found less need for sedation.

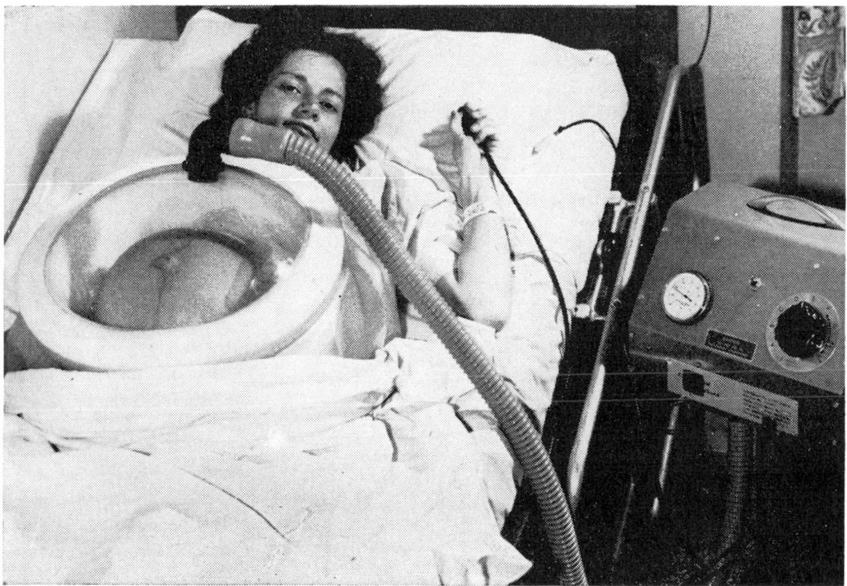

Figure 19–1. *Birtheez. (From Wajdorvicz, Elizabeth K.: Abdominal Decompression During Labor.* American Journal of Nursing, *December, 1964, p. 87.)*

Delivery

Anesthesia may be given by many methods. If natural childbirth is to be practiced, the mother has learned ahead of time to concentrate upon the baby rather than upon herself. She works very closely with her physician who must have spent time with her during her pregnancy and during her labor to guide her and give her adequate support. Hypnosis is used by some physicians who are specially trained in the procedure and know how to select patients on an informed basis. Anesthesia may be given by inhalation, by vein, by caudal injection, by perineal infiltration and various types of regional block.

One new instrument, the vacuum extractor is worthy of mention. Suction is applied to the infant's head and traction is then synchronized with the contractions of the uterus. It is likely that this instrument will be used more commonly. In certain institutions, it has virtually replaced the use of forceps.

Once the infant has been delivered, the baby is turned upside down to allow for drainage of mucus from the mouth and respiratory tract, the cord is clamped, tied and cut, and two drops of 1% silver nitrate solution are dropped into each eye. Some form of identification must be applied to the infant immediately after birth. One of the safest methods is the use of prenumbered bands, one for the mother and one for the baby. The name is written in on the bands in the delivery room and applied to both the mother and the baby before they leave the delivery room. Both the name and number are the same so that the bracelets can be used for identification checks throughout the hospitalization.

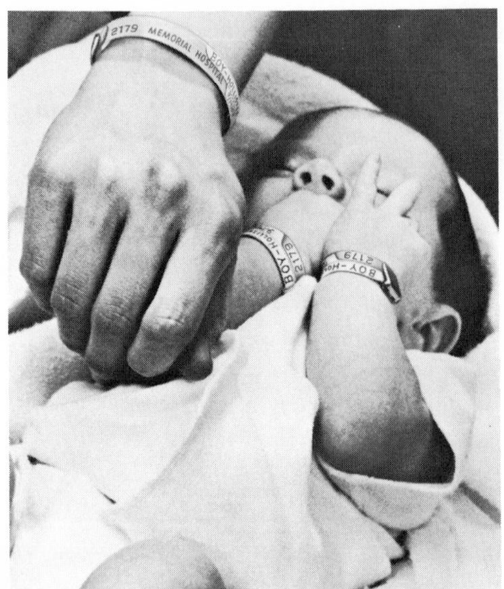

Figure 19–2. *Mother-infant Identabands are applied in the delivery room. (Hollister, Inc.)*

Another means of identification is the footprint or fingerprint. The F.B.I. states that in order for a means of identification to be effective, it must have "individuality," "continuity," and "immutability." Footprints and fingerprints are the only means of identification which have these three qualities, and footprints are becoming not only an aid to identification but may become a requirement for identification of infants in hospitals.

The infant is evaluated before being taken to the nursery. Aside from the usual general observation of the infant, the Apgar scoring system is used in many places. It encourages a keener appraisal of the infant's condition at birth by scoring five signs after observing each for one minute. The heart rate, color, muscle tone, respiratory effort and reflex irritability are observed. Each item is rated 0, 1 or 2. A score of ten is the highest possible score on the Apgar rating scale. Nursing observations are continued in the nursery and a complete physical examination is done later unless there is indication of need for immediate attention.

APGAR RATING EVALUATION OF THE NEWBORN INFANT (method of scoring)

Sixty seconds after the complete birth of the infant (disregarding the cord and placenta) the following five objective signs are evaluated and each given a score of 0, 1 or 2. A score of 10 indicates an infant in the best possible condition.

TOTAL rating: ____________

Sign	0	1	2
Heart rate	Absent	Slow (below 100)	Over 100
Respiratory effort	Absent	Slow - irregular	Good crying
Muscle tone	Limp	Some flexion of extremities	Active motion
Response to catheter in nostril (tested after oropharynx is clear.)	No response	Grimace	Cough or sneeze
Color	Blue Pale	Body pink Extremities blue	Completely pink

Figure 19–3. *Apgar method of evaluating newborn infant.*

POSTPARTUM CARE

Immediate Care

The mother must be checked frequently for one to two hours immediately after delivery. It has been found that a postpartum recovery room or something similar to it provides the mother with the constant vigilance during these hours which are most critical for her welfare. If an obstetric department is large enough, a postpartum recovery room may be set up and staffed around the clock, giving care much like the recovery room associated with operating rooms. When a hospital does not have enough deliveries to make this feasible, an adaptation of the idea is often made. The newly delivered mother may be returned to a bed in the labor room where the labor and delivery room nurse will be able to observe her frequently, or she may be returned to a room where one nurse is assigned to this concentrated care.

During this time, blood pressure, pulse and respirations are taken every 15 minutes. At the same time, sutures are checked for possible hematomas, the perineal pad is checked for bleeding, and the fundus is checked for firmness. The fundus is massaged if there is any evidence of relaxation. The patient receives only clear liquids during the first few hours in case there is any necessity of returning to the delivery room due to bleeding. Incidentally, fundus measurements can now be made more accurately by the use of a disposable paper measuring tape.

Succeeding Care

Early ambulation has contributed to shortening the patient's stay to about four or five days. The patient is usually allowed to get out of bed six to eight hours after delivery. Early ambulation is considered beneficial because it contributes to a psychological sense of well-being, increases circulation, promotes healing and prevents embolism.

Because of early ambulation and the natural excitement of family and friends, the mother is often deprived of one of the most important elements of postpartum care, that of mental and physical rest. The mother is usually besieged with telephone calls and visitors in addition to nursing her new infant, attending classes concerning home care and talking to her physicians. Because hospital rules often seem to be more helpful to the hospital than to the patient, visiting hours have been greatly liberalized at most institutions. In many hospital areas this has been beneficial to the patient. However, in the area of obstetrics, many institutions are going back to shorter visiting hours because their patients become exhausted from so many well-wishers and need more time for rest.

Other vital elements of postpartum care include the prevention of infection, especially of the breast and pelvic areas, the maintenance of an adequate diet, the maintenance of general body functions and education for care of the mother and child in the home.

Instructions Concerning Self-care of the Mother

Many more liberal techniques are being used. Perineal care by an external douche is usually given only the day of delivery. It is often replaced by sitz baths which are given two or three times a day, and the mother is taught to use proper technique when she dries herself or goes to the toilet.

The mother is also taught how to bathe and how to prepare her breasts for nursing. Such instructions are given verbally by the nurse, but they may also be given in writing so that the mother can review them.

Rooming-in

Rooming-in has been used at many institutions. It gives the mother an opportunity to get to know her infant and to learn to handle him before she goes home. Total adoption of rooming-in has not been widely accepted. Therefore, many hospitals either permit a mother to take advantage of rooming-in if she so desires, or they offer a modified version of it. In the latter case, the mother can have her baby in her room when she desires, but the infant is returned to the nursery for the night. Some hospitals are built so that the mother and infant are in adjoining rooms and the mother can always see her child.

Rooming-in may be confined to private rooms. Whether or not rooming-in is used, private rooms are sometimes used for a modified version of family-centered care. In the latter case, the father is allowed to hold and feed the infant when private room facilities are available.

Another modification of rooming-in is known as terminal rooming-in. In this case the infant is brought to the mother on the day of discharge, and the mother cares for the baby until she takes him home with her. All of these plans have the advantage of giving the mother an opportunity to care for her baby while she has professional persons available to her to guide and instruct her.

Care of the Mother With a Defective Baby

Special care and attention must be given to the mother with a defective baby. Such a mother is usually told as soon as possible so that she does not overhear comments or merely go through a period of anxiety while personnel avoid mentioning the offspring.

Such a mother can actually be said to go through a grief period. She mourns the expectations of the kind of life she had hoped for her child. Jane Kallaus describes three phases experienced by these mothers: first, that of numb disbelief; second, the awareness and sense of disappointment and loss; and third, the period of re-experiencing the memory of her expectations.

These mothers will need special attention to rest and quiet. The nurse will want to be available to give accurate information when they need it and ask for it.

They will be overwhelmed at first and it will take time for them to be able to talk about it. To show interest in their feelings, to allow an expression of disappointment and to be available for discussion and emotional support is a vital part of the care of these women who must rally their strength for many difficult adjustments in the future.

Care of the Mother on the Medical-Surgical Station

Once in a while a patient may ask to be cared for in a medical-surgical station rather than the obstetric division. The physician sometimes allows this if he feels it is better for the mother who has lost her baby or who is unmarried and not planning to keep her baby. This is not a rare situation. It is vital that personnel on the station caring for the patient confer with obstetric nursing personnel about the proper care of the patient if they see these patients infrequently. In some institutions, nursing personnel from the maternity section instruct both the patient and the nursing personnel caring for the patient.

INFANT CARE

General Care

Careful observation of the newborn is a must. Color, mucus, voiding, elimination, inspection for any change or possible abnormality, condition of the cord, strength and pitch of the cry and quality of the sucking reflex all must be noted. Any nurse who will become a part of a nursery staff will need to study and review nursing care of infants before she tries to learn procedures and routines of a nursery.

Good medical asepsis is vital to the care of the infant. Prevention of infection is a continuous part of daily care and can never be relaxed. Disposables are used in the nursery for many items. Disposable diapers, disposable crib sheets and disposable wash cloths are only a few of the many possibilities.

Formula Preparation

Formula preparation may no longer be done in the hospital. Milk laboratories are found in larger institutions in many cases, but a formula delivery service from an outside company or ready-to-use formulas may be used instead. Many of the new products, while somewhat more costly to use in the home, are not always more costly to use in an institution because there may be a reduction in the number of personnel needed for formula preparation. Some of the newer products are ready for use and do not require refrigeration; therefore, they do not require warming, as they are already at room temperature. The bottle and nipple may be thrown away. Ready-to-use preparations now include many special formulas as well as regular nursery formula.

Most mothers are encouraged to breast-feed their infants. Even if a mother nurses her infant, she will usually learn to make formula. Some pediatricians allow their mothers to make one bottle of formula at a time, using a well-washed bottle and nipple, powdered formula and tap water at each feeding. This reduces the necessity for refrigeration, heating formula and the worry about spoiled milk. However, pediatricians select the patients they advise to do this. If a mother is careless in her home and in her washing procedures, she should probably be asked to carry out a more rigid technique which will more likely assure cleanliness. Such decisions are up to the physician. Formula preparation of 1891 was a different story!*

Have ten nursing bottles prepared clean every morning. Take 5 ounces of cream and 2-½ ounces of milk. Put in skillet; add pancreatin powder; heat over alcohol flame for 6 minutes; stir and sip constantly; do not overheat.

Of this mixture, put in each bottle 6 drachms (to make 2 ounce bottle). Use funnel. Add to each bottle 10 drachms sugar solution.* Stopper the mouth of each bottle with dry, baked cotton and sterilize for 20 minutes. Set aside to cool. Before use, put bottle in warming cup; apply nipple immediately before giving it to infant.

*Make sugar solution by dissolving one ounce of milk sugar in a pint of warm water. The pancreatin powder, for the quantity indicated, consists of pancreatin, two and a half grain, and bicarbonate of sodium, five grains.

The Nursery

The nursery will have emergency equipment available as well as incubators which are designed to give the infant an environment with temperature and humidity control. Larger hospitals have premature nurseries which may also be used as an intensive care unit for infants who need more constant vigilance and care.

Multiple nurseries are built into new maternity wings. This is to provide rotation of infants and regular cleaning of nurseries. One advantage of such a system is that only a few infants are exposed should one infant become infected. A small observation nursery is also built into nursery units. This provides a place for an infant with a suspected infection where individual technique can be used. Such an area should be visible to the nursery staff even if the room is separate.

Before the infant goes home, he will have a blood specimen taken (a Guthrie test) for the possible diagnosis of phenylketonuria (PKU.) (see Chapter 10). The urine may be examined for possible galactosemia.

*Hirst, Dr. B. C.: An Effort to Obtain a Perfect Substitute for Human Milk. *Medical News*, Philadelphia, 1891, viii, 5.

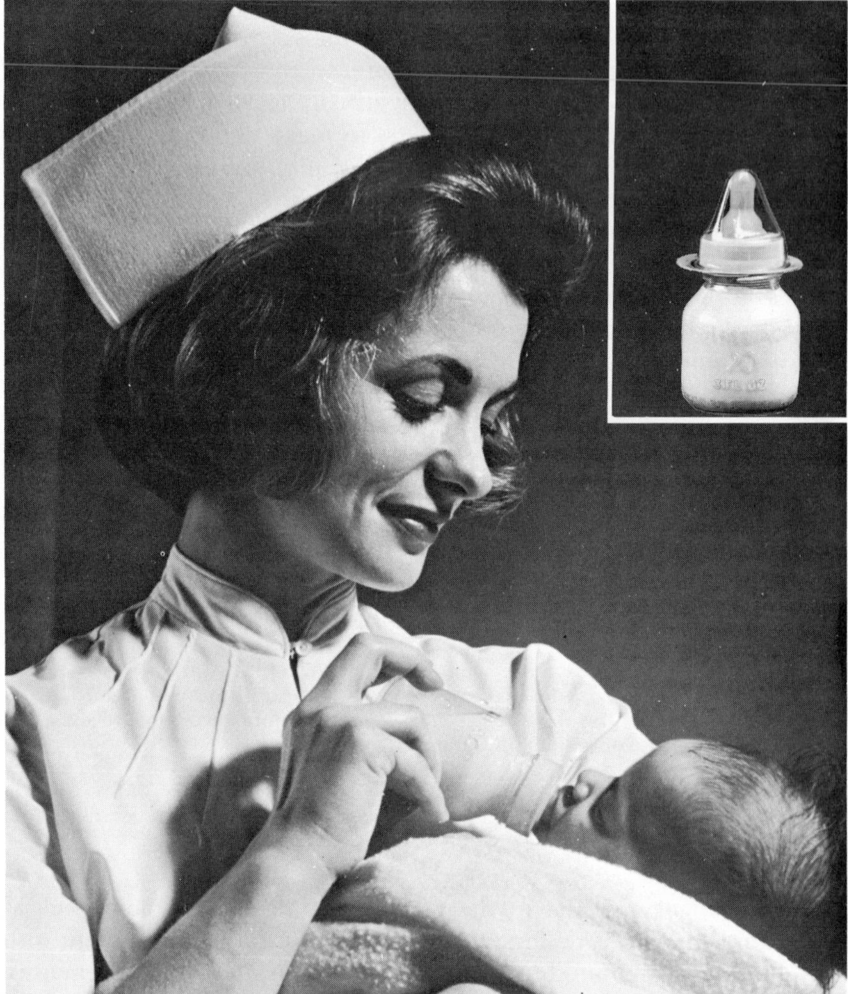

Figure 19–4. Today, ready-to-use formula preparations in disposable containers are used in many hospitals. (Similac; Ross Laboratories.)

These examinations may diagnose two metabolic defects which cause mental retardation and which can be prevented by therapeutic diets if an early diagnosis is made.

NURSE-PATIENT RELATIONSHIPS

Marion Lesser and Vera Keane conducted a study at New York Hospital which provides many insights which nurses could utilize to improve their practice. This study was conducted around obstetric patients so it is included in this chapter, but the findings are applicable to the care of all patients.

Patients were interviewed concerning their concept of the nurse, and nurses were interviewed concerning their concept of their own role. Patients were asking for a "supportive, informative situation," with "fear-dispelling" assistance and "reassurance." It was found that patients took technical competence of nurses for granted. They often viewed the nurse as the doctor's assistant and therefore not accessible to them.

Three types of patients were identified. All had the same needs (knowledge about labor, anesthetics, hospital procedures and a fear of betraying ignorance which needed to be dispelled), but the degree to which their needs were met varied greatly. The "information seeker" was described as the more aggressive individual who reads, attends classes and asks questions. Her needs were met the best because of her active pursuit in obtaining knowledge. The second type of person identified was the "information acceptor" who reads, accepts what she

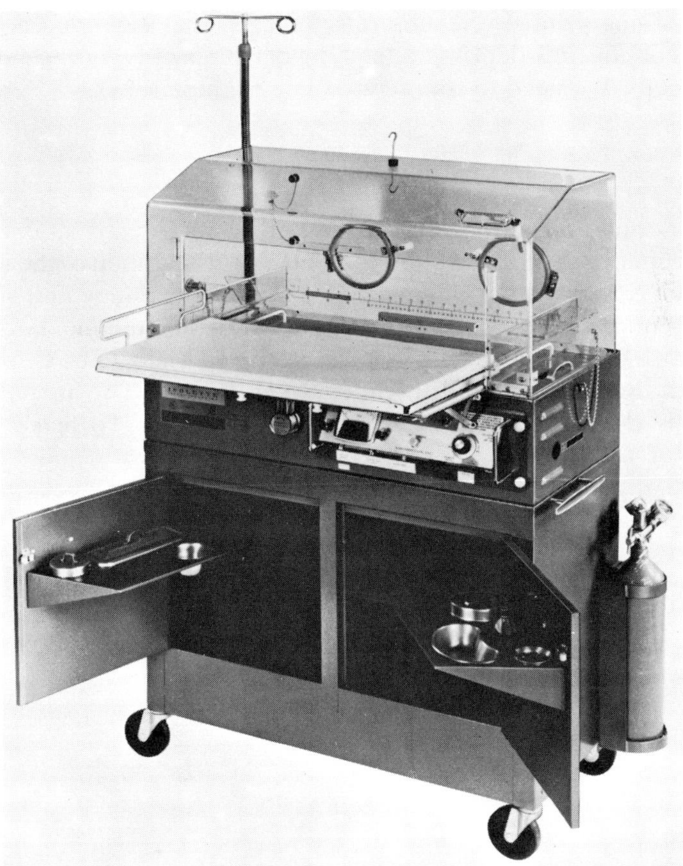

Figure 19–5. *Isolette used for care of the premature infant. (Courtesy Air Shields, Inc., Hatboro, Pennsylvania.)*

gets, but does not bother nurses or doctors who appear to be busy. She feels that they will tell her if it seems important. The third type of individual was the "information resistor" who does not read or attend class and who fears that information might arouse anxiety.

There are many important findings in this study, which is recommended reading for refreshers and practicing nurses alike. One of the most interesting facets of the study is the pinpointing of the kind of barriers which nurses set up between themselves and their patients. A busy, doctor-oriented nurse appears to the patients as uninterested and unavailable. With so many duties delegated to nonprofessional personnel, the nurse seems even further removed.

While it may not be possible for one individual nurse to change an entire system, it is helpful for all of us to see and try to counteract things which are within our province. If a nurse is warm, friendly, inquires about her patients' feelings and makes herself available to them for teaching, patients are at least not discouraged from turning to her for help. Because of early ambulation, more self-care and delegation of many duties, the nurse often forgets that the reduced number of patient contacts deprives our patients from satisfying their dependency needs. We need to counteract some of these losses.

SUMMARY

Maternal and infant nursing cannot be considered an entity separate from the life of a family. Thoughtful consideration of the family is a part of caring for any one person in that family. Many new concepts and inventions make maternal nursing safer, easier and more satisfying. The nurse's role as a teacher in this area is especially to be emphasized for both the educated and the uneducated patient. The area of public health is closely related to mother and child care. To make parents ready for the birth of their child, to make them ready and confident about taking their child home and to provide services as needs arise are major goals in this field of nursing.

SUGGESTED READINGS

Bookmiller, Mae M., and Bowen, George L.: *Textbook of Obstetrics and Obstetric Nursing.* Ed. 4, Philadelphia, W. B. Saunders Co., 1963.

Lesser, Marion A., and Keane, Vera R.: *Nurse-Patient Relationships in a Hospital Maternity Service*. St. Louis, C. V. Mosby Co., 1956.

REFERENCES

American Academy of Pediatrics, *Standards and Recommendations for Hospital Care of Newborn Infants.* Evanston, Ill., 1964.

Apgar, Virginia: Drugs in Pregnancy. *American Journal of Nursing,* March, 1965, p. 105.

Assumpta, Sister M., and Howard, Margaret: Abdominal Decompression During Labor. *Canadian Nurse,* December, 1961, p. 1132.

Bookmiller, Mae M., and Bowen, George L.: *Textbook of Obstetrics and Obstetric Nursing.* Ed. 4, Philadelphia, W. B. Saunders Co., 1963.

Chacon, Adel: Updating Maternity Services. *Nursing Outlook*, August, 1964, p. 47.

Chesterman, Helen: The Public Health Nurse and Family Planning. *Nursing Outlook*, September, 1964, p. 32.

Feeding Solids to Newborns. *OB Yearbook from Hospital Topics*, 1962, p. 59.

Fitzpatrick, Elise, and Eastman, Nicholson J.: *Zabriskie's Obstetrics for Nurses.* Ed. 10, Philadelphia, J. B. Lippincott Co., 1960.

Freda, Vincent J., and Robertson, John G.: Amniotic Fluid Analysis in Rh Iso-Immunization. *American Journal of Nursing*, August, 1965, p. 64.

Glynn, Elizabeth M.: Nursing Support During Intra-Uterine Transfusions. *American Journal of Nursing*, August, 1965, p. 72.

Halliday, Claire: A Decompression Dome Aids Childbirth. *Hospital Management*, March, 1962, p. 6.

Harpine, Frances: Concepts in Maternal and Child Health. *American Journal of Nursing*, December, 1961, p. 84.

International Childbirth Education Association, Inc., *Abstracts*, Third Biennial Convention June 25, 26, 27, 1964. Compiled and printed courtesy of Natural Childbirth Association, Milwaukee.

Iorio, Josephine: Culdoscopy: Nursing Care. *Nursing Outlook*, September, 1964, p. 35.

Irene, Sister: Doctor Researches New Procedures for Saving Doomed 'Rh Babies.' *Hospital Management*, November, 1964, p. 47.

Kallaus, Jane: The Child With Cleft Lip and Palate—The Mother in the Maternity Unit. *American Journal of Nursing*, April, 1965, p. 121.

Knight, Eulalie: Conference for Pregnant, Unwed Teen-Agers. *American Journal of Nursing*, July, 1965, p. 123.

Lesser, Marion A., and Keane, Vera R.: *Nurse-Patient Relationships in a Hospital Maternity Service.* St. Louis, C. V. Mosby Co., 1956.

Maternal, Child Health-Care Congress Proves a Pace-setter. Prepared in cooperation with the American College of Obstetricians and Gynecologists, *Hospital Topics*, April, 1965, p. 89.

McLenahan, Irene G.: Helping the Mother Who Has No Baby to Take Home. *American Journal of Nursing*, April, 1962, p. 70.

Meyer, Herman F.: Survey of Hospital Nursery Ready-to-Feed Milk Mixtures. *Hospitals*, January 1, 1965, p. 60.

Minkler, Donald: Public Policy in Family Planning. *Nursing Outlook*, September, 1964, p. 28.

Owens, Charlotte: Parents' Reactions to Defective Babies. *American Journal of Nursing*, November, 1964, p. 83.

Queenan, John T.: Intra-uterine Transfusion for Erythroblastosis Fetalis. *American Journal of Nursing*, August, 1965, p. 68.

Read, Grantly Dick: *Childbirth Without Fear*, New York, Harper & Brothers, 1944.

Robinson, Alice M.: The Principle, Not the Method. (Editorial). *Nursing Outlook*, September, 1964, p. 27.

Rubin, Reva: The Family-Child Relationship and Nursing Care. *Nursing Outlook*, September, 1964, p. 36.

Seide, Diane: New Help for Habitual Aborters. *Registered Nurse*, November, 1961, p. 73.

Smith, Christine Spahn: *Maternal-Child Nursing*, Philadelphia, W. B. Saunders Co., 1963.

Ulin, Priscilla Richardson: The Exhilarating Moment of Birth. *American Journal of Nursing*, June, 1963, p. 60.

Wajdowicz, Elizabeth King: Abdominal Decompression During Labor. *American Journal of Nursing*, December, 1964, p. 87.

Wooden, Howard E.: Family-Centered Maternity Care at St. Mary's Hospital, Evansville, Indiana, *OB Yearbook from Hospital Topics*, 1962, p. 66.

CHILDREN'S BUREAU PUBLICATIONS FOR PARENTS

The following may be obtained by writing to the Superintendent of Documents, U.S. Government Printing Office, Washington, D. C. 20402.

Title	*Pamphlet No.*	*Price*
Prenatal Care	4	.20
Infant Care	8	.20
Your Child From One to Six	30	.20
Home Play and Play Equipment	238	.15
Your Child From Six to Twelve	324	.20
A Healthy Personality for Your Child	337	.20
The Adolescent in Your Family	347	.25
Your Gifted Child	371	.20
The Mentally Retarded Child at Home	374	.35
A Look at Juvenile Delinquency	380	.25
Your Children and Their Gangs	384	.20
When Your Baby is on the Way	391	.15
Your Baby's First Year	400	.15
A Creative Life for Your Children	Headliner series 1	.35
Pogo Primer for Parents (TV Division)	Headliner series 2	

20

Major Changes in Pediatric Care

Further extension of family-centered nursing focuses on care of children as they grow, develop and mature from infancy through adolescence. Pediatric nursing implies care of the child within a frame of reference that includes his parents, siblings, school, church and other community organizations. It also relates illness to personality, previous experiences and individual reactions. Public health nursing is linked to pediatric nursing as intimately as it is to obstetric and psychiatric nursing.

Changes in pediatric nursing are mostly due to changes in emphasis resulting from disease prevention, better utilization of psychological insights and better medical care in the community in general. With the advent of antibiotics, immunization measures, dietary information and more educational resources, more and more children are being treated in the clinic and the home.

There are anatomical, physiological and psychological differences between adult and pediatric illnesses. Children become ill more suddenly. They require immediate medical attention when they show signs of being sick. The major causes of death between the ages of one and 14 years of age are accidents (excluding motor vehicle), motor vehicle accidents, neoplasms, congenital malformations, influenza and pneumonia.

Sudden death in infants is increasing and the cause is not always clear. Some are due to aspiration, viremia and milk allergy, but many deaths are not understood. Optimum medical care to prevent causes which are known is the best answer we have.

Attention to emotional disorders is vital. All degrees of neurosis, psychosis and psychosomatic ailments can occur in children. Parents may accept a given kind of behavior in themselves but criticize the same behavior in their child. "Failure to thrive"—malnutrition causing lack of physical and emotional development—can be due to a seriously disturbed mother-child relationship. It cannot be overemphasized that early diagnosis can prevent or reduce problems in later years.

TRENDS IN HOSPITAL CARE

Overall Changes

Pediatric services have become more humanized by permitting parents to visit with fewer restrictions and allowing children to have more freedom to enjoy play, recreation and diversion as an integral part of their care. In fact, aside from psychiatric and rehabilitation units, diversional therapy is better provided for children than for any other group of patients.

Research into the care, treatment and prevention of disease has altered the type of conditions seen in today's hospitalized children. More chronic diseases are seen, more emotional and psychosomatic disturbances are recognized and cared for, and the number of acute infections has been reduced. The area of psychology is intimately tied to the care of children. Physical, mental and emotional disturbances are less likely to be considered separately in the care of children than in the care of adults. A modern concept of care considers the whole child and is based on the interaction of all these elements.

The nurse working in a hospital may find herself caring for children with diseases of which she has never heard, or she may see children being treated for conditions for which there was no treatment when she last worked. Agammaglobulinemia is an example of the former. This is a rare disease in which antibodies cannot be formed because of a lack of gamma globulin. Since these patients are unable to fight off infection, they will require monthly injections of gamma globulin throughout their lives. Surgical intervention for increased kinds of congenital defects is possible. Patients requiring open heart surgery are likely to be congregated in a medical center where medical and nursing personnel have the necessary knowledge and equipment. Better education and knowledge has greatly increased the life span of the diabetic child. Better diagnostic methods will continue to change the nature of pediatric conditions seen in hospitals.

Pre-admission Orientation

One of the most important trends in alleviating anxiety of the child about his hospitalization is the pre-admission orientation program which is given a week or two before the child is admitted to the hospital. Patients who are scheduled to come to the hospital are invited to visit the hospital with their parents. They are shown the children's section and a film showing areas of the hospital which are difficult to tour, such as the operating room. Simple refreshments may also be served.

These programs serve a second purpose, that of giving parents an opportunity to discuss their questions with the nurse. The nurse is then able to explain what children need to know, and parents can learn more about their role before and during the hospitalization. The children can play with hospital toys in another area during this period. Such programs serve a very real purpose in preparing the child honestly and realistically for the hospital environment and for what will happen to him.

One shortcoming of orientation programs is that they are usually limited to the surgical patient who can be contacted ahead of time. The child who comes to the hospital as an emergency patient, with an acute infection or a medical problem cannot be contacted in advance. One way of overcoming this problem is to have the hospital work with the school system or special groups who are interested in having children learn about hospitals at some time in their school or organizational experience. Then, when a child needs to be hospitalized suddenly, the fear of the unknown will not be added to anxiety about his condition and separation from his family.

Growth and Development

The nurse must gear her patient care and teaching to many different age levels. In protecting her patient from harm she must adapt her protective measures to the kind of exploratory efforts which might be expected at a certain age. Aside from the expected age and development of a child, the nurse must learn as much as she can about the individual maturity of a particular child. It is for this reason that most hospitals use an admitting sheet similar to the one found on p. 264. Parents first fill in such a form, then they are interviewed about the child using the findings on the sheet as a guide for the interview. Parents can contribute valuable insights which can enhance the quality of care given by the nursing staff.

The nurse assists the child according to his age, his individual development and his particular disease. While the infant and toddler have obvious dependency needs, she must also be aware that the "good" ten-year-old and adolescent may cover up dependency needs in many different ways. In the case of an accident, older children may feel guilty if the cause was related to their going beyond limits which were set for them by parents. In the case of accidents among toddlers, it is the parents who are likely to have guilt feelings. The nurse must stand ready to assist any member of the family who needs her.

Present-day education in pediatric nursing relates a given period of

Our child at home
(As described by the parents)

Your answers to these questions will help the doctors, nurses, and play teachers in their care of your child during his hospital visit.

Name__________ Nickname________ Age______
Address__________ Religion______
Brothers' names and ages__________
Sisters' names and ages__________

Eating:

Time of meals or feedings__________

Where fed: Lap____ High chair____ Own table____ Family table____

Fed by: Breast______ Bottle______ Cup______ Glass______

Feeds self________ Needs help________

Right-handed________ Left-handed________

Food consists of: Strained______ Junior______ Regular______

Special food likes: __________

Any food dislikes: __________

Favorite juices and other drinks: __________

Sleeping:

Sleeps in room alone__________

Sleeps in own bed__________

Light on or off__________

Bedtime______ Awake______ Up______

Nap during daytime________ When________

Sleeps on back______ Stomach______ Side______

Awake during night for bathroom or feeding________

Takes toy to bed with him________ What________

Bathing and dressing:

Has bath in bath basin______ Sink______ Bathtub______
Bathes alone______ With help______
Usual time of bath______
Brushes teeth alone______ With help______ With reminder______
Dresses self alone________ With help________
Undresses self alone________ With help________

Figure 20–1. *Parents of a hospitalized child can provide valuable information. (From* Care of Children in Hospitals, *American Academy of Pediatrics, 1960, pp. 93–94.)*

Toilet Habits:

Toilet training started________ Complete________

Accustomed to nursery chair______ Potty______ Toilet______

Term used to refer to bowel movement______ Urination______

Taken to bathroom at regular times______ When______

Accustomed to wearing diapers______ Training pants______

Playing:

Accustomed to playing alone______ With other children______ With adults______

Favorite toys________

Special interests________

Favorite pets________

Experiences outside the home

Is this the first experience away from home________

In hospital before______ When______ Age at time______

Talks about previous experience________

Told of this hospital visit______ When______ What told________

Has been at camp______ When______

Goes to school______ Sunday School______ Nursery school______ Kindergarten______ Grade______

Likes School________

Teacher's name________

Language used in home: English______ Other______

Shy______ Friendly______ with new people.

Accustomed to baby sitters________

Special friends________

Remarks:

Figure 20–1. (*Continued*)

growth and development with conditions of that period so that disease is related to the maturity of the child both physically and emotionally. Students rarely have milk laboratory experience, yet they learn to teach formula preparation. Where a pediatric census is not high enough to give the student adequate observational opportunities, the student may spend time outside the hospital to learn about the well child, the sick child in the home and public health and psychiatric facilities used for the care of children. The student may spend time with the school nurse, at a nursery school, working at a well baby clinic, in a pediatrician's office or in a specialized clinic. She may attend P.T.A. meetings and Girl Scout meetings or spend a day with a "home-bound" teacher. With proper correlation of learning on the part of the instructor, care of the hospitalized child can be enriched by giving the student such experiences.

The Uniform: White? Colored? Street Clothes?

Should the nurse wear white? This question is often asked, but nurses caring for children have experimented with a departure from the conventional white uniform more often than any others. Some have worn pastels; some have worn colored aprons; some have worn street clothes. Nurses caring for children with psychiatric conditions are especially likely to wear street clothes. If there is a garden project, the nurse may wear blue jeans. In many instances parents, doctors and nurses like the change because they feel that patients respond better when this is done. Some hospitals recommend that nurses relate their apparel to the type of care they give but also permit them to wear white if they wish to do so. The amount of flexibility in this respect varies greatly among institutions.

Play

Books, games, toys and occupational activities appropriate for the age and condition of the child are provided in one degree or another for all hospitalized children. Depending upon the size of the area serving children, such a program may be handled by a volunteer group or a trained recreational therapist. In any case, complete pediatric care includes attention to a child's play needs. Some toys must be modified or restricted for the sake of safety. Balloons are not considered safe. Dolls and animals with dresses or suits should be checked to make sure that they have no pins in them. Sparking toys should not be used near oxygen. In most cases the child will want to bring something from home with him. This is especially important for the toddler who may not be able to sleep without his blanket, doll or whatever he has chosen as a source of comfort.

Sometimes clay, crayons and paints are appropriate. If the pediatric nurse needs to work in an orderly environment, she will be frustrated to find that she is expecting something of children that is neither conducive to their welfare nor even possible in some cases. Play is a means by which a child can learn as well as work out his feelings.

Rooming-in

Rooming-in on a pediatric service is relatively new. Exceptions used to be made only in case of terminal illness. It is a known fact that children show signs of regression or emotional disturbance as a result of hospitalization. It is up to the hospital to provide an atmosphere which will reduce this as much as possible. Greater emotional dependence upon the mother, fear of leaving home, fear of having the mother leave home, poor appetite, fussiness about foods, regression of bowel or bladder training and sleep disturbances are some of the reactions that children have during or after hospitalization. Some children do not manifest their anxiety about their hospital experience and separation from family until after they have gone home, and so the nurse may not actually see some of the reactions to hospitalization.

Many studies have been concerned with this particular reaction. One such study involved three-year-olds who were hospitalized where rooming-in facilities were provided for mothers. They were studied before and after hospitalization. These children not only had no regression but they tended to have a spurt of development immediately following hospitalization.

One large children's hospital provides 22 private rooms where mothers are admitted with their children. The unit is concerned with family care. When a child is in surgery, parents have special attention and orientation. This provides an opportunity to teach parents and to attend to their needs. In such a setting the nurse learns to gain satisfaction from attending to the needs of both mother and child. Even when rooming-in facilities are not regularly available, most hospitals have private rooms so that a parent or child with special needs can be accommodated upon request.

Liberal Visiting Hours

Unless there is some reason why a parent should not visit a child, as in the case of a severely disturbed child who reacts to parental visits with anxiety, the more a hospitalized child knows that his parents are concerned and can visit frequently, the better it will be for the child. Liberal visiting hours are common in most hospitals.

Liberal visiting hours also permit the nurse to provide family care as well as child care. In the past, the nurse often regarded the presence of a parent as an intrusion into patient care and hospital routines. Today this attitude is demonstrated when the nurse stays away from the patient when the parents are there. Parents assume that their child receives the kind of care and attention that they see. If a nurse thinks that she need not see the child as often when parents are there, she is not only giving a false impression of the care being given but is depriving parents of attention that they deserve. Children should receive the same attention during visiting hours as they do at any other time. It is also vital that this time be used to talk to parents so that they are included in the care of their children and are being prepared for home care. Parent education is a major role of the pediatric nurse. A nurse who withdraws from her patients may be considered hostile, unfriendly or indifferent. Such impressions, whether real or not, must be prevented.

Dorothy Geis, who interviewed parents of dying children, reports that parents wanted to participate in the care of their children. They felt less like excess baggage when they were able to contribute to their comfort. In spite of this, they felt a real need for the nurse to do treatments and special procedures, to give emotional support and to interpret various aspects of care of their children. These parents stated that the "little things" were very important; permission for a visit from a sibling, coffee for the mother, encouragement to call the ward if they were worried and many other gestures, however small, demonstrated that the nurse cared.

The responses that were elicited from these mothers could undoubtedly be elicited from mothers of other children. Because of the gravity of their circumstance, nursing measures took on a more lasting impression. The thoughtful, helpful nurse who sees herself considering the needs of all members of the family will certainly be taking full advantage of more liberal visiting hours regardless of the patient's degree of illness.

Care of Children With Communicable Diseases

The American Academy of Pediatrics no longer recommends special hospitals for communicable diseases. As a result, children are either cared for at home or placed in isolation in a general hospital if they are too sick to be cared for at home. Immunizations and better control of communicable diseases have caused a reduction in the size of contagion sections in city hospitals. Children can now be protected against poliomyelitis and measles, two of the most serious diseases which have confronted them. Parents need to see that their children are initially protected as well as currently protected against these diseases as well as diphtheria, tetanus, pertussis and smallpox. It is ironic that parents see that their children are protected but do nothing about keeping their own protection up to date. As a result, a large segment of our population is susceptible to preventable diseases. If the refresher has not recently had a vaccination, a diphtheria-tetanus booster, a polio booster or influenza protection, she might ask her physician about this on her next visit.

Adolescence

By 1970, 10 per cent of our population will be in the adolescent age range. Greater attention and understanding have been given to the adolescent in recent years. Basically this is a healthy age group, but in spite of the general lack of illnesses, the giant spurt in physical and emotional growth causes many problems. Alternating needs for dependence and independence are manifested in behavior which often seems contradictory. They have skin problems, social problems, weight problems, decisions to make about their futures and any number of adjustments to make before they can feel comfortable about entering into the role of an adult.

Parents and nurses can help this age group by avoiding ridicule or intimation that their fears or worries are infantile. They need reassurance and an interested person in whom they can confide while they strive toward a "sense of identity."

Some children's hospitals and pediatric units have planned special areas to serve these youngsters, for one of their special needs is contact with their peer group. Such units provide a day room where there are

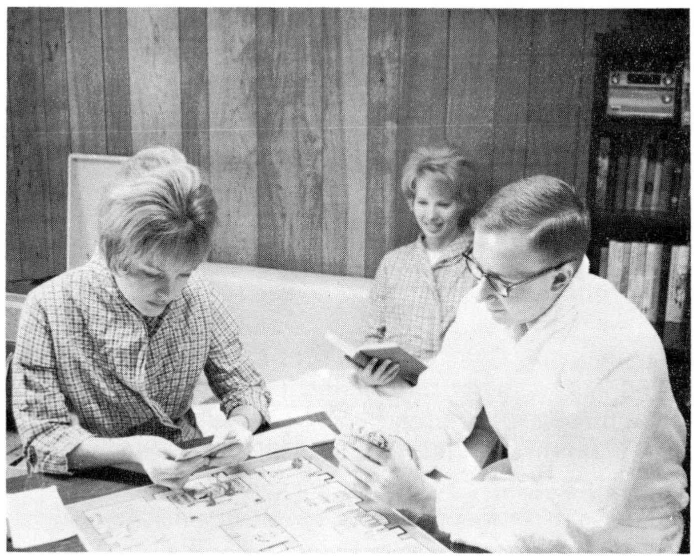

Figure 20–2. *"Teen den" provides for diversional activities of teen-age patients. (St. Barnabas Hospital, Minneapolis, Minnesota.)*

T.V., games, books, phonographs and general diversional facilities. Nurses caring for adolescents are often very near their age, and so they have some understanding of their problems and behavior. They need, however, special in-service education in how to handle them and how to set certain limits for these patients, who are less averse to rules and regulations than is often supposed.

NEW SPHERES OF COMMUNITY ACTION

The Battered Child

Results of child neglect in the form of cruelty, abuse and willful disregard have been termed the "battered child syndrome." There has been increased attention given to this difficult problem and the nurse needs to be aware of this possibility when she sees a child with physical injury of undetermined cause.

There may be certain indications observed in the parents, such as irritability when a history of the child's condition is being taken, contradiction of stories about the cause of the condition or a demonstrated lack of interest in the child. Parents may not visit the child even when it is convenient for them to do so. They may not inquire about the child or even look at him when they do visit.

The nurse may have an opportunity to urge psychological evaluation, but she must never demonstrate a critical attitude, as this may only result in further hostilities aimed at the child. Public health nursing or social agency follow-up should help to determine whether removal from the home becomes necessary. Because these children are not always hospitalized, community workers, such as a public health nurse or social worker, may be the first to see them.

State legislatures are beginning to pass laws requiring the reporting of battered children. Over one third of the states now have mandatory reporting laws. As more states pass such laws, these children will be better protected.

Poison Control Centers

Throughout the United States, Poison Control Centers have been set up to aid in the emergency treatment of patients who have ingested a foreign substance. Previously a physician was faced with the time-consuming gathering of information while the victim waited for the outcome of his findings. These centers contain information about the ingredients of and antidotes for thousands of substances and in many centers, telephones are answered 24 hours a day. Poison Control Centers have saved countless lives by having information immediately available so that the patient can be treated with a minimum of delay. A *Directory of Poison Control Centers* may be obtained from the Superintendent of Documents in Washington, D.C., for 20 cents.

Economic Opportunity Act of 1964

It is a well-recognized fact that environmental factors influence the health of an individual. Poverty and its underlying causes are closely related to the health of the mother and child. The fact that there are about ten nations with a lower infant mortality rate than the United States demonstrates that more can be done in this country. Because an attack on poverty and its causes is being made with the involvement of many disciplines, improvement in maternal and child health can be expected.

Day care centers are needed, not only for working mothers but also for deprived children. Upgrading the environment by enriching it with stimulating experiences in the preschool years is an important feature of these programs. The influences of this act will not be fully recognized for another generation. It is hoped that these efforts will minimize the perpetuation of poverty and its attending problems, which will in turn affect the physical and mental health of the individual as well as the sociological health of our communities.

Mental Retardation

In 1963, the Maternal and Child Health and Mental Retardation Planning Amendments to the Social Security Act and the Mental Retardation Facilities and Community Mental Health Centers Construction Act were passed. These two pieces of legislation have had a profound influence on the study of mental retardation and the care of mentally retarded individuals.

Comprehensive projects to reduce mental retardation by better prenatal, parturitive and postpartum care in the slum areas of large cities were initiated. Research into the causes and prevention of mental retardation, cerebral palsy and other neurological and sensory disorders has expanded. Early diagnosis of potentially retarded children is essential so that, whenever possible, preventive measures may be started before damage occurs, as in the case of phenylketonuria (PKU.). Investigations of population control and better family histories for genetic studies are important approaches to the problem also.

Diagnostic clinics, treatment centers, day care centers and educational facilities have expanded dramatically. Money is also available for the training of members of the many professions which are concerned with these children. Future work of the same magnitude is still needed for the handicapped child.

When mental retardation is suspected, the child is usually evaluated about four or five times during the first 18 or 24 months of life while he is being cared for at home. This gives parents time to make plans in relation to the total family, and it prevents mistakes when a child has pseudo-retardation. While most mental retardation is not preventable with our present knowledge, methods of educating even the most severely retarded have improved. This can make home care possible for a longer period of time as well as upgrade institutional living for more patients.

The White House Conferences on Children and Youth

A major impetus to the care of children has been the White House Conferences on Children and Youth which meet every decade. The first one was held in 1909 and was particularly concerned with the exploitation of children for cheap labor. It is interesting to note the recommendations arising from these conferences, as they reflect the problems of the decade and point to the efforts which will be made during the following decade. In 1960, some of the problems which were considered were poor coordination of public and private agencies, special needs of minority children, juvenile delinquency and health services to children who are poorly served. The aim of many disciplines, to contribute to helping the child develop his full potential, is embodied in these conferences.

SUMMARY

Attention to intrauterine development, physical and emotional growth and development, early diagnosis of congenital defects, along with treatment whenever possible, increased immunization measures, improved treatment methods, better application of psychological insights and legislative measures for improved health services to the community continue to promote better social, emotional and physical health for children and their families.

SUGGESTED READINGS

Leifer, Gloria: *Principles and Techniques in Pediatric Nursing*. Philadelphia, W. B. Saunders Co., 1965.

NOTE: This book would be helpful to a nurse returning to pediatric nursing.

Marlow, Dorothy R.: *Textbook of Pediatric Nursing*. Philadelphia, W. B. Saunders Co., 1965.

NOTE: "Teaching Aids and Other Information," found at the end of many chapters of this pediatric text, lists hundreds of free or inexpensive resource materials concerning specific diseases, growth and development, nutrition, mental health, etc., which would be helpful to parents and nurses alike.

Spock, B. M.: *Baby and Child Care*. Ed. 3, New York, Duell, Sloan and Pearce, Inc., 1957.

REFERENCES

Burn, Mary Ann: Pediatric Nursing Includes Well Children. *Nursing Outlook*, July, 1956, p. 391.

Care of Children in Hospitals. American Academy of Pediatrics, 1960.

Cheng, Nancy, and others: A Second Look at Nurses in Color. *Hospitals*, June 16, 1965, p. 59.

Cholcher, Mary, and Burtis, Mary: Teens Together. *American Journal of Nursing*, July, 1964, p. 104.

Creighton, Helen, and Richard, Sister Gabriella: When You Are Scared. *American Journal of Nursing*, January, 1963, p. 61.

Davens, Edward: A View of Health Services for Mothers and Children. *Children*, March-April, 1965.

Directory of Poison Control Centers. Public Health Service Publication No. 1278.

Dolch, Elaine T.: Books for the Hospitalized Child. *American Journal of Nursing*, December, 1961, p. 66.

Durocher, Mary Ann: Parent Educator in the Outpatient Department. *American Journal of Nursing*, June, 1965, p. 99.

Erickson, Florence: When 6- to 12-Year-Olds are Ill. *Nursing Outlook*, July, 1965, p. 48.

Fagin, Claire: The Case for Rooming In When Young Children Are Hospitalized. *Nursing Science*, August, 1964, p. 324.

Fulk, Delores Leusby: The Battered Child. *Nursing Forum*, Vol. 3, No. 2, (1964). p. 10.

Geis, Dorothy P.: Mothers' Perceptions of Care Given Their Dying Children. *American Journal of Nursing*, February, 1965, p. 105.

Harris, Martha Ray: Mary's Doll Has a Gastrostomy, Too." *American Journal of Nursing*, April, 1957, p. 487.

Herzog, Ruth H.: A Unique Nursing Role. *Nursing Outlook*, November, 1958, p. 622.

Hohle, Bertha M.: We Admit Parents Too. *American Journal of Nursing*, July, 1957, p. 865.

If Your Child Has a Congenital Heart Defect. American Heart Association, 44 E. 23 Street, New York 10, New York, 1960.

Jacobziner, Harold: Rescuing the Battered Child. *American Journal of Nursing*, June, 1964, p. 92.

Jeans, Philip C., Wright, F. Howell, and Blake, Florence G.: *Essentials of Pediatrics*. Ed. 7, Philadelphia, J. B. Lippincott Co., 1963.

Koch, Richard, and Gilien, Nancy Ragsdale: Diagnostic Experience in a Clinic for Retarded Children. *Nursing Outlook*, June, 1965, p. 26.

Marlow, Dorothy R., and Sellew, Gladys: *Textbook of Pediatric Nursing*, Philadelphia, W. B. Saunders Co., 1965.

Miller, Ann: Care for Children of Working Mothers. *American Journal of Nursing*, May, 1965, p. 94.

Nelson, Alice C.: Why Won't Stevie Drink? *American Journal of Nursing*, July, 1961, p. 44.

Roberta, Sister Mary: A Doll Goes to Surgery. *American Journal of Nursing*, November, 1963, p. 82.

Stanley-Brown, Edward G.: *Pediatric Surgery for Nurses*. Philadelphia, W. B. Saunders Co., 1961.

Steele, Shirley: Not Wisely But Too Well. *American Journal of Nursing*, July, 1965, p. 100.

Stryker, Ruth: They Can Take It With Them. *The Minnesota Registered Nurse*, April, 1951, p. 52.

Wheatley, George M.: Poison Control Centers. *Hospitals*, January 16, 1958, p. 38.

21

Changes in Care of the Psychiatric Patient

We are living in an era when mental health and the treatment of mental disease are fortunately beginning to interest both the individual and the community. The field of psychology has made inroads into every facet of our lives. Better understanding of the reasons for the plight of unfortunate persons as well as knowledge of their needs has brought about many kinds of improved facilities. All over the United States many problems are awaiting solutions pending greater citizen interest and understanding.

The field of psychology has affected all branches of medicine and nursing. Previous chapters have stressed present-day emphasis on understanding the behavior of patients and their needs as opposed to 25 years ago. In 1935, only 50 per cent of all nursing students had a psychiatric affiliation during their education, and now almost all schools have such an affiliation. This provides the nurse not only with basic knowledge about care of the psychiatric patient but also with understandings which will assist her in caring for patients in other settings. In spite of present educational trends, only 5 per cent of all nurses work in psychiatric settings, most of whom function in the area of administration or teaching in urban centers (which is not where the majority of psychiatric patients are hospitalized). This is contrasted with the fact that 50 per cent of all hospital beds on any given day are occupied by psychiatric patients. Besides this, many physicians feel that half the patients they see in their offices and admit to general hospitals are afflicted with diseases which have psychological implications. It is also a well-known fact that "tension accentuates physical disease." The nurse, therefore, cannot escape her responsibility in learning interpersonal skills which she can use to assist any patient as much as possible. Her settings will vary and the depth of her knowledge will vary, but she will have a contribution to make even if she is not working directly with psychiatric patients. It is also possible that the nurse who becomes more comfortable and familiar with psychological insights will become more interested in working with the mentally ill.

It is interesting to note that care of patients with mental illness is very closely related to attitudes of the public toward mental illness. People are beginning to learn that childhood trauma and abuse cause adult illness. A larger percentage of the population has a better knowledge of the field of psychology than that of a generation ago. This, together with better methods of treatment, has helped the patient to get help earlier, to obtain therapeutic assistance rather than custodial care and ultimately to be released from a hospital. Although many new facilities and types of care have been created, it is necessary to emphasize that such care is not available to everyone. There is a great lag between what we know is needed in a community and what we do in a community. The reader, therefore, is encouraged to find out what types of care are available in her community.

This is an area in which the nonpracticing nurse might contribute to the health of her community even if she does not go back to nursing. Her well-informed influence might be a very great force in planning with community leaders for better facilities. This in turn could be a very satisfying use of one's professional knowledge. Mental health is not just an individual problem; it is a social problem when one considers how mental retardation, alcoholism and delinquency—to mention only a few conditions—directly influence the health of our society.

TYPES OF FACILITIES

"Distrust all in whom the impulse to punish is powerful."* With all our knowledge we rarely grasp the significance of Nietzsche's statement, which was made in 1883. For many centuries persons with socially unacceptable behavior were grouped together in prisons where they were punished for any outburst in conduct. Eventually the criminal was separated from the mentally ill. However, the old pattern of care (which is still with us) consisted of building institutions in the country away from treatment centers and trained personnel. This is usually interpreted as a continued rejection of the mental patient by society. Erich Fromm states that "man is more afraid of rejection than he is of punishment." It would seem, therefore, that our more humanistic approach to caring for the mentally ill was no more effective in terms of patient treatment.

Aside from mere buildings, the vital part of any facility is its atmosphere, which must contribute to the health of its patients. A purely humanistic approach may not be therapeutic. Kindness and mere social pleasantries may increase dependence upon the institution when,

*_Thus Spake Zarathustra_. Nietzsche, Friedrich Wilhelm, Chapter 29.

at the same time, there is no attempt to develop insight and independence. Fashionable facilities may not satisfy the requirements for a therapeutic environment. As an example, I know one patient who voluntarily went to a modern private psychiatric hospital which faced a cemetery and cost more than the bridal suite at a large nearby hotel. In addition, nursing personnel performed only in the areas of procedures and recreation. The already upset patient became more upset and left the hospital at the end of ten days having spent his energies on his environment rather than on his problems. Most patients are already angry. It is a part of their illness. They are reacting, often subconsciously, to something in their past for which there is good reason to be angered. It is vital that a therapeutic environment is one in which the patient feels comfortable with personnel who are qualified to help locate the original source of the anger. Ingredients of a therapeutic milieu will be discussed later.

Hospitals

Most psychiatric institutions are administered by the state, city or Veterans Administration. Aside from these, there are private psychiatric facilities of various sizes. The majority of psychiatric hospitals have traditionally been custodial in nature, authoritarian and controlled with liberal use of restraints, locked doors and rigid routines which patients were expected to follow. Until recently, exceptions to this type of hospitals were few. Some state institutions and some private hospitals have changed drastically in this respect. The nurse will have to find out about the practices of the facilities in her community.

There will always be some chronically ill patients who have brain damage or a severe psychosis which either was not treated or did not respond to treatment. Custodial care of patients will be based on diagnosis and response to treatment. Even for these patients newer treatments will make them more comfortable and improve their institutional life.

General hospitals are adding psychiatric units to their buildings. These units provide acute care to the patient who needs hospitalization. Intensive therapy is given by members of several disciplines, such as the psychiatrist, the psychologist, the social worker, the nurse, the recreational therapist and nonprofessional attendants. The goal is to treat the patient as quickly as possible so that he can return to his normal environment and continue treatment outside a hospital. This dynamic approach, which utilizes persons who are trained in interpersonal skills, emphasizes mental health rather than mental disease. Such an approach is also utilized at other kinds of hospitals. Rather than expanding facilities which are geared to the care of chronically ill patients, the trend is to increase the number of smaller facilities for the acutely ill and those requiring intensive care so that the need for chronic facilities is lessened.

Most hospitals have a section which can be locked if a particular patient requires it. However, many units are completely unlocked. Patients reflect the way they are treated. Whenever it is possible to show patients this kind of confidence, it will contribute to their welfare.

Day Centers and Night Centers

When day centers exist, they can often be used as an alternative to hospitalization. Patients live at home and come to the center during the day for individual therapy, group therapy, work therapy and resocialization. When these centers operate Monday through Friday, patients interact with the same staff each day, and there are fewer persons to communicate with. Such centers may be used as a transition period after discharge from the hospital, or the patient may be admitted directly to the center for care. Again, the aim is to return the patient to the community as soon as possible.

Day center facilities may become night centers after 5:00 P.M. In this case, the patient continues with his job and comes to the center for treatment after work. Counseling sessions, group programs, etc., are planned before and after supper hours. Patients may not come to such centers five days a week. They may only come two or three times a week. If at any time it is felt that a patient is a suicidal risk, he will be hospitalized until this danger is considered to no longer exist.

One other advantage of day centers and night centers is that patients seem to seek help at an earlier stage of illness when such facilities are available. This advantage may well prevent the development of more severe conditions because patients are allowed a great deal of self-direction, they are not isolated from the community, and their dependency is minimized.

Foster Homes

Some institutions use foster homes in the community for patients who are being released from hospitals. There are two principal reasons for foster home care. First, a patient can continue his care outside a hospital when his own home is not conducive to his health or when he has no home. It also permits patients to stay in the community where follow-up facilities are available. There are many foster homes in Topeka, Kansas, where patients come to the Menninger Clinic from all over the United States. A foster home placement may also prevent the need for hospitalization.

The use of foster homes has been existent for centuries in Gheel,

Belgium, where people once came to worship at the shrine of a saint. This particular pilgrimage was supposed to effect a cure for patients with mental illness. When this first started in the thirteenth century, patients who did not recover immediately wished to stay in Gheel until the visit had a happy outcome. Families of these persons had to return to their homes to continue their daily occupations. As a result, the families of Gheel began to open up their homes to these persons.

Today the mentally ill still live with families in Gheel. Sometimes several placements may be necessary before the appropriate family is found. Patients see a physician once a month and a nurse visits frequently. Because of careful observation, acute attacks are prevented. Gheel residents do not fear the mentally ill. They have lived among them for centuries. The reaction of the residents undoubtedly affects the behavior of the patients. The attitudes of this community are indeed enviable.

Halfway Houses

A halfway house is usually run by professional personnel. Patients who have been discharged from a hospital may live in such a house to determine how well they can relate to persons and to determine how ready they are to return to their own setting. Individual and group therapy may be continued.

It is often difficult to find a community or neighborhood willing to permit the use of a home for such purposes. There is also difficulty in obtaining financial assistance for such projects. Because of this, one halfway house was located on the grounds of a hospital and run by hospital personnel. Patients worked in the town nearby, learned to mix better socially, had an opportunity for recreation and had time to save a little money so that they could return home without financial dependence.

Mental Hygiene Clinics

Mental hygiene clinics may be totally private, totally public or endowed so that the patient pays what he can afford to pay for outpatient psychiatric care. Patients come for psychotherapy which may be given by a psychiatrist, a psychologist or a social worker.

Some cities have emergency clinics or so-called walk-in clinics. Patients who become disturbed at hours other than 9:00 through 5:00 P.M. on Mondays through Fridays can obtain emergency care from professional persons who are available. Some cities have emergency telephone numbers which can be called to provide this kind of help.

It is vital that a discharged patient have outpatient facilities or some kind of follow-up care available to him. New adjustments are required, employment must be found, and family and community acceptance will influence the patient's progress. Some of these facilities are called aftercare clinics and may be associated with a hospital or be part of a mental health clinic.

The role of the public health nurse is vital in this area. She may be the one who visits discharged patients. She must learn to recognize problems, counsel families or refer the patient for assistance in dealing with specific problems. The public health nurse with her continued contacts and access to homes may recognize conditions and prevent the establishment of behavior patterns by promoting treatment at a time when it can be most effective. The industrial nurse is in a unique position to identify and assist workers who need guidance. This is also true of the school nurse who may be working with children of hospitalized parents or dealing directly with pupils who need guidance. This is especially common among the adolescent age group. Ultimately it is hoped that people will ask about psychiatric help in the same manner that they do about physical care.

Ex-patient clubs have been organized in some communities. These give ex-patients an opportunity to share adjustment experiences and provide a method whereby continued group therapy is possible. They also furnish a social outlet. It is essential that such clubs have the guidance of a professional individual in order to make them as effective as possible.

METHODS OF TREATMENT

The general aim of treatment is to help the patient to accept himself with both strengths and weaknesses (self-acceptance), to develop some degree of self-realization through his own creativity (self-expression), to possess an adequate contact with reality, to be directed by inner rather than outer values and to have the ability to handle stress from the environment. It is obvious that all of us have varying degrees of these abilities and controls, whether we are patients or not.

Psychotherapy

When psychiatric care is given on a "one-to-one" basis, the patient usually sees either a psychologist or a psychiatrist. Group therapy utilizes one professional person for every five to ten patients. It is not within the province of this book to discuss the various schools of analysis and therapy. However, psychotherapy is aimed at helping the patient to understand the mechanisms behind his behavior and to understand the origins of his behavior in order to learn new behaviors which will be more satisfying and more realistically oriented.

Somatic Therapy

INSULIN SHOCK. Insulin shock therapy is most commonly used for persons who are withdrawn. It is presently being replaced by drug therapy in many cases.

INSULIN SUBSHOCK. Insulin subshock produces hypoglycemia, but not coma. Such treatment often makes a patient more accessible to psychotherapy. Drug therapy is also replacing this form of treatment.

ELECTROSHOCK. This form of therapy is used for patients who are agitated and for those who have retarded depression, manic depression or schizophrenia. Special treatment rooms with an adjoining recovery area may be built for shock therapy, or the institutional philosophy may be that this treatment seems less "special" if the equipment is brought to the patient's room.

PSYCHOSURGERY. Psychosurgery, usually a prefontal lobotomy in which the association fibers between the frontal lobes and the thalamus are severed, was first done in 1935, in Portugal. This procedure is usually done after other forms of therapy have failed. Drug therapy has replaced the need for surgery in many cases.

NARCOANALYSIS. During World War II, intravenous Sodium Amytal and Pentothal Sodium were used as first-aid treatment in combat traumas. Since then it has become helpful in overcoming resistance to therapy in the suspicious and inaccessible patient.

PSYCHOPHARMACOLOGY. Besides the usual sedatives, stimulants and anticonvulsants used in the treatment of psychiatric patients, there are many new drugs used in what is commonly called the chemical assault on mental illness.

There are two main kinds of antidepressants. One type inhibits mono-amine oxidase in the brain. These so-called MAO inhibitor drugs include Marsilid, Marplan, Nardil, Niamid and Parnate. These drugs have a tendency to affect the action of other drugs, such as tranquilizers, narcotics, sedatives and several home remedies which might be bought without prescription at the neighborhood drug store. They also have a cumulative action so that the effect of the drug can be expected to continue from three to seven days after it has been discontinued. It is, therefore, vital to carefully watch patients who are taking other drugs with these antidepressants and immediately following their discontinuance.

The other group of antidepressants are nonenzyme inhibitors, such as Tofranil, Elavil, Petofrane, Aventyl and Vivactil. These drugs are short-acting, do not accumulate in the system and rarely affect the action of other drugs. It is important that the nurse observe for side-effects whenever either type of drug is being administered. Patients should be especially watched for the release of aggressive impulses which were not previously overt.

There are also two general categories of so-called tranquilizers.

These drugs have different chemical structures which have different side-effects and different indications. One group is especially indicated in the treatment of psychoses. Some of the trade names of these drugs are Permitil, Stelazine, Trilafon, Compazine, Thorazine and Sparine. Side-effects such as dermatitis, jaundice (on occasion), agranulocytosis and neurological reactions occur sometimes. For chronic psychiatric patients it is necessary that drug therapy be continued or symptoms will recur and readmission to an institution may be required.

The other group of tranquilizers are milder in action and include such drugs as Miltown, Equanil, Atarax, Vistaril, Librium and Valium. These drugs are mainly used in the treatment of psychoneuroses and have few side-effects. They, too, are palliative and not curative.

OTHER TREATMENTS. Additional physical treatments for psychiatric conditions include hydrotherapy, cold body packs, sleep therapy, carbon dioxide inhalation and others.

THE ROLE OF THE PSYCHIATRIC NURSE

"Psychiatric nursing practice is the provision of nursing care to patients where the major therapeutic goal is the prevention, detection, treatment and rehabilitation of psychiatric disorders. In providing such care, the function of the nurse is not different in nature from nursing in other clinical fields, but does differ in its primary focus on interpersonal one-to-one and group relationships."* While it is difficult to find complete agreement on the exact role of the psychiatric nurse, this definition certainly draws a picture of the nurse as a dynamic influence in psychiatric care with a therapeutic role.

Hildegard Peplau describes six subroles of the nurse working in the psychiatric unit. The nurse may function in the role of mother-surrogate, in the technical role by performing skills needed for procedures, in the role of unit manager, in a socializing role and in the role of health teacher. The "counseling or psychotherapeutic subrole" is the role which she feels must be emphasized by the psychiatric nurse. A nurse may function in the first five roles when she completes her basic nursing education, but it is generally agreed that she must have a master's degree to perform adequately at the level of the counselor or psychotherapeutic agent.

Another concept of the role of the nurse is something between the psychotherapeutic and the traditional one which emphasizes being kind, adhering to rules and doing what is ordered by the physician. That is the collaborative role. When the nurse functions in this role, she works directly with individual patients. She makes observations and helps to find meanings of behavior, which she discusses with the patient's

*Matheney, Ruth V., and Topalis, Mary: *Psychiatric Nursing*. Ed. 4, St. Louis, C. V. Mosby Co., 1965, p. 13.

therapist. Because of her relationship with the patient, she may contribute valuable help to the patient's ultimate cure. She also works with the family and may coordinate the general program of patient care.

The nurse might also work in group therapy either alone or as a co-therapist. The nurse learns how to encourage patients in self-expression and to guide a group in constructive outlets. Intensive in-service education in group therapy methods has been conducted where there is a shortage of nurses with postgraduate education in psychiatric nursing.

The various roles of the nurse are determined by the personnel around her, her education and ability, the philosophy of the organization and the condition of the patient. The psychiatrist or psychologist may be the major person functioning in the therapeutic role. The nurse may be the most active person working with the patient, especially when intensive insight therapy is not needed. Nursing roles range between these extremes, and careful communication and clearly defined areas of responsibilities are vital.

When a medical-surgical patient is admitted to a hospital, the nurse is likely to begin to get to know her patient by asking about his job, family and home. In a psychiatric setting, these questions are likely to produce anxiety as the patient's problems are undoubtedly associated with one or more of these relationships. The nurse in a psychiatric setting aids her patient best by letting him talk, listening and seeking clues to the reasons for his behavior. If a patient makes a statement about the reason for his behavior, it is wise for the nurse to validate it from the patient to find out whether she understood his statements correctly.

The nurse does not need biographical data from the patient nor should she talk about herself. Her patient contacts are not social exchanges. The nurse must learn to see whether she can identify the existence of fear, ways of relieving anxiety and precipitating situations before a spell of rising anxiety. By these methods, the nurse might prepare the patient for the doctor, or she may reinvestigate understandings to see if they are correct. She helps her patient to see his environment more clearly. All of this requires an education which teaches the nurse to use an explorative approach in order to make nursing care a part of therapy.

It is vital for the nurse to understand that she must not interpret patient behavior to the patient. This may add emotional pressures. Insights from psychotherapy are painful experiences which must be timed properly. The patient must not only be ready for painful memories and insights, but he must have support at the time of their revelation. If the patient could tolerate the knowledge, he would already be aware of it. Therefore, the nurse must refrain from interpretive counseling unless it is a joint decision of the treatment team with full knowledge of the patient's condition.

The patient needs care because his self-development was shattered by stress at some period in his life, usually during his early childhood. The development of his self-concept was based upon the way others responded to him as an infant or child. As a result, his adult behavior is affected by reactions to his past of which he is unaware. When a nurse understands this, she will see patient behavior not as good, bad or indifferent but as an expression of illness. The very heart of therapy is the degree of success with which a patient is reeducated to value himself and others. Therefore, the reaction of persons in his environment toward him will be vital.

The nurse who works with psychiatric patients must learn to make certain distinctions. She will be asked to accept her patient whether he is vulgar, angry or whatever. Acceptance does not mean approval of either a patient's behavior or his acts, but the nurse must learn to accept her own feelings, and she must not make the patient feel that he offended her or that he needs punishment. He needs to feel safe to express his feelings.

Patients need emotional experiences, which will help them to change their behavior, not lectures or reasons why they should feel differently. All of us have had the experience of knowing we should not feel angry at the very moment of feeling irate. This is the situation in which a patient finds himself. If someone tries to reason him out of a certain feeling, it often makes it worse, as he is forced to justify his feeling. A nurse may increase patient anxiety by telling him to cheer up. When he cannot do this, he experiences an all too familiar feeling—failure.

There are various ways in which nursing personnel can support their patients. Aside from the avoidance of punishment, which can be very subtle, such as merely avoiding a patient after a certain outburst, the nurse can try to see things from the patient's point of view. If a patient has hallucinations, she must try to look at the meaning through his experience rather than hers. He needs relationships which will not confirm his feeling of worthlessness. Much patient behavior has the purpose of distracting attention from a fear. The patient might criticize personnel, fight with other patients or become preoccupied with physical symptoms.

The nurse should focus upon meanings of patient behavior especially when it is hard to accept. She must listen, avoid platitudinous reassurance and try to ask questions which cannot be answered by a mere yes or no. Consistency helps patients as they learn what is expected of them and what to expect from their environment. Reassurance is best shown by understanding and interest demonstrated by increasing the number of patient contacts when no particular treatment is needed.

The nurse needs to consider her own reactions when she is caring for patients who exhibit strong emotions. She must accept her own reactions as well as those of the patient. If a nurse feels guilty because she does not feel sympathy for a patient whom she knows is mentally disturbed, she is not likely to be in a position to help him. If she realizes that the patient needs her help and that her reaction is acceptable, she is less likely to demonstrate it to the patient. The nurse must also realize that to have a patient dislike her rather than admire her may actually be helpful to the patient. This is especially difficult for the young nurse who has just been in the throes of adolescent needs for popularity. To be able to put herself into this kind of therapeutic position, she needs proper guidance in her education.

The nurse must learn to observe the effects of her other actions, such as the use of her voice and the use of body movements. She, in turn, can learn that these communicate things to her about her patients. Patients may react to specific words, to music or to certain pictures. An awareness of these things is vital.

The nurse must provide a patient with a relationship which does not become intimate, which can be ended without the patient feeling any sense of betrayal and one in which the nurse does not attempt to fulfill any of her own emotional needs. Such complications do not help the patient. One of the important things about a nurse-patient relationship is that it can be terminated when the therapeutic reason for its existence has ceased. This makes it clear that objectivity is not a cold appraising attitude. When a patient is concerned, objectivity produces the ability to think clearly in the presence of varying degrees and kinds of emotions.

THE THERAPEUTIC ENVIRONMENT

A great deal is being written about providing the psychiatric patient with a therapeutic milieu. This may range from the cheerful aspect of room colors to the education and performance of personnel. Many persons feel that hospitals have actually contributed to making the patient worse.

In order to make the environment more therapeutic, certain goals are strived for. The general attitude of personnel must show that patient improvement is expected. They must provide the patient with a feeling of dignity. In order to accomplish these goals, staff and patients must be closer and patient tasks must have some meaning other than mere activity.

Locked doors may serve the purpose of protecting a patient from suicide or protecting the public from homicide, but few patients can be expected to do either one. It is, therefore, necessary for the dignity of patients not to be locked up unless their behavior patterns indicate such a need. Even in large state institutions, it has been found that three fourths fewer patients need to be in locked areas.

The hospital may develop a social setting where the patient plays a part in decisions about his therapy and about government of the ward. Ward meetings where patients and personnel meet to discuss problems of the institutional setting provide the patient with a sense of responsibility even when he is upset. This also enables patients to help one another. Patients may wear their own clothes. Nurses may wear street clothes. Better food served in dignity is more common today.

The authoritarian role of personnel is eliminated. This removes the necessity for personnel to play a police role and keeps them from being the withdrawn observer. Changing the attitude and role of personnel is part of improving the therapeutic role of the environment. Healthy relationships between personnel is also considered important to patient therapy.

A recent study comparing the background of patients with that of the environment of the institution showed a conflict in terms of therapeutic effect. It compared the two cultures in an institution: the culture within the institution and the culture which was brought in by the patients. If patients from a fundamentalist religious background enter an institution which provides dancing in the evening and smoking rooms, there is a conflict between the culture of the patient and his environment which may not necessarily be therapeutic.

A therapeutic environment should provide experiences which will minimize the patient's distortion of reality, facilitate communication with others, reduce anxiety, increase his self-esteem and help him to realize his full potentialities. The latter is perhaps one of the more difficult things to fulfill because of the cross section of patients in any given hospital. If patients have similar backgrounds, this may not be difficult. However, if the hospital setting includes a patient who is an electronic genius and one who is a gardener in the city park, it becomes obvious that their needs are similar only in very general terms. Both may be withdrawn and need to externalize their emotions, but it is highly unlikely that the stimulus will be the same. Even when patients are of similar backgrounds and intelligence, wide differences in individual needs will exist.

Continued attention to patient reactions to environment is needed. Whether the institution serves chronically ill and/or acutely ill patients, it must function so that the illness is not affected adversely.

SUMMARY

The rapid gains in treatment measures and gradual change in attitudes toward mental illness are beginning to change the types of facilities available, the use of facilities at an earlier stage of illness and the therapeutic quality of the environment in which a patient is cared for. The psychiatric nurse may function in a traditional, a collaborative or a therapeutic role. While the functions of the psychiatric nurse are not clearly identified, she can always contribute to the patient's welfare. Those with advanced degrees will not only help patients directly but also instruct and assist other nursing and nonprofessional personnel to work with patients in a more meaningful way. Up-to-date facilities are aimed at early treatment, fast and intensive treatment and early return of the patient to his family, job and community.

SUGGESTED READINGS

For All

Gregg, Dorothy E.: The Therapeutic Roles of the Nurse. *Perspectives in Psychiatric Care*, January-February, 1963, p. 19.

Matheney, Ruth V., and Topalis, Mary: *Psychiatric Nursing*. Ed. 4, St. Louis, C. V. Mosby Co., 1965, Chapter 8.

Textbook for Those Working With Psychiatric Patients

Matheney, Ruth V., and Topalis, Mary: *Psychiatric Nursing*. Ed. 4, St. Louis, C. V. Mosby Co., 1965.

REFERENCES

Amendt, Janet A., and White, Reginald P.: Continued Care Services for Mental Patients. *Nursing Outlook*, July, 1965, p. 56.

Angrist, Shirley S.: The Mental Hospital: Its History and Destiny. *Perspectives in Psychiatric Care*, December, 1963, p. 20.

Ayd, Frank J., Jr.: The Chemical Assault on Mental Illness, the Antidepressants. *American Journal of Nursing*, June, 1965, p. 78.

Ayd, Frank J., Jr.: The Chemical Assault on Mental Illness, the Major Tranquilizers. *American Journal of Nursing*, April, 1965, p. 70.

Ayd, Frank J., Jr.: Chemical Assault on Mental Illness, the Minor Tranquilizers. *American Journal of Nursing*, May, 1965, p. 89.

Baker, Joan M., and Estes, Nada J.: Anger in Group Therapy. *American Journal of Nursing*, July, 1965, p. 96.

Belcher, John C.: Background Norms of Patients and the Therapeutic Community. *Journal of Health and Human Behavior*, Spring, 1965, p. 27.

Berne, Eric: *Games People Play*. New York, Grove Press, Inc., 1964.

Briggs, Dennie L., and Wardell, Marion F.: A Locked Ward Was Opened. *American Journal of Nursing*, September, 1961, p. 102.

Bueker, Kathleen, and Warrick, Annette: Can Nurses Be Group Therapists? *American Journal of Nursing*, May, 1964, p. 114.

Chamberlain, Amparo S.: Visit to Gheel. *American Journal of Nursing*, January, 1959, p. 68.

Christ, Adolph E., Critchley, Deane L., Larson, Margaret L., and Brown, Myrna L.: The Role of the Nurse in Child Psychiatry. *Nursing Outlook*, January, 1965, p. 30.

Clarke, Eric Kent: *Mental Hygiene for Community Nursing*. Minneapolis, University of Minnesota Press, 1942.

The Community Health View of Mentally Ill and Mentally Restored Patients as reflected in abstracts of papers presented at the 1964 meeting of the American Public Health Association; *Perspectives in Psychiatric Nursing*, Vol. III, No. 1, 1965, p. 9.

A Day Hospital for Psychiatric Patients. *American Journal of Nursing*, September, 1962, p. 80.

Duran, Fernando A.: The Clarinda Plan. *American Journal of Nursing*, August, 1965, p. 77.
Fromm, Erich: *The Art of Loving*. New York, Harper and Brothers, 1956.
Fromm, Erich: *Man for Himself*. New York, Rinehart and Company, Inc., 1947.
Gregg, Dorothy E.: The Therapeutic Roles of the Nurse. *Perspectives in Psychiatric Care*, January-February, 1963, p. 19.
Hale, Shirley L., and Richardson, Julia H.: Terminating the Nurse-Patient Relationship. *American Journal of Nursing*, September, 1963, p. 116.
Heckel, Robert V.: The Nurse as Co-Therapist in Group Psychotherapy. *Perspectives in Psychiatric Care*, Vol. II, No. 4, 1964, p. 18.
Holmes, Marguerite: The Need to be Recognized. *American Journal of Nursing*, October, 1961, p. 86.
Hurley, Elizabeth A.: Some Requirements for Therapeutic Nursing Care. *Perspectives in Psychiatric Care*, March-April, 1963, p. 23.
Matheney, Ruth V., and Topalis, Mary: *Psychiatric Nursing*. Ed. 4, St. Louis, C. V. Mosby Co., 1965.
Menninger, Karl: *Love Against Hate*. New York, Harcourt, Brace and Co., 1942.
Mereness, Dorothy: Problems and Issues in Contemporary Psychiatric Nursing. *Perspective in Psychiatric Care*, Vol. II, No. 1, 1964, p. 15.
Meyers, Jerome K., Bean, Lee L., and Pepper, Max P.: Social Class and Psychiatric Disorders: A Ten Year Follow-up. *Journal of Health and Human Behavior*, Summer, 1965, p. 74.
Paquette, Arleen, and Lafave, Hugh: Halfway House. *American Journal of Nursing*, March, 1964, p. 121.
Peplau, Hildegard E.: Interpersonal Techniques: The Crux in Psychiatric Nursing. *American Journal of Nursing*, June, 1962, p. 50.
Peplau, Hildegard E.: Principles of Psychiatric Nursing *in* Arieti, S. (ed.): *American Handbook of Psychiatry*. New York, Basic Books, Inc., 1959, Chapter 92.
Peplau, Hildegard E.: What is Experiential Teaching? *American Journal of Nursing*, July, 1957, p. 884.
Robinson, Alice M.: Creativity Takes Courage. *Nursing Outlook*, July, 1963, p. 499.
Robitaille, Normand D.: The Organization of Nursing Service for the Establishment of Nurse-Patient Relations. *Perspectives in Psychiatric Care*, Vol. II, No. 3, 1964, p. 30.
Siegel, Nathaniel H.: What Is a Therapeutic Community? *Nursing Outlook*, May, 1964, p. 49.

22

Back to Nursing

At the age of 80, Sarah Colvin, a graduate of Johns Hopkins University, recalled the words of Isabel Hampton Robb, her superintendent of nurses, "Miss Hampton used to say to us when we were in training that we would never find any kind of life more interesting or more absorbing than the life of a nurse, because it combined so many different activities." This timely reflection was made in 1892, and it becomes more appropriate with each passing decade. The nurse has challenges, responsibilities and stimuli which are unique. Many nonpracticing nurses maintain interest in their profession.

Sarah Colvin was an example. She was the wife of a surgeon, participated in women's rights movements, was a governor's appointee to the Minnesota Board of Education, was the first president of the Minnesota Nurses' Association and was active in working with nursing organizations to promote standards of nursing education. She is an example of the kind of nurse who remained active in nursing although she was a nonpracticing nurse.

If you are one who contemplates going back to the practice of nursing, you will find that the challenges and responsibilities will not be overwhelming if you take them in sensible stages. You did not become a nurse overnight, and you will not become "refreshed" overnight. Take a refresher course if one is available. It will provide you with an opportunity to observe and to practice both manual and interpersonal skills in an unhurried manner as well as guide you in review and study of present concepts. Familiarity with functions and trends will begin to give you a feeling of security which will replace your fear of the unknown. Routines and procedures are the easiest things to learn and therefore should be considered last.

It would be unfair to give the refresher the idea that returning to work is easy. It is not. Only another refresher can know how really difficult it is. The difficulties in adjustment are more than compensated for, however, because the goal is so satisfying. Each nurse who returns to work will do so for a different reason. I know one nurse who does it purely because she wants to. In fact, she gives the financial remunerations she receives to charity. Another woman may be helping to educate her children and find that her life is fuller because of it. Still another nurse may do it purely for the "extras" she enjoys so much. Most nurses work because they have to and later find they also want to. Whatever the reason satisfaction can be the same.

WHERE TO WORK

Since almost every hospital in the country needs nurses, the refresher will be welcomed with rare exceptions. It is important to keep this in mind. Because you will feel somewhat useless, you may feel so grateful to any director who will have you that you may accept the job at the first place to which you go. This would be a mistake unless you live in an area where there is only one hospital within a 50-mile radius. Even then, you need to have certain information to help you make a decision. It is very important to find an atmosphere in keeping with your needs. All institutions are not alike and, as a refresher, you will want as pleasant a first work experience as possible. This is most likely if you go to two or three different places and make your decision upon the things you learn about each institution.

Selecting the Hospital

There are many ways to find out about a hospital. You may have friends who work there, you or your family may have been a patient there, it may be affiliated with your church, or your family physician may have a suggestion. Modern facilities are important and desirable, but they should be only one of several factors contributing to your decision. Distance from home is a factor some people need to take into account if they are needed at home immediately before or after work.

One word of caution is needed about working at the neighborhood hospital. The nurse is likely to be continuously exposed to questions whenever she personally knows patients, their family and their friends. She needs to be able to say, "I do not discuss my work," and mean it. If the nurse can do this and not become trapped into revealing information which comes to her confidentially as a result of her work, this will be no problem to her. In smaller areas this can become a serious problem. More than one rural hospital prints its surgery schedule without the name of the procedure to be performed, because it is so difficult to protect the privacy of patients. In any case many nurses drive long distances and pass many other hospitals in order to work at the hospital which they consider the best. Even then, it is necessary to remember the confidential nature of patient information whether it concerns neighbors, public figures, locally prominent persons or John Doe.

The Job Interview

After you have evaluated factors such as facilities, distance from home and general reputation for care, your next step is the job interview. The job interview is a *two-way* conversation. You must remember that it is as necessary to ask questions of the person interviewing you as it is for the interviewer to ask you questions. This is why it is wise to apply at several institutions. In this way you will learn to detect differences in general tone, atmosphere and attitudes. As a matter of fact, the job interview might well be considered a part of being refreshed.

You will need time to ask your questions, and the person who interviews you will need time to ask questions, also. This cannot be done hurriedly at a spur-of-the-moment visit. Plan ahead by calling the hospital to find out who you are to see, and make an appointment with that person or his secretary. In a larger institution, you will find a personnel department where initial screening interviews are done and where job applications are made out. Afterwards you will usually be interviewed by the Director of Nursing or one of her delegated assistants. By calling the hospital ahead of time, you will find out whom to see and be able to arrange an appointment. Time will have been set aside for you, and the interview will not be affected by the irritation of your having interrupted other work.

Some Things the Hospital Wants to Know

For the purpose of this chapter, we will assume that you are to see the Director of Nursing Service. This may not be true if the hospital is large or its organizational plan assigns selection of nursing personnel to someone else.

First of all, the director will want to know what things have contributed to your desire to return to work. She will want to know what area of nursing interests you. Remember, the hospital may have vacancies, but they may not necessarily be in the area of your choice or there may be a more urgent need on one station than on another. Nonetheless, she will want to place you in the area of your choice if at all possible. She will want to know what arrangements you have made for your children if this is a factor. She will want to know how your family feels about your return to work. All these things will help her to know you and the kind of nonworking factors which you will be experiencing.

She will want to know what your previous work history consisted of, regardless of how old it is. She is unlikely to follow up on work references over five years old. Anything older than that, whether good or bad, deserves a certain amount of reservation. Individual problems and responsibilities change. Even for a nurse who has never stopped practicing, only the most recent work references are usually studied by a potential employer. In lieu of this, the director may wish to talk to the instructors of a refresher course, if you took one, or she may be content with several character references.

Your license to practice nursing will need to be verified by some evidence of licensure. Nurses who have become inactive or who are registered in another state need to become currently licensed in the state in which they are employed. If this is a need, you should contact the Board of Nursing in your state to initiate the proper procedure. If you are not currently licensed, you will probably be allowed to practice if you obtain a permit and show evidence of original licensure. This will not delay your plans to go to work under ordinary circumstances.

The director will also describe what she expects of you in terms of reliability, hours, tenure and general responsibilities. She will need to know if you have any health problems which might interfere with your work. Each director will desire other information which she finds helpful in assessing individuals. In general, you will find that the director is seeking nurses and is most hopeful that she can hire you.

Some Things You Will Want to Know

Among other things, you will want to know about salary, days off, holidays, shifts, retirement plans, vacation time, leave of absence policies and all the things which come under the heading of personnel policies. These vary greatly from one part of the country to another. At best, one could only describe the situation in a particular locale. Generally speaking, salaries and personnel policies have improved in the past 20 years, but not at a rate which is always consistent with the times. Because of this, labor unions have tried to organize nurses in many places. The state Economic Security programs of the American Nurses Association have been a moving force in improving salaries and benefits in some areas of the country. In the latter case the organization may negotiate a contract with one or more hospitals in a particular area. If this is true, the nurse will find that contracting hospitals in her area have similar salary ranges, benefits, etc.

If you wish to work only part time, you will want to know what days you are expected to work, how many and how often. Because most personnel work a five-day week, a two-day part-time nurse is invaluable to the necessary seven-day coverage. Sometimes a part-time nurse and a full-time nurse can work out a rather regular pattern of days on and off. This is helpful, as everyone can plan his life around such a schedule and alter it only when special occasions arise. Once in a while the hours of two part-time nurses complement each other, i.e., when one works four days a week and one works three days a week. You will not be able to set these schedules, but these are the kinds of possibilities which you may encounter.

The part-time nurse and the full-time nurse should always share week-ends and holidays. Some nurses say they will only work on Tuesdays and Wednesdays or they will not work at all, and some institutions accept such persons because they are short of help. This may, in reality, contribute to a shortage of help. When such demands are made, there is an adverse affect on morale. Other personnel must then work around the so-called "plum days and hours" of such an individual. This causes resentment among personnel and often results in turnover of the full-time nurse who literally finds herself penalized for working full time.

It is hoped that you as a refresher will expect to share week-ends and various shifts with other workers and that the institution where you work will expect the same, not only of you but of all its employees.

You will want to know what the institution expects of its registered nurses. Undoubtedly, it will expect you to function as described in Chapter 7. In any case, it is imperative that you and the director come to a decision about WHEN you will be expected to assume these responsibilities. If I were a refresher, I would select an employer for several reasons, but the content and individualization of the orientation would influence me more than any other single factor.

Does the hospital have a formal orientation program? If so, how long is it and what is included in it? If not, what kind of an orientation will they plan? Aside from the formal orientation program, how much time will they allow before full responsibilities must be assumed? Will they adjust the overall plan if it becomes necessary? The answers to these questions should help you to select your employer. A nurse who will be working in a small, isolated hospital, may not have the benefit of a formal orientation program. She still has a need, however, for time to work with other employees to learn the routines of the particular hospital and to regain skills.

One of the greatest fears of the refresher is that of being plunged into work before learning where the dietary dumbwaiter is located, what the visiting hours are, how to work the oxygen apparatus and all the many details which are needed before feeling comfortable at work. These are things which should be included in an orientation program, formal or informal. Most refreshers have experienced inadequate orientation in the past, and it is such experiences which may deter them from working. Every nurse, whether a refresher or not, needs orientation, but you, the refresher, may need it more and at a somewhat slower pace. There is no reason to apologize for this, and you have every right to ask for time to learn.

After the interview, go home and consider the pros and cons of your interviews. Discuss it with your family, but remember, it is your life and the conversation should center on this aspect of the situation. If your family encourages you to try it, they can be your best cheering section. Many skeptical families have ultimately been convinced of the desirability of such a pursuit.

Once you make your decision, call the director of your choice and buy yourself one of the stunning new drip-dry uniforms now available. It will be worth every penny of it. If you can no longer buy your school cap, get a permastarch cap which can be washed with a brush. Put on a comfortable pair of shoes, and you will be ready to take the road back to nursing.

ORIENTATION

Even if you plan to go back to nursing only part time, it is strongly recommended that you work full time during your first two or three months of employment in order to get firmly grounded and thoroughly oriented to your job. If it takes you eight weeks to assume full responsibilities of a registered nurse comfortably on a full-time basis, it will take you more than twice that long on a part-time basis, and you may never feel really comfortable in your work. Therefore, plan to work full time the first few months no matter what your later plans are. Be sure to discuss this with your employer before you start so that you have a complete understanding about this. You will find that most employers consider a thorough orientation very much worthwhile.

Orientation can be divided into four rather distinct parts. First, the new nurse needs to know about her physical surroundings. She needs to learn the physical layout of the hospital and more detailed information about the location of things on her particular station. Where is the medication room? Where is the emergency equipment? Where are the charts kept? It is most disconcerting to spend hours looking for something as simple as a urine specimen container or a safety pin.

Second, new employees in all hospital departments, whether it be the laundry, the lab or the nursing department, need certain information. What is the procedure in case of fire? What kind of hospitalization and other insurance benefits are available? Where do I pick up my pay check? Where is the parking lot? Where is the locker room? Where do I go if I become ill or am injured while I am working? All these things need to be known by all employees.

Third, if there is a formal orientation program, it will include general policies and procedures of the nursing department and provide for brief introduction to other departments. During this time, the nurse becomes acquainted with the chaplaincy service, the volunteer service, duties of personnel in the nursing department and the aims of whatever educational programs exist. The nurse is introduced to the isolation policy and procedure, the routine for operative patients, the various printed forms used, the methods of ordering tests and supplies for patients, admission and discharge procedures and the most commonly used equipment. The formal orientation program may last anywhere from a few days to a few weeks, depending upon its content and sequence. Information which is given in the formal program at one hospital may be given informally at another. The content of the program is far more important than the length of it.

Fourth, the nurse needs individualized help geared to her particular needs as related to the expectancies of her employer. For instance, if the hospital asks its nurses to start intravenous fluids, a head nurse, supervisor or instructor needs to be available to teach the procedure. If this is not expected of the R.N., then obviously she need not learn it. If the nurse has not catheterized a patient in 15 years, she needs the opportunity to observe the performance of this procedure as well as an opportunity to do the procedure under supervision the first time she does it. Some nurses have never learned to take blood pressures. If they have not, then they need to be taught. The individualized portion of the orientation program dovetails the needs of the hospital with the needs of the nurse. It provides her with time for observation and practice and allows her confidence to grow at about the same pace as her responsibilities.

Some nurses feel comfortable in their work within six to eight weeks. Some do not feel comfortable for three months or more. This varies not only with the individual's temperament but with her previous experience. Two nurses may have been away from nursing for 15 years, but there is a difference between the nurse who married immediately after graduation and the nurse who worked for ten years before marriage. It also makes a difference whether the experience was in a doctor's office, a public health agency or a hospital. What is important is that both the nurse and the employer see progress during these first weeks.

One other interesting factor is common among refreshers. That is, the performance of a refresher is often far better than the refresher thinks it is. In other words, you are likely to find yourself doing satisfactory work before you actually feel secure and comfortable in the performance of your work. You may not always receive the amount of encouragement you really need because those around you are seldom aware of this. It is important, therefore, that you have an opportunity to discuss your work and your feelings about your work with your immediate superior every week or two during the first three months of employment.

CONTINUING IN-SERVICE EDUCATION

Once you have been "refreshed" and oriented to your new job, you will find that new developments continue to occur. Some of this information is provided through in-service education programs at the hospital. In-service education is not a refresher course. It is not a post-graduate course in nursing. It is, however, a program which your employing institution provides to improve patient care and to make it possible for you to use newly purchased equipment and to adapt to new procedures. In-service education is mainly aimed at the needs of personnel at a particular institution or in a specific area of an institution.

SOME TRICKS OF THE TRADE

Procedures Have Common Elements

If you read a procedure book, you are likely to find that there is much repetition among procedures concerning aseptic technique, care of equipment, patient privacy and other things. It is helpful to learn some of the common elements of procedures so that it will then be easier to get to the meat of a new procedure without reviewing a great deal of repetitious material. Whether a nursing procedure is performed to provide comfort, to aid in diagnosis or to provide a therapeutic effect, it needs to be performed with asepsis, minimal discomfort to the patient, safety and accuracy. It must then be recorded properly.

PREPARATION OF PATIENT AND EQUIPMENT. (1) Order necessary equipment and take it to the bedside. (2) Wash hands thoroughly. (3) Explain the purpose and basic steps of the procedure to the patient. (4) Provide the patient with privacy. (5) Protect the patient's bedding from becoming wet with a bath blanket on top and a plastic or rubber sheet underneath whenever necessary.

CARE OF THE PATIENT DURING THE PROCEDURE. (1) Observe the general and local effects of the treatment or procedure. (2) Discontinue the procedure if untoward effects occur, and notify the charge nurse. (3) Remain with the patient if it is essential to his peace of mind or his safety, or required for continuous observation. (4) If it is not necessary to remain with the patient continuously, place the signal cord within his reach so that he can summon you when he so desires.

AFTERCARE OF THE PATIENT AND EQUIPMENT. (1) Replace bedding as necessary. (2) Make patient comfortable and attend to his needs before leaving the room. (3) Rinse off all re-usable equipment, safely discard disposable equipment and place all soiled linen in a hamper. CAUTION: Soiled dressings should be wrapped in a moisture repellent bag. (4) Wash hands thoroughly. (5) Make out a charge slip if this is applicable. (6) Label any specimens clearly and see that they are sent to the laboratory promptly.

CHARTING. Charts no longer contain trivia, repetition and general routines at most institutions. Only pertinent changes in the patient are expected to be entered on Nurses' Notes. In the case of a procedure, you might chart the following:

1. Clinical Sheet: Enter the name of the procedure, the time and your initials. Enter medications, the time and your initials. Enter any specimens collected and the time.
2. Nurses' Notes: Enter reactions and observations of the patient, a description of any specimen and your name.
3. Intake and Output Slip: Use if applicable.

Advice From a Successful Refresher

One of the most outstanding nurses I have ever known happens to have been a refresher. She used a great deal of initiative in her own learning, was 57 years old when she went back to nursing and is admired by everyone who has ever been fortunate enough to work with her. She has been a source of inspiration to other refreshers, but she also has some very good advice which may be of help to others. Here is her advice in brief.

Think of yourself as having a reorientation to nursing. Part of this reorientation consists of emphasis on patients to care for, rather than things to do. Once you start seeing patients, supposedly forgotten things will surprisingly begin to come back to you.

Set reasonable goals for yourself. Do not expect to learn everything in a week. Use every opportunity to observe care which is unfamiliar to you. Naturally, someone else can do things better. Remember, experience and time will give you the proficiency you observe in others. As an aside, it might be worthwhile to observe the performance of others, knowing that everything you see may not be an example of the highest standard of care. If you observe carefully, you may learn how to do things better by seeing them done poorly or only moderately well. All of us can improve our standards of care and many persons tend to become careless as time goes on. It is something to prevent in yourself at a later time.

Do not compare yourself with others, not even with other refreshers. Compare yourself with yourself. In this way, you will see progress and be less easily discouraged. Golfers see personal improvement by comparing their own previous scores with present scores, not by comparing their score with that of Arnold Palmer. Everyone's background and experience is different. Successful refreshers include former teachers, public health nurses, office nurses, as well as women who had no work experience at all.

The first month is very difficult. Ultimately, however, the rewards of staying, are commensurate with how much of yourself you invest. Those who have invested a great deal of themselves find a sense of self-identity and an opportunity for self-growth as well as monetary advantages.

Take time to review policy and procedure books and patient information pamphlets. The latter will tell the patient how to obtain a haircut and what the visiting hours are. You will want to know as much as the patient, and patient information pamphlets are an excellent resource.

Listen to everyone in your environment. Read charts, attend in-service programs, refer to procedure books frequently and above all do not be afraid to say "I don't know." You can always add "but I'll find out." Ask questions. If you feel that you are interrupting the head nurse too often, carry a notebook and jot down questions which do not require immediate answers. In this way, you can accumulate questions and talk to the head nurse at a convenient hour. Remember, the head nurse wants you and needs you. It is in her interest to help you as much as possible.

Other personnel will also be very helpful. Old timers enjoy helping a new person. They were new once, and they know that no one learns by osmosis. Keep in mind that, within three months, you will be showing a new employee where the linen chute is located and you will recall your own orientation which you got through after all!

Finally, do not adjust by blaming others or by fault-finding. Use praise both for yourself and for others. When you are new, co-workers will not be too anxious to help you if you continually compare the past with the present and criticize their methods. Later on, when you become part of the particular unit in which you work, you can better evaluate the pros and cons of the new and then lend your influence to improved care. By that time, you will be admired by your colleagues, and your opinion will be properly valued.

ADJUSTMENT STAGES

Marcella Davis wrote an interesting article which is a suggested reading for all refreshers. She describes four phases of adjustment. It would be helpful for refreshers as well as for those who work with refreshers to understand these changes.

The first stage is the intrusion into one's previous way of life. This comes before new contacts have been established. A 60-year-old refresher acquaintance of mine said that she had the greatest problem with an afternoon bridge club to which she belonged. Although she readily gave up morning coffee gatherings with her neighbors, she was not happy to give up her bridge group. As time went on, it was convenient for her employer to give her Wednesdays off regularly. The club changed the day and she did not have to give up bridge. The refresher will find herself sorting these interferences and find that she need not give up things having a high pleasure priority.

The second stage identified by Marcella Davis is the launching, when you begin to feel involved with the new adventure. After a little more time the third stage, the fitting, occurs. During this time, you will begin to take issues and identify with your peers. This kind of involvement leads to the fourth stage, the arrival, when you enjoy chit chat after work and find yourself accepted by your peers and comfortable in your daily work.

SUMMARY

Going back to nursing is an adventure. It has its ups and downs, but the new knowledge is stimulating, the new adjustments are a challenge, and the new life will be rewarding and worth every effort you put into it.

SUGGESTED READINGS

Davis, Marcella Z.: The Return Phenomenon. *Nursing Forum*, Vol. II, 1963, p. 58.
Kelly, Cordelia W.: *Dimensions of Professional Nursing*. Section X, Career Opportunities in Nursing, New York, Macmillan Co., 1962.
Seidman, Joel: The Trend Among Professional Groups Today. *American Journal of Nursing*, January, 1965, p. 72.

REFERENCES

Colvin, Sarah Tarleton: *A Rebel in Thought*. New York, Island Press, 1944.
Davis, Marcella Z.: The Return Phenomenon. *Nursing Forum*, Vol. II, 1963, p. 58.
Kelly, Cordelia W.: *Dimensions of Professional Nursing*. New York, Macmillan Co., 1962.

23

Beyond the Present

"Every ultimate fact is only the first of a new series. Every general law is only a particular fact of some more general law presently to disclose itself."*

Whether you are a graduate of a modern, up-to-date program of nursing education or a refresher, Ralph Waldo Emerson's observation is pertinent. One's education is never complete regardless of the academic degree attained. Knowledge which is new to us as individuals and knowledge which is new to the world will unfold throughout our lives.

Although no one can be informed about all new advances, each of us can stay generally informed of many things and specifically informed about things affecting the care we give to our own patient. What then are the resources available to help us to stay refreshed and to continue our education either formally or informally? Resources mainly consist of in-service education programs, collegiate courses, clinical conferences, workshops and many varied reading materials.

IN-SERVICE EDUCATION

In-service education was briefly described in the last chapter, but a few more general comments are indicated. In-service education programs can only help those who attend them. The nurse needs to take some initiative in getting herself there. She needs to plan her patient care so that she may attend on duty time or she may need to stay an extra half hour to attend a program if the former is impossible.

If the nurse does not attend because program subjects do not interest her, she should talk to someone about it. Most in-service education directors welcome an expression of the desires of personnel

*Emerson, Ralph Waldo: Circles in *Essays* (first series). Boston, Houghton, Mifflin and Co., 1889.

so that it is possible to have a hand in selecting subjects for programs.

Most in-service programs are 30 to 60 minutes in length, are usually repeated several times during a day or over a period of several days, are work-oriented and are given in the institution. It is, therefore, possible for most employees to attend conveniently.

WORKSHOPS

Workshops, clinical conferences, conventions and institutes are the most usual ways of gaining up-to-date information. They also provide opportunities for exploration of new ideas and concepts. A workshop or similar type of program may last anywhere from several days to several weeks. It may be sponsored by an organization such as the American Nurses' Association, the National League for Nursing, the American Hospital Association, the American Public Health Association, a private foundation, a health department, a hospital or a college or university. Topics vary widely. Clinical subjects such as care of the cardiac or diabetic patient, management of personnel, new medical treatments, educational methods, human relations, nursing roles and nursing organizational structure are only a few topics taken from recent program announcements. Professional magazines and newspapers will announce most of these programs in advance. Program attendance is sometimes limited to membership of the sponsoring organization.

COLLEGIATE COURSES

Local colleges and universities may be an excellent resource for the refresher. Courses in the physical and biological sciences as well as in the social sciences such as anthropology, sociology and psychology may be of particular interest. Although most refreshers are unlikely to return to school formally, local educational facilities may provide a source of enrichment to a former education which should not be missed.

If a refresher is interested in continuing her formal education she should go to the college in her community to find out what programs are available. She may find that she is eligible for a traineeship or scholarship through the government or a private organization.

READING MATERIALS

The number of excellent periodicals and books available to nurses is too numerous to list. Hospital and nursing school libraries are excellent resources. It is always important to have at least a few resources available in one's home. An up-to-date textbook and a subscription to at least one nursing journal is essential. The following is a list of magazines that have a major emphasis on nursing:

Magazine	*Address*	*Rate*
The American Journal of Nursing (Official magazine of the American Nurses Association, published monthly)	The American Journal of Nursing 10 Columbus Circle New York, N. Y. 10019	$5.00, with a reduced rate for members
Nursing Outlook (Official publication of the National League for Nursing)	Nursing Outlook 10 Columbus Circle New York, N. Y. 10019	$5.00, with a reduced rate for members
R. N.	R. N. Oradell, N. J. 17649	$3.50
Nursing Forum	Nursing Publications, Inc. P.O. Box 218 Hillsdale, N. J.	$6.50
Nursing Science (F. A. Davis Co.)	Subscr. Address: Nursing Science 1323 Greenwood Road Baltimore, Md. 21208	$5.00
Journal of Psychiatric Nursing	Journal of Psychiatric Nursing Box No. 204 Bordentown, N. J. 08505	$3.00

NURSING ORGANIZATIONS

In 1952, six independent nursing organizations were restructured to become the two major nursing organizations of today. They are the American Nurses' Association and the National League for Nursing. The A.N.A. and N.L.N. provide opportunities for the nurse to contribute to her profession and to be exposed to the many advantages which come from membership. Refreshers often have the misconception that there is no point in belonging to an organization unless they are employed. This is not true. In fact, membership in an organization is an excellent means of keeping in contact with nurses and nursing whether or not you are employed.

American Nurses' Association (A.N.A.)

The A.N.A. is the professional association of registered nurses. Members must be R.N.'s. When you join the A.N.A., you automatically become a member of your state and district nurses' associations. A nurse who is not employed may join the organization as an associate at reduced dues. Associates have the same privileges as members except that they cannot vote, hold office, serve as delegates or serve as chairmen of standing committees.

A.N.A. accomplishes many objectives through its major programs. It works to protect nurses and the public from undesirable and unqualified persons by promoting licensure laws and standards of practice. It conducts a public relations program to interpret and to disseminate information about nursing. It works to promote improved salaries and conditions of employment for nurses. National, state and district associations contribute to improved nursing care by dissemination of information through meetings, workshops, institutes, clinical conferences, etc. Through its legislative program, it promotes federal and state legislation which protects nursing and the public health. The Professional Counseling and Placement Service (P.C. & P.S.) will assemble and keep a confidential cumulative record of your education and experience, which can be sent to a potential employer at your request. Some states also provide counseling and job referral services.

National League for Nursing (N.L.N.)

Members of N.L.N. may be nurses, members of allied professions or lay persons who are interested in nursing. The individual joins the state or local league, as the case may be in the individual community. This organization is principally concerned with fostering improvement in nursing service and nursing education "through the coordinated efforts of nurses, allied professional groups, citizens, agencies and school."

Six of the major N.L.N. programs include accreditation of professional and practical schools of nursing, recruitment of nursing students, test services and State Board Test Pool Examinations for both practical and graduate professional nurses, research studies and advisory service for those in tuberculosis nursing and mental health and psychiatric nursing.

OTHER NURSING ORGANIZATIONS

American Association of Nurse Anesthetists

This organization serves professional nurses employed in the field of anesthesiology.

American Association of Industrial Nurses

The majority of the members of this organization are professional nurses in the field of occupational health.

Association of Operating Room Nurses

This organization, started in 1957, serves professional nurses engaged in or formerly engaged in operating room nursing.

International Council of Nurses

The I.C.N. is a federation of national nurses' associations. Each country is represented by its officially designated nursing organization. Individuals cannot join, but A.N.A. members are represented in the I.C.N. through A.N.A. Aside from the benefits of international exchange of ideas and nurses, the I.C.N. has divisions concerned with nursing service, nursing education and economic welfare.

American Nurses' Foundation (A.N.F.)

The A.N.F. is devoted to research in nursing. Gifts to this organization are tax free and are used for research projects.

SUMMARY

With every advance comes a new opportunity and a new satisfaction. Since an achieved goal ceases to motivate, refreshers are indeed fortunate to belong to a profession which is so dynamic and one which provides many resources to meet its challenges.

REFERENCES

Dreves, Katharine Densford: 1933-1952 Measuring Up. *Three Score Years and Ten 1893-1963*, National League for Nursing, 1963.

Emerson, Ralph Waldo: Circles in *Essays* (first series). Boston, Houghton, Mifflin and Co., 1889.

Kelly, Cordelia W.: *Dimensions of Professional Nursing*, Section VII, New York, Macmillan Co., 1962.

N.L.N. Biennial Reports 1963-1964, National League for Nursing, May, 1965.

Index

Page numbers set in italic type refer to illustrations

Abbreviations, for hospital use, 203
Acid-base balance, 214–215
Acidosis, metabolic, 215
  respiratory, 214
Adaptors, plastic, 229
Addressograph, 233
Adolescent, hospital service for, 269, *269*
Adrenal glands, 215
Aftercare clinics, 278
Air exchange, 146
Alkalosis, metabolic, 215
  respiratory, 214
American Association of Industrial Nurses, 302
American Association of Nurse Anesthetists, 302
American Nurses' Association, 301
  Statement of Functions of Licensed Practical Nurse, 71–73
  Statement of Functions, Standards and Qualifications of the Director of Nursing Service, 33–36
  Statement of Functions, Standards and Qualifications of General Duty Nurses, 44–46
  Statement of Functions, Standards and Qualifications for Head Nurse, 39–44
  Statement of Functions, Standards and Qualifications for Supervisor, 36–39
  Statement on Auxiliary Personnel in Nursing Service, 67–69
American Nurses' Foundation, 303
Anemic anoxia, 147
Anesthesia recovery period, 168–169
Anesthetists, nurse, association of, 302
Anoxia, manifestations of, 147–148
  patient care in, 146–160
  types of, 146–147
Antidepressant drugs, 280
Apgar rating scale, 251, *251*
Aquamatic K pad, 234
Architectural designs, for nursing units, 22, *24–25*
  infection control and, 188
Arithmetic, practice problems in, 209
Asepsis, 295
Assignment, of ward duties, 78–80
Assignment form, for delegation of duties, 82, *83*
Assistant director of nursing, 30. See also *Supervisor.*
Associate degree program, 49–50
  baccalaureate education following, 52
Association of Operating Room Nurses, 303
Associations, nursing, 301–303
Atrophy, bed rest and, 178
Auto-analyzer, 15
Automation, mechanical devices and, 16–18
Auxiliary personnel, functions of, 67–69. See also *Hospital personnel.*
  supervision by registered nurse, 63–75
Auxiliary services, of hospital, 14–15

Baccalaureate education, for nursing, 51–52
Bacteria. See *Infection control.*

Barium enema, 114
Bath, sitz, disposable, 229, *237*
Bathing, of patient, 137–139
Bed boards, 178
Bed rest, disadvantages of, 178
Beds
  circle, 234
  CircOlectric, *241*
  components of, 231
  electric, 17, 154, *241*
Bedside unit, electronic, *240*
Bennett respirator, 150, 155, 235
Bird respirator, 150
Birth control, 243–244
Birtheez, *249*
Bladder and bowel training, 180
Blanket, thermal, 234, *240*
Blood analysis, 15
Blood transfusion, 155–156
  reactions from, 220
Bowel and bladder training, 180
Breathing, labored, 147. See also *Dyspnea* and *Anoxia.*
Bronchogram, 114

Cannula, nasal, 150, *151*, 154, 155
Cardiac resuscitation, 157, *158–159*
Cardiopulmonary arrest, emergency care in, 156–160
  resuscitation for, 157, *158–159*
Cardiovascular disease, 176
Case method, of duty assignment, 79
Catheter, nasal, 150, *151*, 154, 155
Catheterization sets, 230, *238–239*
Central service department, 22
Chapels, 15
Chart nurse, 74–75
Charting, 88, 295
Chest x-ray examinations, 115
Child. See also *Pediatric care.*
  battered, 270
  mentally retarded, 271
Child care. See *Pediatric care.*
Childbirth. See *Labor and delivery.*
Clinics, mental hygiene, 278
Closed-chest cardiac resuscitation, 157, *158–159*
College courses, for nurses, 300
Colon, x-ray examination of, 114
Communicable diseases. See *Diseases.*
Communication system, in hospital, 232
Community colleges, nursing programs in, 49
Computers, in nursing, 10, 18, *19*, 233
Contamination. See *Infection control.*
Convalescence, 170–171
Conveyor belt, 16
Croupette, 235, *241*
Cultures, infection control and, 192
Curricula, regrouping of, 57

Davis, M., 297
Day centers, 277
Decompression, for labor, 249
Decubitus ulcers, sites for, 142
  treatment of, 144
    nursing accessories for, 143
Dehydration, 219
Delivery. See *Labor and delivery.*
Diabetic exchange system, 129, *130–131*
Diagnosis, laboratory and x-ray examinations in, 107–117. See also *Laboratory examinations* and *X-ray examinations.*
  radioactive materials in, 115
  ultrasonography in, 116
Dictating machines, 18
Dietary service
  changes in, 15, 118–133
  decentralized, 119
  infection control and, 191
  new equipment in, 121
  selective menus of, 119, *120*
  snack carts in, 123
Diets
  diabetic, 129, *130–131*
  for metabolic disorders, 132
  hospital, 124–125
  low cholesterol, 129
  low sodium, 128
  skin care and, 143
  therapeutic, 125–132
  weight-reducing, 125
Director of nursing service, assistant, 30. See also *Supervisor.*
  functions, standards and qualifications of, 33–36
  role of, 29
Diseases, communicable, 268
  requiring rehabilitation, 176–177
Disposables, 225–230
  paper, 226
  plastic, 228
Dosage, of drugs, 198, 202
Drainage, skin care for, 139
Dressings, 229
Drug(s)
  action of, 197
  administration of, 195–211
    by nurse, 205
    by patient, 204
    by physician, 205
    changes in, 206
    reminders for, 206
    routes of, 198
  antidepressant, 280
  arithmetic conversions for, 199
    sample problems in, 201
  charting of, 208
  dosage of, 198, 202
  intravenous, 202
  study of, 197
  study sheet for, 199
  weights and measures for, 199

Dumbwaiters, 16
Duogram, 114
Duties, assignment of, 78–80, 82, *83*
Dyspnea, patient care in, 148–150. See also *Anoxia.*

Economic changes, affecting nursing, 5–7
Economic Opportunity Act of 1964, 271
Education, hospital programs of, 23
  in-service, 294–295, 299–300
  nursing. See *Nursing education.*
Electric beds, 17, 154, *241*
Electrolytes. See *Fluid and electrolyte balance.*
Electronic bedside cabinets, 232, *240*
Electronic ovens, 121
Electronic thermometer, *242*
Electroshock, 280
Emergency care, for cardiopulmonary arrest, 156–160
Employment, job interview for, 290
Enema, barium, 114
Equipment and supplies
  care of, 295
  cloth and other materials for, 229
  for hospital kitchen, 121
  for laboratory, 15
  for oxygen administration, 150, 228
  for positioning of bed patient, 178, *178*
  for treatment, 233–235
  in nursing station, 232–233
  in patient's room, 230–232
  miscellaneous, 235–236
  new, 225–242
  paper, 226
  plastic, 228
Examinations, laboratory. See *Laboratory examinations.*
  prenatal, 246
  preoperative, 165
  review of, 99
  x-ray. See *X-ray examinations.*
Expenses, hospital, 6, *8*
Extractor, vacuum, 250

Family planning, 243–244
Federal funds, for nursing education, 11
Fluid and electrolyte balance, 212–223
  body regulators of, 215
  in infants, 216
  intake and output records of, 220, *221*
  problems in, 216
Fluid therapy, 217–223
  intake and output records in, 220, *221*
  signs and symptoms in, 219
Fluids
  body, 213–214
    cellular or intracellular, 213
    extracellular, 214
Fluids, body (*Continued*)
    interstitial, 214
  intravenous, 219
  oral, 217
  parenteral, administration of, *222*
  subcutaneous, administration of, 218
  vascular, 214
Foley catheterization sets, 230, *239*
Food(s), maintaining temperatures of, 120, *122*
  preparation of, 121
Food groups, 124, *126–127*
Food service. See *Dietary service.*
Footboard, 178, *178*
Formula preparation, 254, *256*
Formulary, 196

Gallbladder, x-ray examination of, 114
Glands, endocrine, fluid balance and, 215
Growth and development, pediatric care and, 263

Halfway houses, 278
Head nurse, functions, standards and qualifications of, 39–44
  role of, 30
Health care, community services for, 9–10
  hospital contributions to, *8*
  legislation affecting, 10–12
Hematologic diseases, 177
Hemiplegics, bladder and bowel training for, 180
Hexachlorophene soap, 137
Histotoxic anoxia, 147
Hospital(s)
  architectural designs for, 22, *24–25*, 188
  as treatment center, 187–188
  description of, 14
  education programs in, 23, 294–295, 299–300
  employment information for, 290
  expenses of, 6, *8*
  health contributions of, *8*
  income of, 7, *8*
  infections in. See *Infection control.*
  major changes in, 14–26
    affecting personnel, 7
    of attitudes, 28
  paramedical services of, 15–16
  personnel turnover in, 64
  psychiatric care in, 276
  research in, 16
  rooms in, 230–232, *240*
  satellite, 22
  selection of, for nurse, 289
  visiting hours in, 267
Hospital administration, 18–20
Hospital beds. See *Beds.*

Hospital brochure, for patient orientation, *94–98*
Hospital formulary, 196
Hospital personnel, 7–9
auxiliary, 67–69. See *Auxiliary personnel.*
evaluation of, 89
individual roles of, 29–32
team approach for, 23–26
turnover rates of, 64
Hospital volunteers, 75
Housekeeping department, 15, 190
Hydration, excessive, 220
Hyperbaric chamber, 23, *26*
Hypertonic solution, 213
Hypotonic solution, 213
Hypoxia. See *Anoxia.*

Identabands, *250*
Income, of hospitals, 7, *8*
Incontinent patient, drainage in, 139
Industrial nurses, association of, 302
Infant, care of, 254–256. See also *Maternal and child care.*
defective, mother with, 253
fluid and electrolyte requirements of, 216
formula preparation for, 254, *256*
premature, apparatus for, *257*
rating scale for, 251, *251*
Infection control, 187–193
architectural designs and, 188
dietary department and, 191
housekeeping department and, 190
interrelated services and, 188–192
laboratory and, 192
laundry and, 189
nursing department and, 191
Infertility, 244
Inhalation therapist, 151–152
In-service education, 294–295, 299–300
Insulin, dosage of, 202
Insulin shock, 280
Insulin subshock, 280
Insurance coverage, for intensive care, 21
Intercommunication system, 232
International Council of Nurses, 303
Intravenous fluids, 219
Ionization, 212
Isolette, 155, *257*
Isotonic solution, 213

Job interview, 290
Junior colleges, nursing programs in, 49

Kidneys, fluid balance and, 215
Kitchen, decentralized, 119
new equipment for, 121

Labor and delivery, 248–251, *249*
anesthesia for, 250
decompression apparatus for, 249, *249*
identification bands for, 250, 251
vacuum extractor for, 250
Laboratory
description of, *96*
education programs and, 57
infection control and, 192
new equipment for, 15
Laboratory examination
order for, 108
preparation for, 108
reports from, 110
specimen collection for, 109
Lamaze method, 249
Laundry, infection control and, 189
Legislation, affecting health care, 10–12
Levine, E., 64
Library resources, for refreshers, 3
Linen. See *Laundry.*

Mammograms, 115
Maternal and child care. See also *Prenatal care.*
changes in, 243–258
family-centered, 244–245
nurse-patient relationships in, 256–258
Mattress, alternating pressure, 234
Meal hours, in hospitals, 123
Medical records department, 18
Medical-surgical station, care of mother on, 254
Medicare, 12
Medication. See *Drug(s).*
Medication technician, 205
Mental hygiene clinics, 278
Mental retardation, of child, 271
Menus, selective, 119, *120*
Metabolic acidosis and alkalosis, 215
Metabolic disorders, diets for, 132
rehabilitation for, 177
Metrology, 199
Meyer, G., 29
Microorganisms. See also *Infection control.*
mutation of, 188
Mobility, loss of, 178
Monitoring devices, 10, 18, *19*, 233
Mouth-to-mouth resuscitation, 157, *158–159*
Mother, care of. See *Maternal and child care.*
on medical-surgical station, 254
postpartum care of, 251–254. See also *Postpartum care.*
unwed, 247
Moving, of patients, 179
Muscle tone, loss of, 178
Myelogram, 115

Narcoanalysis, 280
Narcotic pill counter, 228, *236*
Nasal cannula, 150, *151*, 154, 155
Nasal catheter, 150, *151*, 154, 155
National League for Nursing, 302
Needles, disposable, 228
Night centers, 277
Nosocomial infections. See *Infection control.*
Nurse
  appraisal of patient needs by, 85
  as team leader, 80–88. See also *Team leader.*
  assignment methods of, 78–79
  chart, 74–75
  college courses for, 300
  dietary service and, 118–119
  drug administration by, 205. See also *Drug(s).*
  employment of, 290
  evaluation of care by, 89
  general duty, functions, standards and qualifications for, 44–46
  head. See *Head nurse.*
  industrial, association of, 302
  operating room, association of, 303
  patient chart and, 88
  personnel supervised by, 63–75
  practical. See *Practical nurse.*
  psychiatric, 281–284
  public health, 279
  reading materials for, 300
  responsibilities of, 76–90
    administrative, 88
    charge, 89
  role of, 31
  teaching of patient by, 92–104. See also *Teaching, of patient.*
  vocational. See *Practical nurse.*
  workshops for, 300
Nurse aide, background of, 65
  duties of, 32, 65, 66
Nurse Training Act of 1964, 10
Nursery, 255
Nursing
  abbreviations used in, 203
  adjustment stages in, 297–298
  assistant director of, 30
  continuing education and activities in, 299–303
  future changes in, 32–33
  history of, 86
  obstetric. See *Maternal and child care.*
  of patients receiving fluid therapy, 217–223
  procedures in, 295
  psychiatric. See *Psychiatric care.*
  refreshing in, 288–298
    library resources for, 3
    orientation for, 293–294
    stages of, 1–4
  rehabilitation, 177–184
Nursing (*Continued*)
  sociological, economic and technical advances affecting, 5–12
  values in, 29
Nursing accessories, for skin care, 143
Nursing associations, 301–303
Nursing care conference, 87
Nursing care plan, 87, *87*
Nursing department. See *Nursing service.*
Nursing education
  associate degree in. See *Associate degree program.*
  baccalaureate, 51–52
    for graduates of diploma and associate degree programs, 52
  clinical experience in, 57
  curriculum regrouping in, 57
  diploma school of, 50–51, 52
  federal funds for, 11
  postgraduate, 53
  practical, 48–49
  programs of, 48–61
    selection of, 54
  tape recorder in, 56
  teaching methods in, 54–60
  television in, 56
Nursing organizations, 301–303
Nursing procedures, common elements in, 295
Nursing service
  auxiliary personnel in, 67–69
  director of. See *Director of nursing service.*
  division of labor in, 29
  infection control and, 191
  new insights in, 27–29
  present patterns of, 27–46
Nursing station, 232–233
Nursing units, architectural designs for, 22, *24–25*, 188

Obstetric nursing. See *Maternal and child care.*
Occupational therapy department, 16
Operating room, 21
Operation
  nursing care during, 167–168
  preparatory care for, 163
    legal aspects of, 166
    physical, 165
    psychological, 163
  recovery period following, 168–169
Orderlies, 32, 67
Organisms. See *Infection control.*
Orientation, of nurse, 293–294
  of patient, 99, 262
Osmosis, *213*
Outpatient department, 16
Ovens, electronic, 121
Overhydration, 220

Oxygen
administration of, equipment for, 150
precautions during, 152–155
air exchange and, 146
supplies for, 228
Oxygen cylinders, 152
Oxygen mask, 150, *151*, 154, 155
Oxygen tent, 150, 153, 155
Oxygen wall gauge, *153*

Pacemaker, 10, *11*
Paging system, closed circuit, 17, *17*
Paper products, disposable, 226
Paramedical services, in hospitals, 15–16
Parathyroid glands, 215
Parent classes, 247
Parenteral fluids, record of, *222*
Patient
bathing of, 137–139
care of, common elements in, 295
progressive stages of, 20–21
convalescence of, 170–171
drug administration by, 205
follow-up of, 184
hemiplegic, 180
incontinent, drainage in, 139
information for, after discharge, 101
concerning condition of, 100
concerning hospital routine, 99
insurance coverage for, 21
moving of, 179
needs of, appraisal of, 85
nurses' expectations of, 78
of today and yesterday, 92
operative care of, 162–172. See also *Operation.*
orientation of, 99
pediatric. See *Pediatric care.*
postoperative care of, 169–170
preoperative care of, 163
previous knowledge of, 101
psychiatric. See *Psychiatric care.*
receiving fluid therapy, 217–223
receiving hot and cold treatments, 140
rehabilitation of, 174–185. See also *Rehabilitation.*
skin care of, 135–144. See also *Skin care.*
teaching of, 92–104. See also *Teaching, of patient.*
with anoxia, 146–160. See also *Anoxia.*
with drainage, 139
with dyspnea, 148–150. See also *Dyspnea.*
Patient care conference, 87
Patient chart, 88
Patient room, 230–232, *240*
Pediatric care
changes in, 261–272
community services for, 270
for communicable diseases, 268

Pediatric care (*Continued*)
growth and development and, 263
information form for, *264–265*
play activities and, 266
pre-admission orientation for, 262
rooming-in and, 267
trends in, 262–270
uniform for, 266
visiting hours and, 267
Peplau, H., 281
Personal property, hospital liability for, 167
Personnel, auxiliary. See *Auxiliary personnel.*
Personnel, hospital, 7–9. See also *Hospital personnel.*
Physical examination, preoperative, 165
Physical therapy department, 16, *95*
Physician, drug administration by, 205
Physician's order, for laboratory examinations, 108
x-ray examinations, 111
Pill counter, 228, *236*
Pituitary gland, 215
Plasma, 214
Plastic bags, 229
Play activities, 266
Pneumatic tube, 17, 232
Pneumoencephalogram, 115
Poison control centers, 270
Poliomyelitis, rehabilitation from, 176
Positioning, of bed patient, 178, *178*
Postanesthesia room, 21, 22, 168–169
Postgraduate nursing education, 53
Postoperative care, 169–170
Postpartum care, 251–254
immediate, 251
self-care in, instructions for, 252
succeeding, 252
Practical nurse
background of, 69
drug administration by, 205
duties of, 70
education for, 48–49
functions of, 71–73
Premature infant, apparatus for, *257*
Prenatal care, 245–248
first examination in, 246
follow-up examinations, in 246
of unwed mother, 247
parent classes in, 247
Pressure chamber, hyperbaric, 23, *26*
Pressure sores, 142. See also *Decubitus ulcers.*
Proctoclysis, 218
Programed learning, 55, *55*, *60*
Pruritus, 140
Psychiatric care
changes in, 274–285
day centers and night centers for, 277
facilities for, 275–279
foster homes and, 277
halfway houses for, 278

Psychiatric care (*Continued*)
  mental hygiene clinics for, 278
  nurse's role in, 281–284
  therapeutic environment in, 284–285
  treatment methods in, 279–281
Psychiatric nurse, 281–284
Psychopharmacology, 280
Psychosurgery, 280
Psychotherapy, 279
Public health nurse, 279
Pyelogram, intravenous, 114

Radio, 230
Radiography, vascular, 115
Radiology department, *96*
Range of motion, passive, 180
Recovery room, 21, 22, 168–169
Referral form, sample, *182–183*
Refresher, advice for, 296
Rehabilitation
  care during, 174–185
  diseases requiring, 176–177
  explanation of, 174
  following surgery, 171
  follow-up after, 184
  possible team members for, 174–176
  psychological consideration in, 181
Rehabilitation nursing, 177–184
Research, in hospitals, 16
Respirator, Bennett, 150, 155, 235
  Bird, 150
Respiratory acidosis and alkalosis, 214
Resuscitation, for cardiopulmonary arrest, 157, *158–159*
Retardation, mental, 271
Rh factor, prenatal care and, 246
Rooming-in, 253, 267

Services, auxiliary, of hospitals, 14–15
Shifts, of personnel, responsibilities of R.N. and, 89
Shock, 220
  insulin, 280
Sitz bath, disposable, 229, *237*
Skin
  anatomy and function of, 135–136
  breakdown of, 141
  dry, 139
  problems of, reduction of, 139–144
  sensitive, 140
Skin care, 135–144
  general purpose of, 136–137
  in wound areas, 141
  nursing accessories for, 143
  for drainage patients, 139
  for patient receiving hot and cold treatments, 140
  turning schedule in, 142
Skin closure, nonsutural, 229, *237*
Smoking, oxygen administration and, 152
Snack carts, 123
Soap, with hexachlorophene, 137
Sociological advances, affecting nursing, 5–12
Sodium restricted diets, 128
Solutions, hypertonic, 213
  hypotonic, 213
  isotonic, 213
Somatic therapy, 280
Spinal cord, diseases of, 177
Spinogram, 115
Staffing secretary, 32
Stagnant anoxia, 147
Station manager, 74–75
Steri-Strip, *237*
Stomach, x-ray examination of, 114
Suction bottle, wall, *242*
Supervisor, functions, standards and qualifications for, 36–39
  role of, 30
Supplies. See *Equipment and supplies.*
Surgery. See *Operation.*
Syringes, disposable, 228

Tape recorder, 56
Teaching
  of nursing students, 54–60
  of patient, 92–104
    aids for, 103
    assessment of needs for, 103
    by example, 103
    hospital brochure for, *94–98*
    major areas of, 93–101
    objectives of, 93
    of activities of daily living, 181
    planning activities for, 102
    ways of improving, 102–104
  of personnel, for team system, 84
Team conference, 87
Team leader
  administrative responsibilities of, 88
  appraisal of patient needs by, 85
  delegation of care by, 82, *83*
  functions of, 80–88, *81*
  plan of care of, 86
  teaching personnel by, 84
Team system
  assignment form in, 82, *83*
  delegation of care in, 82
  for hospital personnel, 23–26
  for rehabilitation, 174–176
  of assignment of duties, 79–80, *81*, *83*
Technical advances, affecting nursing, 10
Technician, medication, 205
Teenager, hospital service for, 269, *269*
Television, in nursing education, 56
  in hospital room, 230
Therapist, inhalation, 151–152

Thermal blanket, 234, *240*
Thermometer, electronic, *242*
Thrombophlebitis, 179
Time clocks, 18
Toys, for pediatric patients, 266
Transfusion, blood, 155–156
  reactions from, 220
Transistor radio, for paging, 17, *17*
Tubing, 228

Ulcers, decubitus. See *Decubitus ulcers.*
Ultrasonography, 116
Uniform, for pediatric care, 266
Unwed mother, prenatal care of, 247
Urogram, 114

Vacuum extractor, for childbirth, 250
Vascular radiography, 115
Vending machines, 122
Ventriculogram, 115
Visiting hours, in pediatrics, 267
Vocational nurse. See *Practical nurse.*
Volunteer, hospital, 75

Ward duties, assignment of, 79–80
Ward manager, 32
Ward secretary, 73–74
White House Conferences on Children and Youth, 272
Workshops, 300
Wounds, dressings for, 229
  nonsutural closure of, 229, *237*
  skin care of, 141

X-ray department, 15
X-ray examination, 107–117
  examples of, 114
  order for, 111
  preparation for, 111, *112*
  report from, 114
  transporting patient for, 113
X-ray therapy, skin care during, 141